MW01067453

Evidence-Based Approaches for the Treatment of Maltreated Children

Child Maltreatment

Contemporary Issues in Research and Policy

Series Editors

Jill E. Korbin, Ph.D.
Professor of Anthropology
Associate Dean, College of Arts and Sciences
Director, Schubert Center for Child Studies
Crawford Hall, 7th Floor
10900 Euclid Avenue
Cleveland, OH 44106-7068, USA
jill.korbin@case.edu

Richard D. Krugman, MD
Professor of Pediatrics and Dean
University of Colorado School of Medicine
Room C-1003 Bldg 500
Anschutz Medical Campus
13001 E. 17th Place
Aurora, CO 80045, USA
richard.krugman@ucdenver.edu

This series provides a high-quality, cutting edge, and comprehensive source offering the current best knowledge on child maltreatment from multidisciplinary and multicultural perspectives. It consists of a core handbook that is followed by two or three edited volumes of original contributions per year. The core handbook will present a comprehensive view of the field. Each chapter will summarize current knowledge and suggest future directions in a specific area. It will also highlight controversial and contested issues in that area, thus moving the field forward. The handbook will be updated every five years. The edited volumes will focus on critical issues in the field from basic biology and neuroscience to practice and policy. Both the handbook and edited volumes will involve creative thinking about moving the field forward and will not be a recitation of past research. Both will also take multi-disciplinary, multicultural and mixed methods approaches.

For further volumes:
http://www.springer.com/series/8863

Susan Timmer • Anthony Urquiza
Editors

Evidence-Based Approaches for the Treatment of Maltreated Children

Considering core components and treatment effectiveness

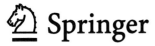 Springer

Editors
Susan Timmer
Department of Pediatrics
CAARE Center
Sacramento, CA, USA

Anthony Urquiza
Department of Pediatrics
CAARE Center
Sacramento, CA, USA

ISSN 2211-9701   ISSN 2211-971X (electronic)
ISBN 978-94-007-7403-2   ISBN 978-94-007-7404-9 (eBook)
DOI 10.1007/978-94-007-7404-9
Springer Dordrecht Heidelberg New York London

Library of Congress Control Number: 2013953899

© Springer Science+Business Media Dordrecht 2014
This work is subject to copyright. All rights are reserved by the Publisher, whether the whole or part of the material is concerned, specifically the rights of translation, reprinting, reuse of illustrations, recitation, broadcasting, reproduction on microfilms or in any other physical way, and transmission or information storage and retrieval, electronic adaptation, computer software, or by similar or dissimilar methodology now known or hereafter developed. Exempted from this legal reservation are brief excerpts in connection with reviews or scholarly analysis or material supplied specifically for the purpose of being entered and executed on a computer system, for exclusive use by the purchaser of the work. Duplication of this publication or parts thereof is permitted only under the provisions of the Copyright Law of the Publisher's location, in its current version, and permission for use must always be obtained from Springer. Permissions for use may be obtained through RightsLink at the Copyright Clearance Center. Violations are liable to prosecution under the respective Copyright Law.
The use of general descriptive names, registered names, trademarks, service marks, etc. in this publication does not imply, even in the absence of a specific statement, that such names are exempt from the relevant protective laws and regulations and therefore free for general use.
While the advice and information in this book are believed to be true and accurate at the date of publication, neither the authors nor the editors nor the publisher can accept any legal responsibility for any errors or omissions that may be made. The publisher makes no warranty, express or implied, with respect to the material contained herein.

Printed on acid-free paper

Springer is part of Springer Science+Business Media (www.springer.com)

Contents

Evidence-Based Approaches to the Treatment of Maltreated Children: Considering Core Components and Treatment Effectiveness

Introduction

What is maltreatment, what exactly is it doing to our children, and how can we help them? These are the questions we address in this volume. Thanks to research on the outcomes of abuse and neglect for children, we know that maltreatment has long-lasting, multi-level negative effects. Studies have documented neurological effects (Heim, Newport, Mletzko, Miller, & Nemeroff, 2008; Nemeroff, 2004), hormonal effects related to physiological arousal (Cicchetti, Rogosch, Gunnar, & Toth, 2010) and emotional regulation (Maughan & Cicchetti, 2002), cognitive effects related to attention deficits and hyperarousal (Pollak Cicchetti, Hornung, & Reid, 2000). We have observed that maltreated children also have high rates of physical aggression, noncompliance, and antisocial behaviors (Cicchetti & Toth, 2000; Mersky & Reynolds, 2007). What we are just beginning to investigate is whether there is a difference in the severity of effects of maltreatment depending upon when it occurs. Additionally, and to the point of this volume, there is an accompanying awareness that the interventions we use might need to be differently focused with different aged children in order to most effectively treat them.

In this volume, we will examine the developmental and child maltreatment research literature to help us understand what happens when children are maltreated at different ages, and how the effects of these adverse experiences can snowball, interfering with healthy functioning in many different areas of their lives. We will consider the findings that describe effects of maltreatment on neurobiological and regulatory systems, cognitive, social, and emotional development. We use this context of development to consider the implications of mental health symptoms children display in different stages of development and consider the treatments that address these specific symptoms common to children at each age. During the last two decades there has been a growing trend to develop interventions for children and families who experience the symptoms associated with child maltreatment.

In 1993, the Society of Clinical Psychology (Division 12) of the American Psychological Association (APA) convened a Task Force to examine the use of empirically supported psychological treatments. This task force spawned a growing research movement. In the past few years the terms "evidence-based practice" and "evidence-based treatment" have become more widely used in the field of clinical psychology. Evidence-based practice (EBP) is a broad term for the use of a scientific approach that combines clinical expertise and is informed by best available research evidence (APA Presidential Task Force on Evidence-Based Practice, 2006; Kazdin, 2008). As Kazdin stated in 2009, "evidence-based treatment (EBT) refers to the interventions or techniques" that have been informed by research trials, generally by randomized controlled trials that show a treatment is more effective than another.

Over the past two decades, evidence based treatments (EBTs) have emerged as hopeful pathways to mental health for children. During this time, researchers and policy makers developed strict requirements for being labeled as "evidence based." An intervention is not considered to be evidence based unless it is supported by two or more randomized control trials, with two different groups of researchers evaluating the strengths of the outcomes (Fixsen, Blase, Naoom, & Wallace, 2009). Randomized control trials testing the efficacy of EBTs for treating children's mental health problems have been conducted and replicated; effectiveness studies also have been conducted, testing their usefulness among diverse populations of children. But what is the evidence for applying them to maltreated children? Do the interventions need to be "tailored" for these populations? Can an intervention be used for any child that meets its inclusion and exclusion criteria, or are there other considerations? Should the timing, duration, and severity of a child's history of maltreatment, or allostatic load, be considered, in addition to developmental stage, when selecting an intervention? If a child is eligible for more than one intervention, how do therapists decide which to use? And finally, is one intervention sufficient to meet all the mental health problems of maltreated children, or does their history suggest that more than one intervention is needed? The purpose of this volume is to present information that can help us answer these questions.

When we thought about editing a book on empirically based treatments for maltreated children, the evidence based treatment (EBT) movement was already fully launched and gaining momentum. The National Child Traumatic Stress Network had a list of EBTs for traumatized children easily downloadable from the internet; there is an internet-based California Evidence Based Clearinghouse (CEBC) for Child Welfare that lists and describes many different evidence-based treatments used for the population we wanted to write about. There are nearly 300 different EBTs listed on the CEBC website.

As we looked through the lists, it was clear that interventions varied significantly in format and goals according to the age of children for whom they were designed. At first glance, treatments for younger maltreated children often targeted caregivers' parenting attitudes and behaviors, while treatments for older children targeted their affect and cognitions. Many seemed designed for specific traumatizing events (e.g., sexual abuse, domestic violence), or specific diagnoses (e.g., PTSD, substance abuse). Our long history of working with maltreated children has shown us that there are often overlaps in experience with different types of abuse and neglect, and also overlaps in diagnoses. Sexually abused youth can present with PTSD and problems with substance abuse, or they may be suicidal. For this reason, we chose to look more closely at children's emotional, cognitive, and physical (e.g., neurological) development. We hypothesized that recent research on development and developmental psychopathology could help us understand why certain types of interventions might be effective with certain populations, and why others might be less effective. We dug into researching this area with a will, motivated to read, sift, synthesize findings, and present the reader with a coherent, though far from exhaustive, snapshot of how the research describes the effects of maltreatment on development. We quickly realized how much valuable research has been conducted in developmental psychopathology and psychopathology that directly applies to mental health treatment, but that has not reached across the great divide between research and practice.

Following this research, we selected ten well-known EBTs for inclusion in this volume, representing one of four different age categories across the childhood years: infancy, young children, school-aged children, and adolescence. These categorizations represent their match with what we see are the primary developmental issues of each age group, rather than an identification of the ages of the children they serve. We asked either the treatment developer or scholars who had conducted significant research on each EBT to contribute chapters describing the intervention, including a case study description. We asked them to elaborate on any decision-making involving issues of developmental appropriateness, so that the reader could understand the links between development and clinical practice that are rarely articulated and often taken for granted. Additionally, knowing that nearly all EBTs have a specific assessment protocol, we asked each author to include a description of their pre- and post-treatment assessment, including the assessment data – so readers could view the intervention from a similar perspective as the author. We wanted to leave the reader with a belief that once these EBTs were established, life had to improve for maltreated children (the Hollywood ending). Our conscience got the better of us, however. The truth is, that having the EBTs established scientifically is only half the battle. Therapists who provide services for maltreated children have to be able to use these EBTs effectively in order to achieve the promised positive outcomes. Teaching therapists about the EBTs and facilitating their growth and sustainment in community mental health settings is the other half of the battle. To fully explain the entire EBT scenario, we decided to include chapters on dissemination and implementation of EBTs.

Now that we have sketched the big picture describing this volume's goals and purposes, we will describe the parts and chapters in a little more detail. The introductory part of this volume (Chaps. 1, 2 and 3) provides the reader with a framework for using EBTs with maltreated children. In the first chapter, "A Brief History of Identifying Child Maltreatment," groundwork is laid for understanding child maltreatment by describing its history and definitions of different kinds of abuse and neglect. In this chapter, Hollis maps how we arrived at the realization that maltreated children needed mental health services. In Chap. 2, "A Brief History of

Evidence-Based Practices," Forte and colleagues describe the history of their emergence of EBTs, allowing the reader to more fully understand the discontent that spurred their creation and the controversy still surrounding them. In Chap. 3, we discuss our theoretical approach to using EBTs to maltreated children in "Why we think we can make things better with Evidence Based Practices: Theoretical and Developmental Context." We outline the effects of maltreatment on the developing child to emphasize for the reader the unseen ways that maltreatment harms children, believing that understanding the nature of the problem and its effects will help us understand why certain interventions are effective for maltreated children. We portray the effects of maltreatment and treatment choices as defined and guided by children's developmental stage and past experience in a table at the end of Chap. 3.

In Chaps. 4, 5, 6, 7, 8, 9, 10, 11, 12 and 13, we present the EBTs. In each chapter, the authors discuss the evidence base for the intervention and describe the protocol, and illustrate how the intervention works through case description. Interventions for infants and toddlers are described in Chaps. 4 and 5. In Chap. 4, Dozier and colleagues write on their intervention, ABC, in "Attachment and Biobehavioral Catch-up: An Intervention for Parents at Risk of Maltreating Their Infants and Toddlers." In Chap. 5, Van Horn and Reyes describe the process of providing Child-Parent Psychotherapy (CPP) to maltreated children in "Child-Parent Psychotherapy with Infants and Very Young Children." Chapters 6, 7, 8 and 9 present information on interventions for young children. In Chap. 6, Webster-Stratton explains the Incredible Years (IY) intervention in "Incredible Years® Parent and Child Programs for Maltreating Families." In Chap. 7, Pickering and Sanders discuss Triple P in "The Importance of Evidence-Based Parenting Intervention to the Prevention and Treatment of Child Maltreatment." Urquiza and Timmer describe Parent-Child Interaction Therapy (PCIT) and how it is provided to maltreated children, in Chap. 8. In Chap. 9, Gilliam and Fisher discuss MTFC in "Multidimensional Treatment Foster Care for Preschoolers: A Program for Maltreated Children in the Child Welfare System." Interventions for school-aged children are described in Chaps. 10 and 11. Mannarino and colleagues help the reader to grasp the intricacies of Trauma-Focused Cognitive Behavioral Therapy in Chap. 10. Kolko and colleagues present information on AF-CBT in Chap. 11, "Alternatives for Families: A Cognitive Behavioral Therapy: An Overview and Case Example." Chapters 12 and 13 provide descriptions of interventions for adolescents. In Chap. 12, "MST-CAN: An Ecological Treatment for Families Experiencing Physical Abuse and Neglect," Swenson and Schaeffer provide an overview and description of multisystemic therapy. In Chap. 13, "Dialectical Behavior Therapy for Suicidal and Self-Harming Adolescents with Trauma Symptoms," Berk and colleagues describe the way DBT has been adapted for use with adolescents.

In the two chapters following the descriptions of the interventions for different ages of children, we discuss the intricacies of dissemination and implementation, providing a framework for understanding why this is an important topic for those interested in EBTs. Chapter 14, "Taking it to the Street: Disseminating Evidence-Based Practices," gives the reader a framework for understanding the training process, and how the EBTs described in this volume have trained clinicians to provide their intervention. In Chap. 15, "The Bridge from Research to Practice – Just Leap Across the Last Bit," we elaborate on the process of implementation and the difficulty EBT developers have achieving and maintaining treatment fidelity.

It has been, and continues to be, our mission to provide aid, support, and intervention to children and families where maltreatment has had a destructive influence. We hope readers find this volume interesting to read; and we hope it spurs additional research and scholarship on EBTs for maltreated children.

References

APA Presidential Task Force on Evidence-Based Practice. (2006). Evidence-based practice in psychology. *American Psychologist, 61*(4), 271–285.

Cicchetti, D., & Toth, S. (2000). Developmental processes in maltreated children. In D. Hansen (Ed.), *Nebraska symposium on motivation* (Motivation and child maltreatment, Vol. 46, pp. 85–160). Lincoln, NE: University of Nebraska Press.

Cicchetti, D., Rogosch, F. A., Gunnar, M. R., & Toth, S. L. (2010). The differential impacts of early physical and sexual abuse and internalizing problems on daytime cortisol rhythm in school-aged children. *Child Development, 81*(1), 252–269. doi:10.1111/j.1467-8624.2009.01393.

Fixsen, D., Blase, K., Naoom, S., & Wallace, F. (2009). Core implementation components. *Research on Social Work Practice, 19*(5), 531–540.

Heim, C., Newport, D. J., Mletzko, T., Miller, A. H., & Nemeroff, C. B. (2008). The link between childhood trauma and depression: Insights from HPA axis studies in humans. *Psychoneuroendocrinology, 33*, 693–710.

Kazdin, A. (2008). Evidence-based treatment and practice: New opportunities to bridge clinical research and practice, enhance the knowledge base, and improve care. *American Psychologist, 63*(3), 146–159.

Maughan, A., & Cicchetti, D. (2002). Impact of child maltreatment and interadult violence on emotional regulation and socioemotional adjustment. *Child Development, 73*(5), 1525–1542.

Mersky, J., & Reynolds, A. (2007). Child maltreatment and violent delinquency: Disentangling main effects and subgroup effects. *Child Maltreatment, 12*(3), 246–258.

Nemeroff, C. B. (2004). The neurobiological consequences of childhood trauma. *Journal of Clinical Psychiatry, 65*, 18.

Pollak, S., Cicchetti, D., Hornung, K., & Reed, A. (2000). Recognizing emotion in faces: The developmental effects of child abuse and neglect. *Developmental Psychology, 36*, 679–688.

Part I
Introduction

Chapter 1
A Brief History of Identifying Child Maltreatment

Nicole Hollis

The Child Maltreatment 2010 report estimated that Child Protective Services (CPS) received reports indicating that about 5.9 million children were involved in what callers believed to be child maltreatment in the 50 States, the District of Columbia, and the Commonwealth of Puerto Rico (U.S. Department of Health and Human Services, Administration for Children and Families, Administration on Children, Youth and Families, & Children's Bureau [USDHHS], 2011).[1] According to CPS criteria, 9.1 of every 1,000 children in the population were victims of child maltreatment whose cases were considered valid enough to receive a response from CPS. Most calls (58 %) were made by professionals, such as teachers, police, lawyers, and social services staff members (USDHHS, 2011).

Not every one of these 5.9 million children who were subjects of reports in 2010 had their cases substantiated: 39 % of all referrals were screened out (i.e., not investigated) by CPS. A referral can be screened out for a number of reasons, which include: the referral did not concern abuse or neglect, the referral did not contain enough information to allow for investigation, or the children were the responsibility of a different agency or jurisdiction (USDHHS, 2011). Limited financial resources or limited CPS staff can even cultivate conditions that lead to the investigation of only the most severe child maltreatment cases. The fact that one third of referrals were not investigated signals a likelihood that the actual number of children who suffered maltreatment is far greater than the numbers presented in the Child Maltreatment national reports (Cicchetti & Toth, 2005).

In principle, the experience of maltreatment—not the presence of a substantiated allegation of maltreatment—influences a child's healthy development. Children whose home environments include domestic violence perpetrated by or against a caregiver, caregiver alcohol abuse, or caregiver drug abuse are at higher risk for

---

[1] Hereafter cited as (USDHHS, 2011).

N. Hollis, Ph.D. (✉)
Department of Human Ecology, University of California, Davis, CA, USA
e-mail: ndhollis@ucdavis.edu

S. Timmer and A. Urquiza (eds.), *Evidence-Based Approaches for the Treatment of Maltreated Children*, Child Maltreatment 3, DOI 10.1007/978-94-007-7404-9_1,
© Springer Science+Business Media Dordrecht 2014

maltreatment than other children (USDHHS, 2011). A child may have been exposed to these risk factors but not have a substantiated report of maltreatment. In addition, among children for whom allegations of maltreatment have been made, involvement in child welfare services has been associated with increased likelihood of mental health service utilization (Leslie et al., 2005).

To understand what having a "history of maltreatment" means for the children participating in empirically-based mental health interventions, we will review the emerging history of policy and practice surrounding the concept of child maltreatment.

History of Child Maltreatment in the United States

In America and Europe before the 1800s, childhood and adulthood were not considered separate phases of human development (Scannapieco & Connell-Carrick, 2005) as they are now. The absence of harsh guidance, rather than its presence, was considered child maltreatment. This is because Puritan values included a belief in strong discipline, justifying severe corporal punishment (Barnett, Manly, & Cicchetti, 1993). In the early 1600s, the Protestant church used to send representatives to the homes of pilgrims to make sure they were introducing children to church morals properly. Social control of children was considered very important and people believed that they would gain control of children through beating and whipping them (Scannapieco & Connell-Carrick). During the 1800s, state statutes even called for parental rights to be severed in cases in which parents were shown to endanger their children's morals by not using these methods to gain control (Barnett et al., 1993).

Poor Laws

Before the 1900s, early America had "poor laws," which required that children from poor families be separated from their families with the goal of diminishing their likelihood of future economic destitution. These laws were based on the belief that parents who were poor would raise children who were poor and dependent through their examples of laziness. It was not until the early 1900s that the American government began to distinguish between neglectful parents and those who were impoverished. Interestingly, in the late 1800s, parental poverty was a greater concern than severe corporal punishment, and these concerns were reversed by the end of the 1900s (Barnett et al., 1993).

Shifts in Ideology

In the 1700s, British philosopher John Locke wrote about the innate goodness of children. Jean-Jacques Rousseau, a Swiss-French philosopher, asserted that children should be able to be children before becoming adults—that children were not miniature adults but experience life differently from how adults experience it. He argued that children need education and nurturing and that instead of providing harsh discipline, families should provide support and affection (Scannapieco & Connell-Carrick, 2005).

In the early 1800s, people began to view children as innocent and vulnerable, the public began to condemn the practice of treating children harshly without justification, and cases of exceptionally cruel treatment of children were brought to court (Barnett et al., 1993).

Scannapieco and Connell-Carrick (2005) summarized key elements that contributed to the ideological shift that took place in the 1800s. They emphasized Charles Darwin's developmental view that included the importance of the environment for human growth and behavior, G. Stanley Hall's focus on developmental stages and the importance of parents' understanding of each unique stage, and Sigmund Freud's assertion that infants and children need to be nurtured during infancy and childhood if they are to become healthy and productive adults.

Following this ideological shift, parents were brought to court when it was believed that they had treated their children in an exceptionally cruel manner. A lack of an official definition of physical abuse meant that presence or absence of physical abuse was determined by court precedents. The trying of severe cases of physical abuse marked great progress. However, little consideration was given to the severity of the child's injuries that resulted from this treatment, and rulings were based on the parents' motivation for harming their children. If parents harmed their children because of misbehavior, this was considered acceptable. If parents harmed their children for some other reason, judges tended to rule against them (Barnett et al., 1993).

First Official Case of Child Protection

In 1874, the stepparents of a girl named Mary Ellen severely beat and neglected her. She was likely 8–10 years old and lived in New York City (see Barnett et al., 1993; Scannapieco & Connell-Carrick, 2005). Neighbors heard Mary Ellen screaming during beatings, and contacted a volunteer church worker with their concerns. The church worker contacted the authorities, who told the church worker that they refused to intervene, despite a New York City law allowing removal of children maltreated by caregivers. The volunteer church worker asked the president of the New York Society for the Prevention of Cruelty to Animals (NYSPCA) for help. Acting as a private citizen, the president asked an attorney from the SPCA to petition for the removal of the child from her home so that she would be able to testify about how she had been treated (Scannapieco & Connell-Carrick, 2005). In 1875, the president of the NYSPCA helped found the New York Society for the Prevention of Cruelty to Children (NYSPCC)—8 years after the SPCA was established (Barnett et al., 1993).

Increasing Support for Child Protection Efforts

In 1900, 250 child protection agencies existed in the United States. In the early part of the century, cultural attitudes continued to become more supportive of intervention when families did not show much concern for the wellbeing of their children. However, there was still widespread disagreement about what constituted maltreatment (Barnett et al., 1993). During this time, private charities like the Society for the Prevention of Cruelty to Children (SPCC) were primarily responsible for protecting children (Scannapieco & Connell-Carrick, 2005).

In 1912, the U.S. Children's Bureau was established to represent children's interests. This agency grew out of the recognition that the federal government needed to play a role in child protection and child rights. While this bureau had authority over child protection, it did not handle individual maltreatment cases. In 1935, the Social Security Act was passed, requiring states to strengthen their welfare services for children. While this act mandated intervention for abused and neglected children, it did not address maltreatment identification or prevention (Scannapieco & Connell-Carrick, 2005). As the government increasingly played a role in the welfare of maltreated children, the public relied less on private charities for handling child maltreatment cases. Public attitudes promoted an emphasis on family rehabilitation and assisting parents in keeping child custody. After these changes, provision of services shifted from private citizens to professionally trained mental health workers (Barnett et al., 1993).

Beginning of Research on Child Maltreatment

In the mid-1900s, the medical community recognized and began to define child maltreatment. In 1945, John Caffey from Columbia University wrote about the occurrence of unexplained fractures and subdural hematomas in children, stating the possibility that these injuries were inflicted by parents (Scannapieco & Connell-Carrick, 2005). In 1960, Dr. C. Henry Kempe and colleagues in Colorado first described battered child syndrome. They published an article entitled, "The Battered Child Syndrome," giving a detailed description of characteristics of child physical abuse (see Roche, Fortin, Labbé, Brown, & Chadwick, 2005), and drawing the attention of researchers.[2] In the 1960s and 1970s, researchers began to explore the etiology and extent of the abuse and neglect of children (Scannapieco & Connell-Carrick, 2005); this research continues today.

---

[2] While this was the first research published in the U.S. on battered child syndrome, this syndrome was described in 1860 by the French forensic physician Ambroise Tardieu. One of Kempe's colleagues, Frederic N. Silverman, credited Tardieu as the first to describe battered child syndrome. However, since no English translation of Tardieu's monograph describing the syndrome was yet available, Roche and colleagues provided an English summary of the monograph in 2005 (Roche et al., 2005).

Recent Child Protection Laws

The Child Abuse Prevention and Treatment Act (CAPTA) was signed into law in 1974 (P.L. 93-247) and guides child protection efforts today. The law was amended and reauthorized several times since 1974, and was amended and re-authorized most recently in 2010 (Child Information Gateway, 2011).

Defining Child Maltreatment: Challenges and Inconsistencies

In 1993, the National Academy of Science reported that inconsistencies in definitions often preclude comparative analyses of clinical studies (National Research Council, 1993, p. 5). The National Research Council (NRC) noted that despite two decades of debate in an effort to develop definitions of abuse and neglect that are clear, useful, reliable, and valid, little progress has been made. While the names of maltreatment types are generally consistent across research studies (e.g., physical abuse, sexual abuse), operational definitions differ. Researchers' ability to draw conclusions about the scope of the problem of child maltreatment and its causal factors is limited by these definitional issues (National Research Council, 1993). The state of affairs has not changed much in more than a decade. Heyman and Slep remark that "… most people would be incredulous to learn that there is no accepted operationalized definition of what constitutes child or partner physical, sexual, or emotional abuse or child neglect…clinical decisions about who has and who has not committed… child maltreatment are made every day in the absence of empirically supported definitions," (2006, p. 397). The threshold for what types of parenting practices are considered inappropriate varies across investigators and states (Manly, 2005).

The NRC listed the following as difficulties that face researchers who attempt to define child maltreatment: lack of social agreement on which types of parenting are acceptable versus dangerous; lack of certainty about whether child maltreatment should be characterized by adult behavior, child outcomes, context, or more than one of these factors; disagreement about whether Endangerment or Harm Standards should be included in definitions; and uncertainty about the appropriateness of having similar definitions across the legal, clinical, and scientific fields (National Research Council, 1993). Barnett and colleagues (1993) summarized different fields' definitions of child maltreatment, explaining that the sociological perspective defines child maltreatment as a social judgment that certain acts of parents are not appropriate for cultural standards, and that the legal perspective defines child maltreatment based on documentable physical injuries or emotional harm that resulted from parental actions against the child. Hence, the sociological perspective focuses on parental actions and the legal perspective focuses on the effects of maltreatment (Barnett et al., 1993). Researchers still grapple with this debate (Cicchetti & Toth, 2005).

One can find costs and benefits to a child for each type of approach. If we base the definition of maltreatment on effects on a child, we then focus on evaluating children's wellbeing when considering whether maltreatment has occurred. However, this approach may cause us to disregard cases in which a child suffered maltreatment but shows no evidence of the maltreatment (e.g., sexual abuse that has happened behind closed doors and leaves no physical evidence, emotional abuse that may show harm later in life that is not evident immediately after the abuse takes place). In some cases, if we based definitions of maltreatment on the actions of the caregiver, this could lead our focus away from the wellbeing of the child. However, in cases in which there is evidence of the caregiver's actions against the child but no way to prove evidence of harm, basing definitions of maltreatment on the actions of the caregiver could increase child victims' chances of gaining necessary protection and intervention.

Different Definitions for Different Purposes

With each way that maltreatment is defined, we should ask what purpose the definition serves. A definition that is useful for research may not be appropriate in a legal setting. A definition that is focused on more apparent signs that maltreatment has occurred, such as those used in a medical setting to detect physical maltreatment, may not be useful for detecting subtle types of maltreatment (Cicchetti & Toth, 2005). The debate is made even more complex because child maltreatment includes physical abuse, sexual abuse, emotional maltreatment (sometimes called "emotional abuse" or "psychological abuse"), and neglect (Cicchetti & Toth, 2005; National Research Council, 1993; Scannapieco & Connell-Carrick, 2005).

Legal Definitions of Abuse

The Child Abuse Prevention and Treatment Act (CAPTA) provides the federal definition of child maltreatment: "'child abuse and neglect' means, at a minimum, any recent act or failure to act on the part of a parent or caretaker, which results in death, serious physical or emotional harm, sexual abuse or exploitation, or an act or failure to act which presents an imminent risk of serious harm." (USDHHS, 2003, p. 44).

Defining Neglect

Mennen, Kim, Sang, and Trickett (2010) provide an extensive review of the studies conducted in the past decade that have developed categories of subtypes of neglect within the broader category of neglect to account for the wide variety of experiences of children whose maltreatment is named under the umbrella of "neglect." They conclude that one of the "most important" attempts to classify the types of neglect resulted in the Modified Maltreatment Classification System (MMCS) neglect subtypes. The MMCS subtypes of neglect are Physical Neglect, Failure to Provide; and Physical Neglect, Lack of Supervision (English & The LONGSCAN Investigators, 1997).

"Physical Neglect, Failure to Provide is coded when a caregiver or responsible adult fails to exercise a minimum degree of care in meeting the child's physical needs." (English & The LONGSCAN Investigators, 1997, p. 15). In cases of families who are below the poverty line, neglect is scored when families have failed to access available community resources in order to provide for their children's needs. These needs include adequate food; sanitary, weather-appropriate clothing allowing the child's freedom of movement; adequate shelter; adequate health care for medical, dental, and mental health needs; and adequate hygiene (English & The LONGSCAN Investigators, 1997).

Physical Neglect, Lack of Supervision "...is coded when a caregiver or responsible adult does not take adequate precautions to ensure a child's safety in and out of the home, given the child's particular emotional and developmental needs." (English & The LONGSCAN Investigators, 1997, p. 22). Lack of Supervision is one of the most commonly reported subtypes of neglect even though there are no clear standards for age-appropriate supervision. If a caregiver permits a child's exposure to dangerous circumstances or fails to take sufficient precautions to assess a child's safety, the caregiver may be judged as having physically neglected the child by a lack of supervision (English & The LONGSCAN Investigators, 1997).

While neglect is the most commonly occurring maltreatment type in the United States, it has been studied far less than any of the other types (Mennen et al., 2010) and tends to have a low profile in public awareness (Stone, 1998). It is likely that its status as the most frequently occurring yet probably least understood maltreatment type is due to definitional issues and the difficulty of substantiating any neglect except in the most severe cases (Urquiza & Winn, 1992). Neglect tends to have a low profile in public awareness when compared with abuse. This may be caused by the public's view of abuse as a crisis and by the tendency of neglect to be a long-term issue that affects development over time. This may cause neglect to be less noticeable to the public (Stone, 1998). For over 25 years, researchers have referred to this lack of attention relative to the importance of this type of maltreatment as the "neglect of neglect" (McSherry, 2007; Wolock & Horowitz, 1984).

Another challenge in identifying neglect is that there is a spectrum of parenting quality that ranges from truly excellent care to wholly inadequate care, and neglectful parenting exists on this spectrum. The spectrum includes a grey area, and it is difficult to determine where a line should be drawn to separate adequate from inadequate childcare (Dubowitz, 2007).

Defining Physical Abuse

"Physical Abuse is coded when a caregiver or responsible adult inflicts physical injury upon a child by other than accidental means." (English & The LONGSCAN Investigators, 1997, p. 2). Types of abuse represented by these codes include shaking, throwing, physically dropping a child; hitting a child with a hand or an object; pushing, grabbing, dragging, or pulling a child; and punching or kicking a child (Sedlak et al., 2010). When a caregiver threatens a child but does not make any physical contact with the child, it is considered emotional abuse. When sexual interactions directly cause physical injuries such as vaginal or rectal tears, these injuries are noted solely as having resulted from sexual abuse. Injuries that result from acts such as burning or beating a child in order to force the child into engagement in sexual relations with the abuser are scored as both physical abuse and sexual abuse (English & The LONGSCAN Investigators, 1997).

Defining Sexual Abuse

According to CAPTA, "sexual abuse includes (a) the employment, use, persuasion, inducement, enticement, or coercion of any child to engage in, or assist any other person to engage in, any sexually explicit conduct or simulation of such conduct for the purpose of producing a visual depiction of such conduct; or (b) the rape, and in cases of caretaker or inter-familial relationships, statutory rape, molestation, prostitution, or other form of sexual exploitation of children, or incest with children..." (USDHHS, 2003, p. 44). Sexual abuse includes sex with or without force, child's prostitution or involvement in pornography, molestation with genital contact, exposure/voyeurism, provision of sexually explicit materials, failure to supervise child's voluntary sexual activity, and attempted/threatened sexual abuse with physical contact (Sedlak et al., 2010).

With respect to the most deleterious acts against children, professionals and most families seem to agree on general definitions of what is and is not maltreatment. With respect to what Barnett and colleagues (1993, p. 44) call, "the 'grey area' that lies between insensitive parenting and outright abuse and neglect," Barnett and colleagues say that the definitions of maltreatment are not static, and that there will not ever be a definition of maltreatment that satisfies professionals and families and is relevant to multiple generations.

References

Barnett, D., Manly, J. T., & Cicchetti, D. (1993). Defining child maltreatment: The interface between policy and research. In D. Cicchetti & S. L. Toth (Eds.), *Child Abuse, Child Development and Social Policy* (Advances in applied developmental psychology, pp. 7–73). Norwood, NJ: Ablex Publishing Corp.

Child Information Gateway. (2011). *About CAPTA: A legislative history*. Washington, DC: U.S. Department of Health and Human Services, Children's Bureau.

Cicchetti, D., & Toth, S. L. (2005). Child maltreatment. *Annual Review of Clinical Psychology, 1*(1), 409–438. doi:10.1146/annurev.clinpsy.1.102803.144029.

Dubowitz, H. (2007). Understanding and addressing the "neglect of neglect:" Digging into the molehill. *Child Abuse & Neglect, 31*(6), 603–606. doi:10.1016/j.chiabu.2007.04.002.

English, D. J., & The LONGSCAN Investigators. (1997). *Modified Maltreatment Classification System (MMCS)*. For more information visit the LONGSCAN website at: http://www.iprc.unc.edu/longscan/. Accessed 9 Apr 2012.

Heyman, R. E., & Slep, A. M. S. (2006). Creating and field-testing child maltreatment definitions: Improving the reliability of substantiation determinations. *Child Maltreatment, 11*(3), 217–236. doi:10.1177/1077559506288878.

Leslie, L. K., Hurlburt, M. S., James, S., Landsverk, J., Slymen, D. J., & Zhang, J. (2005). Relationship between entry into child welfare and mental health service use. *Psychiatric Services, 56*(8), 981–987.

Manly, J. T. (2005). Advances in research definitions of child maltreatment. *Child Abuse & Neglect, 29*(5), 425–439. doi:10.1016/j.chiabu.2005.04.001.

McSherry, D. (2007). Understanding and addressing the "neglect of neglect": Why are we making a mole-hill out of a mountain? *Child Abuse & Neglect, 31*(6), 607–614. doi:10.1016/j.chiabu.2006.08.011.

Mennen, F. E., Kim, K., Sang, J., & Trickett, P. K. (2010). Child neglect: Definition and identification of youth's experiences in official reports of maltreatment. *Child Abuse & Neglect, 34*(9), 647–658. doi:10.1016/j.chiabu.2010.02.007.

National Research Council. (1993). *Understanding child abuse and neglect* (p. xiii, 393pp.). Washington, DC: National Academy Press.

Roche, A. J., Fortin, G., Labbé, J., Brown, J., & Chadwick, D. (2005). The work of Ambroise Tardieu: The first definitive description of child abuse. *Child Abuse & Neglect, 29*(4), 325–334. doi:10.1016/j.chiabu.2004.04.007.

Scannapieco, M., & Connell-Carrick, K. (2005). *Understanding child maltreatment: An ecological and developmental perspective*. New York: Oxford University Press.

Sedlak, A. J., Mettenburg, J., Basena, M., Petta, I., McPherson, K., Greene, A., et al. (2010). *Fourth National Incidence Study of Child Abuse and Neglect (NIS-4): Report to Congress*. Washington, DC: U.S. Department of Health and Human Services, Administration for Children and Families.

Stone, B. (1998). Child neglect: Practitioners' perspectives. *Child Abuse Review, 7*(2), 87–96. doi:10.1002/(sici)1099-0852(199803/04)7:2<87::aid-car368>3.0.co;2-7.

U.S. Department of Health and Human Services [USDHHS]. (2003, June 25). *The Child Abuse Prevention and Treatment Act Including Adoption Opportunities and The Abandoned Infants Assistance Act*. Washington, DC: U.S. Department of Health and Human Services.

U.S. Department of Health and Human Services, Administration on Children, Youth and Families, & Children's Bureau. (2011). *Child Maltreatment 2010*. Available from http://www.acf.hhs.gov/programs/cb/stats_research/index.htm#can. Accessed 9 Apr 2012.

Urquiza, A. J., & Winn, C. (1992). *Treatment for Abused and Neglected Children: Infancy to Age 18*. Washington, DC: United States Department of Health and Human Services.

Wolock, I., & Horowitz, B. (1984). Child maltreatment as a social problem: The neglect of neglect. *The American Journal of Orthopsychiatry, 54*(4), 530–543.

Chapter 2
A Brief History of Evidence-Based Practice

Lindsay A. Forte, Susan Timmer, and Anthony Urquiza

While Dr. Archie Cochrane takes most of the credit for today's widespread implementation of Evidence-Based Practice (EBP) in medicine, our story of EBP in psychology dates back to a clash between psychodynamic and behavioral/learning theory in the 1950s. In the 1950s, there was very little evidence to support the use of adult and child psychotherapy. In fact, both Eysenck (1952) and Levitt (1957, 1963) had concluded that "the simple passage of time" could account for any positive effects of psychotherapy. Luckily for the sustainment of this field, these scathing reviews led to more trials, tests, and a general movement towards evidence and research to justify treatment.

In the early 1960s, a clinical child psychologist named Alan O. Ross was staunchly in favor of empirically-based practice. In 1959 he wrote *The Practice of Clinical Child Psychology*, a book that goes into detail about how research is one of the main areas of clinical child psychology. Ross went on to help found and lead the Clinical Child Psychology section (Section 1) of APA Division 12, Clinical Psychology in 1962, which became Division 53 of the American Psychological Association, the Society of Clinical Child & Adolescent Psychology (SCCAP). Today, Division 53 works to bring evidence-based treatment to parents and therapists and sponsors online education and training. Division 53 and the Association for Behavioral and Cognitive Therapies (ABCT), founded under the name Association for Advancement of Behavioral Therapies (AABT) shortly thereafter in 1966, currently help to widely disseminate evidence-based practice by keeping updated research publications listed and available (Erickson, 2011).

The Task Force on Promotion and Dissemination of Psychological Procedures (part of APA Division 12) made a bold move in 1995 by publishing a report that

L.A. Forte (✉) • S. Timmer, Ph.D. • A. Urquiza, Ph.D.
CAARE Diagnostic and Treatment Center, Department of Pediatrics, University of California at Davis Children's Hospital, 3671 Business Dr., Sacramento, CA 95820, USA
e-mail: lindsay.forte@ucdmc.ucdavis.edu; susan.timmer@ucdmc.ucdavis.edu; anthony.urquiza@ucdmc.ucdavis.edu

S. Timmer and A. Urquiza (eds.), *Evidence-Based Approaches for the Treatment of Maltreated Children*, Child Maltreatment 3, DOI 10.1007/978-94-007-7404-9_2,
© Springer Science+Business Media Dordrecht 2014

defined and adopted the term "empirically supported." This report identified four main categories of treatments; "well-established" treatments were those that had been proven effective according to at least one randomized control trial (RCT) following very strict experimental guidelines. In order to be well-established, a treatment must be statistically significantly superior to a placebo or another treatment, or equivalent to (if not better than) an already established treatment. "Probably efficacious" treatments should be proven to be more effective than a no-treatment control group, "possibly efficacious" treatments must have at least one study showing positive results, and "experimental" treatments have not yet been tested in randomized control trials. These terms were general guidelines to categorize the full range of psychotherapy in adults and children. And of the identified and categorized treatments in the report, only three treatments specifically for children were decidedly "well-established." Not one of these acknowledged treatments were specifically designed for maltreated children. By laying out the standards of "empirical support," the APA confirmed its support for evidence-based practice. Evidence-based practice is an approach to clinical practice that calls for research, specifically quantitative experimental designs, to determine the best clinical methods.

In full support of APA's mandate, the very next year, Urquiza and McNeil (1996) published an article pushing for increasing evidence-based practice for a very specific population: physically abused young children. In their thought-provoking article, they suggested that Parent–Child Interaction Therapy (PCIT) could be the go-to treatment for that population. It became clear in the field of child clinical psychology that more research and evidence was needed to prove that treatment was actually making a difference for these children. Around the same time, Cohen and Mannarino (1996) and Deblinger, Lippmann, and Steer (1996) both conducted a randomized controlled trial looking at the effects of very similar interventions, which supported the use of TF-CBT in reducing trauma symptoms in sexually abused children. Cohen and Mannarino found positive results for TF-CBT being more effective than a nondirective supportive therapy, while Deblinger and her colleagues (1996) documented the importance of including parents in treatment with the children. At the time, finding a reliable way to treat the debilitating effects of sexual abuse was an important move forward for supporters of the use of evidence-based practice in clinical psychology. These clinical research scientists were changing the definition of clinical outcomes, from one emphasizing the way people thought about themselves and stressful events to one that depended on measuring changes of symptom intensity (Kazdin, 2008). While evidence-based treatments (EBTs) were gaining research spotlight and advocates in the policy world, many concerns were raised about the quality of EBTs empirical findings.

Opponents of the EBP movement brought up three concerns (Ollendick, 1999). First is the reliance on randomized control trials to establish the empirical base, proving efficacy caused a problem, because not all theories of practice lent themselves well to these types of quantitative experiments. For example, more psychodynamic interventions emphasized clients' changing perceptions of themselves and their social environment, and was less concerned about reductions in symptom levels. But according to the definitions of well-established EBTs these treatments that did not have evidence showing positive "outcomes" through RCTs could not be considered effective. The evidence-based treatment game was being played on a lopsided playing field. Behaviorally oriented interventions, or interventions that aimed to reduce the frequency of discrete behaviors, were easy to research in RCTs and so were "empirically supported." More idiosyncratic psychodynamic approaches that strive for less measurable outcomes were difficult to research and lacked empirical support.

Second, there was a concern that the evidence base was rolling out from the settings that could fund it, and that these interventions would not translate to the "real world." Finally, therapists are concerned that their clinical training and judgment would not be valued if their practice came solely from manualized treatments. They argued that a manual could not contain an answer for every possible scenario that might pop up in a treatment session and that having to maintain fidelity to the treatment would interfere with meeting the needs of each client (Ollendick & King, 2004). Ollendick and King, addressing these concerns, came to the conclusion that there are major arguments for and against using EBTs, and in order to fully address them, clinicians and researchers must communicate about what works and how to streamline translation of empirical evidence to practice. Furthermore, they asserted that "Children and their families presenting at our clinics deserve our concerted attention to further the true synthesis of these approaches and to transform our laboratory findings into rich and clinically sensitive practices." (Ollendick & King, p. 21)

While the number of evidence-based treatments were increasing, national surveys such as those conducted by the U.S. Surgeon General in 1999 (U.S. Public Health Service, U.S. Department of Health and Human Services, & Office of the Surgeon General, 1999) made it clear that many people were not receiving these services. In 2002, President Bush convened the New Freedom Commission on Mental Health to address this problem. After careful study, the Commission issued a report in 2003 recommending the transformation of America's mental health care system. The recommendations suggested that the transformation should involve a push towards making evidence-based practice the foundation of all clinical practice. The report states that it currently takes far too long for research on effective treatments to translate into clinical practice. This transformation was meant to eliminate confusion, and increase effectiveness and efficiency within the overall mental health care system. It was stated that in order to achieve this transformation, more funding from clinical programs would need to go toward supporting evidence-based practice for children, specifically for PCIT, multi-systemic therapy, functional family therapy, and treatment of foster care children. The commission urged the Centers for Medicare and Medicaid Services (CMS) to aid programs in making these financial changes (President's New Freedom Commission on Mental Health, 2003, p. 17). This 2003 President's New Freedom Commission report is an example of how on a national level a light is being shone on evidence-based practice, increasing the pressure on community mental health agencies to provide these services.

With policy makers and government agencies advocating for and funding psychotherapeutic interventions that actually worked for the people they were designed for, treatment developers had strong incentives for conducting research to confirm the efficacy of their interventions. As a result, the number of controlled investigations supporting treatments increased dramatically, although the evidence for some interventions was noted to consist of laboratory analogues, small groups, or using children whose symptoms were non-clinical (Ollendick & King, 1998). Research focused largely on proving efficacy rather than their effectiveness in clinical practice. In 1996, Barlow, sounding a rally cry, wrote an article underlining the concerns the mental health field would face if researchers didn't find more evidence to help create a more comprehensive list of effective psychotherapeutic interventions and establish evidence-based treatments as effective in practice settings. His concern was that government agencies such as the American Psychiatric Association placed too much emphasis and funding on pharmacological interventions over psychotherapy because there was so little evidence that their positive outcomes would generalize in the community (Barlow, 1996). Also responding to the need to establish effective treatments in clinical practice, Brown and colleagues discussed ways in which clinical researchers could begin to bridge the vast gap between research and practice in a 1997 article (Brown et al., 1997). Their article described how multisystemic therapy (MST) was structured in a way that insured communication among clinical researchers, clinical practitioners and stakeholders (e.g., Child Protective Services). While MST serves as a model for optimizing communication between research and practice, the "gap" between evidence-based treatments and the patients who need them in the clinic is a continuing problem in child clinical psychology (Shafran et al., 2009).

In spite of the increasing hope that EBTs would reduce the burden of mental health problems in young children, researchers' ability to demonstrate success in the laboratory continued to outpace their effective use in clinical practice (Weersing & Weisz, 2002). Findings from studies comparing the effectiveness of EBTs in community mental health settings with research settings suggested that their effects were more modest than expected (Weiss, Catron, Harris, & Phung, 1999), not much better than control groups fared in the university setting (Weersing & Weisz). The results of these studies presented a new burden for treatment developers and EBP advocates: to consider how the community practice setting might reduce the effectiveness of the intervention.

The history of evidence-based practice contains important research breakthroughs in the realm of clinical child psychology. It allowed us to move past the question of "if" psychotherapy works for children, and tackle the question of "which one" works best for which children. The push toward evidence-based practice has helped us to make sure that treatment will "have a sound theoretical basis, a good clinical-anecdotal literature, high acceptance among practitioners in the child abuse field, a low chance for causing harm, and empirical support for their utility with victims of abuse" (National Crime Victims Research and Treatment Center & Center for Sexual Assault and Traumatic Stress, 2004).

More recently, research on evidence-based treatment in psychology has shed light on the fact that there are not always tailored interventions for specific underserved populations (APA Task Force on EBP for Children and Adolescents, 2008), such as maltreated children. In 2000, Congress established the National Child

Traumatic Stress Network (NCTSN). Originally developed as part of the Children's Health Act, the NCTSN has helped to develop over 40 evidence-based treatments to date (National Child Traumatic Stress Network, 2012), suitable for treating traumatized children. They are also a large force in providing training resources for clinicians working with maltreated children.

On the journey towards improved mental health for children, the good news is that we have many excellent EBTs that are developed for maltreated children and have demonstrated value – both in university laboratories and in the community – for decreasing child mental health problems resulting from different types of sexual abuse, physical abuse, and neglect. Additionally, these interventions address nearly all of the common mental health problems presented to private practitioners, non-profit mental health agencies, and state and local mental health programs.

References

American Psychological Association Task Force on Evidence-Based Practice for Children and Adolescents. (2008). *Disseminating evidence-based practice for children and adolescents: A systems approach to enhancing care.* Washington, DC: American Psychological Association.

Barlow, D. H. (1996). Health care policy, psychotherapy research, and the future of psychotherapy. *The American Psychologist, 51*(10), 1050–1058.

Brown, T. L., Swenson, C. C., Cunningham, P. B., Henggeler, S. W., Schoenwald, S. K., & Rowland, M. D. (1997). Multisystemic treatment of violent and chronic juvenile offenders: Bridging the gap between research and practice. *Administration and Policy in Mental Health, 25*(2), 221–238.

Cohen, J. A., & Mannarino, A. P. (1996). A treatment outcome study for sexually abused preschool children: Initial findings. *Journal of the American Academy of Child and Adolescent Psychiatry, 35*(1), 42–50.

Deblinger, E., Lippmann, J., & Steer, R. (1996). Sexually abused children suffering posttraumatic stress symptoms: Initial treatment outcome findings. *Child Maltreatment, 1*(4), 310–321.

Erickson, M. T. (2011). *A brief history of the society of clinical child and adolescent psychology (SCCAP) from Section 1, APA Division 12, status through APA Division 53 status. American Psychological Association, Division 53.* Retrieved from https://www.clinicalchildpsychology.org/node/137. Accessed 9 May 2013,

Eysenck, H. J. (1952). The effects of psychotherapy: An evaluation. *Journal of Consulting Psychology, 16*(5), 319–324.

Kazdin, A. E. (2008). Evidence-based treatment and practice: New opportunities to bridge clinical research and practice, enhance the knowledge base, and improve patient care. *The American Psychologist, 63*(3), 146–159.

Levitt, E. E. (1957). The results of psychotherapy with children: An evaluation. *Journal of Consulting Psychology, 21*(3), 189–196.

Levitt, E. E. (1963). Psychotherapy with children: A further evaluation. *Behavior Research and Therapy, 1*(1), 45–51.

National Child Traumatic Stress Network. (2012). History of the NCTSN. *Raising the standard of care.* Retrieved from www.nctsnet.org/about-us/history-of-the-nctsn. Accessed 9 May 2013.

National Crime Victims Research and Treatment Center, & Center for Sexual Assault and Traumatic Stress. (2004). *Child physical and sexual abuse: Guidelines for treatment.* Retrieved from http://musc.edu/ncvc/resources_prof/OVC_guidelines04-26-04.pdf. Accessed 9 May 2013.

Ollendick, T. H. (1999). AABT and empirically validated treatments. *Behaviour Therapist, 18*, 81–82.

Ollendick, T. H., & King, N. J. (1998). Empirically supported treatments for children with phobic and anxiety disorders: Current status. *Journal of Clinical Child Psychology, 27*, 56–167.

Ollendick, T. H., & King, N. J. (2004). Empirically supported treatments for children and adolescents: Advances toward evidence-based practice. In P. M. Barrett & T. H. Ollendick (Eds.), *Handbook of interventions that work with children and adolescents: Prevention and treatment* (pp. 3–25). New York, NY: Wiley.

President's New Freedom Commission on Mental Health. (2003). *Report of the President's new freedom commission on mental health*. Retrieved from http://govinfo.library.unt.edu/mentalhealthcommission/reports/comments_011003.pdf. Accessed 9 May 2013.

Ross, A. O. (1959). *The practice of clinical child psychology*. Oxford, UK: Grune & Stratton.

Shafran, R., Clark, D. M., Fairburn, C. G., Arntz, A., Barlow, D. H., Ehlers, A., et al. (2009). Mind the gap: Improving the dissemination of CBT. *Behaviour Research and Therapy, 47*(11), 902–909.

Task Force on Promotion and Dissemination. (1995). Training in and dissemination of empirically validated treatments: Report and recommendations. *Clinical Psychologist, 48*, 3–23.

Urquiza, A. J., & McNeil, C. B. (1996). Parent–child interaction therapy: An intensive dyadic intervention for physically abusive families. *Child Maltreatment, 1*(2), 124–144.

U.S. Public Health Service, U.S. Department of Health and Human Services, & Office of the Surgeon General. (1999). *Mental health: A report of the Surgeon General*. Rockville, MD: Substance Abuse and Mental Health Services Administration. Retrieved from http://profiles.nlm.nih.gov/ps/retrieve/ResourceMetadata/NNBBHS. Accessed 9 May 2013.

Weersing, V. R., & Weisz, J. R. (2002). Mechanisms of action in youth psychotherapy. *Journal of Child Psychology and Psychiatry, and Allied Disciplines, 43*(1), 3–29.

Weiss, B. H., Catron, T., Harris, V., & Phung, T. M. (1999). The effectiveness of traditional child psychotherapy. *Journal of Consulting and Clinical Psychology, 67*, 82–94.

Chapter 3
Why We Think We Can Make Things Better with Evidence-Based Practice: Theoretical and Developmental Context

Susan Timmer and Anthony Urquiza

The Ecological—Transactional Model of Development

More than 20 years ago, Cicchetti and Lynch (1993) developed a theory to explain how child maltreatment could have such a potent effect on children's development: the ecological-transactional model of development. Ecological-transactional theory is founded on an understanding that different qualities of children's environments—their cultural environments, social resources, family environments, and individual differences all combine to shape the way children respond to the surrounding world. Like Belsky (1980), they called these different types of environments "ecologies": the "macrosystem" (i.e., cultural environment), "exosystem" (i.e., community), "microsystem" (i.e., family system), and at the individual level, a child's ontogenesis. They proposed that characteristics of these environmental systems influence the way children negotiate different developmental tasks, providing foundations of structures at one point in time that influence later development. Cicchetti and Lynch (1993) proposed that these ecologies contain "potentiating factors," or conditions that increase the likelihood that either maltreatment might occur or negatively affect the child, and "compensatory factors," that reduce the likelihood of maltreatment and violence and their accompanying negative effects. For example, the Administration for Youth and Families' 2010 report on Child Maltreatment in the United States showed that 3.9 % of child victims of maltreatment were reported to have behavior problems (U.S. Department of Health and Human Services (USDHHS), Administration for Children, Youth & Families, & Children's Bureau, 2011). While this aggressive behavior is likely a response to problems in their own family, we might also expect to observe higher levels of aggression in children living

S. Timmer, Ph.D. (✉) • A. Urquiza, Ph.D.
CAARE Diagnostic and Treatment Center, Department of Pediatrics, University of California at Davis Children's Hospital, 3671 Business Dr., Sacramento, CA 95820, USA
e-mail: susan.timmer@ucdmc.ucdavis.edu; anthony.urquiza@ucdmc.ucdavis.edu

S. Timmer and A. Urquiza (eds.), *Evidence-Based Approaches for the Treatment of Maltreated Children*, Child Maltreatment 3, DOI 10.1007/978-94-007-7404-9_3,
© Springer Science+Business Media Dordrecht 2014

in cultural environments more accepting of domestic violence (e.g., Guerra, Hammons, & Clutter, 2011; Staub, 1996) or in communities with high levels of violence (Guerra, Huesmann, & Spindler, 2003). In this way, cultural attitudes towards domestic violence and the community experience of violence serve as a *potentiating factor* in the child's exosystem for aggressive behavior in children. However, a family value system strongly advocating self-control and non-violence might serve as a *compensatory factor* reducing the likelihood that a child would be aggressive.

These compensatory and potentiating factors, present in all levels of children's ecologies are also described as varying according to their stability, or enduring quality (Cicchetti & Toth, 2000). Certain risk factors, such as a parent's mental health, may be enduring. Enduring risk factors are considered to be *vulnerabilities*—existing across developmental stages. Other risk factors, such as a child's medical condition, might be a transient challenge—causing stress and *potentiating* the likelihood of abuse until the condition is resolved or managed. Certain compensatory factors like parent intelligence or employment may also be enduring. These are considered to be *protective factors*—protecting the child from abuse or the negative effects of abuse across developmental stages. More transient protective factors, like influential teachers, are referred to as *buffers*, creating a temporary wall against the tides of misfortune. When the potentiating factors and challenges outnumber the protective factors and buffers, theory suggests that the child will display maladaptive behavior, creating developmental vulnerabilities and increasing the likelihood of psychopathology.

So far this model seems simple—the ratio of positives to negatives from different parts of the child's environment should increase the likelihood of maladaptation. However, it is important to point out that the strength of these factors in promoting risk or resilience at any one point in time varies according to both the developmental stage of the child and what has happened to the child at earlier ages (Alink, Cicchetti, Kim, & Rogosch, 2009; Sroufe, Egeland, & Kreutzer, 1990). In other words, the same negative event occurring at two different points in children's development can have different outcomes for children's mental health because of differences in their abilities to understand the event (i.e., differences in cognitive ability), the meaning the event has at the particular point in development that it occurred, and the meaning the event has for the child's ongoing ability to adapt positively, "collecting" protective and buffering factors. For example, Sroufe and his colleagues, using data from a longitudinal study, examined the power of early attachment, adaptation during preschool and kindergarten, and the home environment to affect a child's emotional health in elementary school. They found that earlier positive adaptation and home environment predicted emotional health even when they took into consideration the current home environment. However, the quality of children's attachment at 12–18 months of age did not significantly predict functioning in elementary school when they considered children's adaptation in preschool and kindergarten. The message from this research, taken from the perspective of the ecological transactional theory is that the power of early traumatic experiences to continue to exert negative influences on children's development depends on the degree to which they link to later potentiating factors and maladaptive behaviors.

While the development of mental health problems seems inevitable when considering the trauma of witnessing violence or experiencing abuse, it is difficult to estimate the power that certain experiences or conditions have to build resilience in the child (O'Connor, 2003). Even when you think you know all the salient facts of a child's environment, there is always the mystery of the resilience inherent in the child's physiological, neurological, and cognitive makeup and how they work together in the developing child. From an ecological-transactional perspective, the best that we can say is that the development of psychopathology is probabilistic and not certain. Furthermore, this theory views development as "a series of qualitative reorganizations among and within biological and psychological systems" as children mature (Cicchetti & Toth, 2000, p. 94). In other words, as children mature cognitively they perceive the world around them qualitatively differently. This maturation is thought to drive reorganization of previous experiences, prompting children to adopt a more complex understanding of their environment and life history (Cicchetti & Lynch, 1993).

While cognitive maturation most certainly limits or shapes children's understanding of their worlds, it is also believed that each developmental stage contains different "tasks" considered central to children's ability to successfully negotiate that stage. How well these tasks are resolved determines the quality of the organization and integration of different systems (e.g., neurological, cognitive, social, emotional) in that stage. The network of integrated systems is believed to provide a groundwork upon which subsequent developmental structures are built. In this way, different developmental tasks always retain significance over time, even when other developmental tasks are more salient. In other words, if a developmental task in one system is negotiated poorly or incompletely—this affects not only the quality of that system, but of the whole—as the weakness of one system can limit the strength of other integrated systems, both at that developmental stage and at hierarchically more advanced developmental stages. For example, take the example of an infant boy who experienced chronic domestic violence over several months, and often cried inconsolably when his mother was out of sight. One task of this developmental stage is increased independence from the primary caregiver and tolerance of strangers. This poorly resolved task, connected with heightened activation of the fear response system, might also spill over into the child's ability to reach other developmental milestones. An infant that is hypervigilant to his mother's emotional presence might not be attending fully to other information in his environment important to language or cognitive development. If, as we suppose, these early skills, emotional reactivity, attention, and learning strategies serve as a foundation for higher-level skills, then early chronic activation of the fear-response system could inhibit the optimal development of later cognitive and social-emotional systems.

Two guiding principles of developmental psychopathology are that one should expect many different kinds of outcomes to exposure to a type of event (multifinality) and that there are many paths to a single type of outcome (equifinality). So, in spite of the gloomy forecast one might have for a child exposed to violence or maltreatment at an early age, one would expect that not all of these children end up with problems. In fact, research has supported this expectation (Cicchetti & Rogosch, 1997).

Hence, we can say that negative outcomes are not inevitable, but probabilistic. There is always room to build resilience and improve functioning. The assumption that the development of psychopathology is probabilistic, and that these probabilities are constantly being shaped and reshaped by experience is the most important assumption of this theory for people interested in prevention and intervention for traumatized children. What this means is that changing the trajectory of development is always possible when there is a possibility of accumulating new, more positive experience, particularly when the new experience forces a reorganization of old experiences and thought patterns through the lens of more positive experience. Effective mental health interventions should be able to help modify the negative effects of early trauma on future functioning if, as we believe, there is always a path to a new, more positive way of functioning.

While we understand that theoretically there should be a path to more positive functioning for maltreated children, finding that path is not always simple. What determines the most effective intervention for different children? We believe that to make a proper judgment about which intervention to use, it is important to understand what is happening to children neurologically, physiologically, cognitively, emotionally, and behaviorally.

Maltreatment and Development

Ecological-transactional theory (Cicchetti & Lynch, 1993) would suggest that the younger a child is when he or she experiences an adverse event such as maltreatment, the more far-reaching its effects would be, since these same systems affected by the stress of maltreatment rapidly develop in the early years of life. While this makes logical sense, we know that infants will not remember their preverbal experience, and think that they are probably safe from the most devastating effects of maltreatment. These adverse events do not generate memories and learning in the way it might in a 5-year old. And yet, accumulating evidence from research on animals and humans suggests that chronic exposure to fear and anxiety, and abusive caregiving leave a neurological footprint (e.g., Cicchetti, Rogosch, Gunnar, & Toth, 2010; Sanchez et al., 2010) that underpins the shape of their attachment to primary caregivers (Cicchetti, Rogosch, Toth, & Sturge-Apple, 2011), determine which events in their environment are perceived, how they are interpreted (Pollak, Cicchetti, Hornung, & Reed, 2000), and which events are remembered (Goodman, Quas, Batterman-Faunce, Riddlesberger, & Kuhn, 1997).

Neurological Effects

Chronic or acute stress resulting from maltreatment or other adverse early life experiences can cause different types of neurological responses in infants: (1) through the sympathetic adrenomedullary system they can cause a release of norepinephrine and epinephrine (flight or fright response); (2) or through the locus coeruleus they can cause increased neural activity in the amygdala (Ellis, Jackson, & Boyce, 2006). These neurological responses cause two types of onward physiological effects. They can stimulate corticotropin-releasing hormone (CRH) production, which increases hypothalamic-pituitary axis (HPA) activity (Herman et al., 2003). They can also directly excite the HPA axis by activating the hypothalamus and thus stimulate the release of cortisol. A stress hormone, cortisol activates or inhibits other physiological systems involved in promoting survival in response to acute stress. When infants are chronically exposed to stress hormones, the body's feedback systems for managing and regulating their production can become dysregulated, showing a hyperresponse to stressors (i.e., greater than expected) followed by a period of hyporesponsiveness (i.e., less than expected) (Heim, Ehlert, & Hellhammer, 2000). Animal studies have shown that high levels of cortisol in the system have been found to have harmful, even toxic effects on neural tissue (Zhang et al., 2002). When levels are high, cortisol can regulate gene transcription (McEwen, 2000) and is related to specific patterns of gene expression (Yehuda et al., 2009). HPA-axis dysregulation resulting from early adverse care or maltreatment has the potential for disrupting healthy development, because it increases allostatic load—the physiological vulnerability from chronic exposure to stressful adverse experiences and their accompanying neuroendocrine responses (McEwen & Stellar, 1993). Increased allostatic load may cause dysregulation in the physiological stress management system (e.g., Juster, McEwan, & Lupien, 2009) and impair emotional, cognitive, and physical health (Felitti et al., 1998). The take-away message of this research is that early trauma affects the way children respond to future stressful events; and the way they respond makes them vulnerable to difficulties and delays that create other problems later in development.

While any infant's first experience with an extreme threat is likely to result in the "high-cost" endocrine response described above (e.g., Lupien et al., 2006), subsequent encounters (or anticipated encounters) with the threat should result in the infant seeking out their primary caregivers for help in modulating their anxiety and fear (Heim, Newport, Mletzko, Miller, & Nemeroff, 2008). Infants are dependent on their caregivers for help in soothing, and their soothing helps regulate the infant's stress response system. These social and behavioral solutions have been termed "low-cost" solutions for the infant because of the relatively low expenditure of neurobiological resources needed to accomplish system regulation (Lupien et al.). As an example, maternal separation can cause considerable anxiety for infants once they reach about 8 months of age. When an infant cries inconsolably upon separation from the mother, the baby's HPA axis kicks into gear and sends cortisol into the blood stream. However, one study found that cortisol levels did not increase in 1-year olds who interacted with their babysitters when faced with a separation from their mothers, although it did increase in infants who withdrew and in those who fell asleep (Gunnar, Larson, Hertsgaard, Harris, & Brodersen, 1992). It is interesting that even when the child reacted in a way that would seem benign to an observer— falling asleep or withdrawing rather than engaging with a strange caregiver—there were still signs of increased physiological stress. The strong message of this study was that children who received caregiving presented a more regulated stress response system.

Other related investigations have further shown the power of sensitive and responsive caregiving in promoting children's emotion regulation, stress responsivity, and healthy development (e.g., Bugental, Martorell, & Barraza, 2003; Sroufe, 2005). In fact, the quality of the parent–child relationship, which includes both the child's attachment style and parenting quality have been shown to play important roles in determining the effect of children's early experience of maltreatment on later development of psychopathology.

Sensitive Periods

There is thought that some of maltreatment occurring in infancy may have long-lasting consequences for children because these early negative experiences occurred at a *sensitive period* of development (Knudsen, 2004). In a *sensitive period*, the effects of experiences on the brain are particularly strong for a brief period of time (Knudsen). In infancy, where many neurological and biological systems are growing and changing, early maltreatment might have a particularly strong effect, increasing the chances that a child's future healthy growth and development might be compromised. Alternately, early maltreatment could be particularly devastating for children because there may be *critical periods*, where certain positive experiences are necessary for optimal, healthy development to occur (Knudsen), so that when children experience maltreatment, their developmental trajectories are irrevocably altered. There is no doubt that when maltreatment occurs early, children's likelihood of later exposure to risk is also heightened (Appleyard, Egeland, van Dulmen, & Sroufe, 2005), which naturally increases the likelihood of seeing long-term negative outcomes for these children. But does early maltreatment that results in dysregulation of the stress response system doom the child to a future of psychological problems?

Results of studies comparing children adopted out of Eastern European orphanages at different ages give some evidence for sensitive periods. These studies typically compare the cognitive functioning and attachment styles of children who have spent varying amounts of time in environments of neglect with non-institutionalized children, allowing the investigator to test the notion that if social deprivation occurs before a certain age, it is less likely to cause permanent psychological damage. Several studies' findings suggest that in fact, if children are adopted out of the institution within the first 6 months of their lives, they are indistinguishable from non-institutionalized infants and fare better than their later-adopted counterparts across a range of developmental outcomes (e.g., Beckett et al., 2006; Fisher, Ames, Chisholm, & Savoie, 1997). A meta-analysis of adoption studies conducted by Bakermans-Kranenburg, van IJzendoorn, and Juffer (2008) reported no significant differences in the probability of secure attachment in children adopted before they reached 1 year of age compared to non-adopted children. In addition to studies of institutionally raised children, scholars investigating the effects of maltreatment on neural circuitry have described results in which early maltreatment (before 5 years of age) appeared to be associated with more negative outcomes than maltreatment that occurred later in childhood (Cicchetti et al., 2010), supporting the idea that there is a sensitive period to the effects of maltreatment.

In spite of these convincing findings supporting the existence of sensitive periods, it is important to remember the principle of *multifinality*, one of the guiding theories of developmental psychopathology. This principle asserts that given a similar history, many outcomes are possible, since many environmental events and internal psychophysiological strengths and challenges work together to forge a particular outcome. Given the complex array of behaviors associated with attachment, it is difficult to accept that it could be subject to a sensitive period. According to Knudsen (2004), sensitive periods are properties of neural circuits, not complex behaviors, even though they tend to be defined in terms of behavior and are dependent upon experience. When a neural circuit is repeatedly and intensely activated during a sensitive period, the synapses associated with the neural circuit consolidate, and the architecture of the circuit stabilizes a "preferred" pattern of connectivity (Knudsen). Afterwards, the circuits retain some plasticity, but Knudsen asserts that the plasticity is limited by the architecture established during the sensitive period. At the same time, it is also important to remember that the brain is organized so that higher order circuits can compensate for maladaptive neural circuits at lower levels, supporting our theoretical belief in the probabilistic nature of the outcomes associated with maltreatment.

The Role of Attachment

John Bowlby, who first wrote on attachment, observed that infants appeared driven to form attachment relationships, but that the quality of these relationships might vary considerably (Bowlby, 1969/1982). He believed that the quality of infants' attachment provided a foundation for later personality development, in particular the growth of self-reliance and emotional regulation (Bowlby, 1973). For example, Bowlby believed that when caregivers successfully helped regulate infants' emotions, infants would discover through experience that they could regulate their own emotions, growing increasingly more confident in this ability.

Later research found that infants displayed one of three different consistent, organized strategies to get a particular parent's help when they were anxious or perceived a threat (Ainsworth, Blehar, Waters, & Wall, 1978). Some infants showed secure attachment, displaying an easy ability to use their caregivers for help in regulating distress. Some were anxious-avoidant, where they behaved as though they did not need help. Others displayed anxious-ambivalence, not responding quickly to parents' attempts to soothe, and often seeking help. Later research found that not all infants had an organized attachment (Main & Solomon, 1986). These infants were categorized as having disorganized attachment.

Unlike organized attachment (e.g., insecure and secure attachment), children with disorganized attachment displayed multiple qualities in the same interaction. For example, an infant approaching a caregiver when agitated, then turning away or freezing might be classified as disorganized because it is both secure and avoidant in equal measure. Main and Hesse (1990) proposed that when caregivers were a source of fear and anxiety in addition to being a protective source, this created a psychological contradiction for the infant and would increase the likelihood of developing insecure or disorganized attachment. In fact, Carlson, Cicchetti, Barnett, and Braunwald (1989) noted a higher incidence of disorganized attachment among maltreated than non-maltreated children.

Alan Sroufe and his colleagues at the University of Minnesota began exploring the role of attachment in child development in a longitudinal study in 1975, testing this hypothesis. In a 2005 article, Sroufe confirmed Bowlby's hypotheses that attachment is linked with critical development pathways like arousal modulation and emotional regulation, but also described considerable complexity in the attachment system over the course of development. Outcomes were probabilistic, not definite, and subject to the influences of a changing environment. A secure infant attachment strategy, occurring when the caregivers were a source of comfort and emotional regulation, "promoted" the likelihood of future adaptive responses (Sroufe, 2005). Luijk and her colleagues (2010) tied attachment strategies together with variations in stress response in a study of 369 infants and their mothers. They found that infants with an insecure- anxious strategy showed increasing stress in an assessment exposing them to multiple separations from their caregivers (i.e., Strange Situation Procedure) and a flattened, shut down response to the same assessment among infants showing disorganized attachment (Luijk et al.). Trying to discover what disorganized attachment meant for ongoing development, Lyons-Ruth, Alpern, and Repacholi (1993) found that 71 % of preschoolers who showed high levels of hostile behavior toward classroom peers had been classified as showing disorganized attachment at 18 months. Even more convincingly, Sroufe reported that the disorganized attachment was a strong predictor of later disturbance: the degree of disorganization in infancy correlated strongly ($r = .40$) with the number and severity of psychiatric symptoms at age 17.5.

Taken together, the evidence suggests a strong connection between early attachment and stress response systems, particularly those of emotional regulation during infancy. In general, researchers have found considerable flexibility in the degree to which attachment predicted outcomes as infants matured, confirming the idea that many environmental and family factors play a part in ongoing personality development. However, researchers have found repeatedly that disorganized attachment seems to be accompanied by greater ongoing vulnerability.

Maltreated children's vulnerability to disorganized attachment, and the subsequent negative outcomes associated with this lack of organization (including accompanying risks), suggest that the ingredients of attachment—the infant-caregiver relationship, and particularly caregiver responsiveness and warmth—would be excellent targets for early intervention.

The Role of Parenting

In addition to the clear effects of violence and trauma on children, results of numerous studies have also illustrated different effects of harsh and coercive parenting both on children's stress response system (Blair et al., 2008; Bugental et al., 2003; Hill-Soderlund et al., 2008), as well as the subsequent likelihood of observing aggression (e.g., Denham et al., 2000; Gershoff, 2002), anxiety (McLeod, Wood, & Weisz, 2007), depression (McLeod, Weisz, &Wood, 2007), withdrawn behavior (e.g., Booth-LaForce & Oxford, 2008) and other mental health problems (e.g., Cicchetti & Toth, 2000; Patterson, 1982; Schechter & Willheim, 2009).

Why does harsh parenting have such a toxic effect on young children? Evolutionary psychologists might argue that infants are attuned to threatening tones of voices and behaviors, and react as they would to any other high stress situation, usually with distress (e.g., screaming, crying, and other dysregulated behavior). Over time, they may learn other ways of managing their emotional dysregulation through observing others' behaviors when they are distressed. In some ways, infants' and young children's aversive behavior can be thought of as strategies for adapting to frightening, threatening environments (Ellis, Boyce, Belsky, Bakermans-Kranenburg, & van IJzendoorn, 2011). While these behaviors might be considered "adaptive" responses, they can also be considered as cogs in a larger family mechanism that sustains a cycle of violence (Patterson, 1982).

Parenting does not have to be harsh or coercive to cause problems in the parent–child relationship or to be associated with problem behaviors in children. Children of depressed mothers also are reported to have more behavior problems (e.g., Gartstein, Bridgett, Dishion, & Kaufman, 2009) and a higher risk of later psychopathology (e.g., Downey & Coyne, 1990; Goodman & Gotlib, 1999). Some of the most dramatic findings illustrating the importance of sensitive parenting for children's healthy development have emerged in studies of children who experienced neglect or inconsistent caregiving. In 1951, John Bowlby first reported to the World Health Organization that even when all their physical needs were met, children still showed serious negative effects from institutional care, which he attributed to their inability to form stable, continuous attachment relationships with a primary caregiver.

Recent studies have also documented effects of inadequate caregiving on attachment security, finding even higher rates of disorganized attachment strategies than among maltreated children (Cyr, Euser, Bakermans-Kranenburg, & Van Ijzendoorn, 2010). Researchers have also explored the effects of institutional care on children and have found that children who spent their first few years in institutions showed delayed physical (Van Ijzendoorn, Bakermans-Kranenburg, & Juffer, 2007) and cognitive growth (e.g., Zeanah, Smyke, Koga, & Carlson, 2005). Atypical diurnal cortisol patterns have also been noted in these children (Carlson & Earls, 1997), similar to the pattern found in children in foster care (Fisher, Gunnar, Chamberlain, & Reid, 2000). In sum, studies of children who spend their early years in institutions show disruptions in most areas of development, suggesting that neglectful caregiving also undermines the foundations of healthy physical, neurological, and psychological development.

Taken all together, research suggests that in the early years, emotional dysregulation resulting from attempts to manage the anxiety of perceived threats is at the root of many mental health problems in young children. Furthermore, parenting seems to directly influence children's stress response system. The stress response system, in turn, is central to children's developing capacity for emotional regulation. When parenting is sensitive, it appears to buffer the effects of stress on children (Dozier, Lindheim, Lewis, Bick, & Bernard, 2009), promoting more healthy responses to stress. When parenting is ineffective and non-optimal, it magnifies the stressfulness of early traumatic experiences, possibly by increasing their perceived threat (Martorell & Bugental, 2006). Improving the quality of parenting would seem to be a promising and productive focus for intervention through early childhood.

The Role of Cognition

Executive functions are cognitive skills associated with frontal lobe operations (Rubia et al., 2001), that help to control and coordinate our thoughts and behavior, by aiding in planning and sequencing a set of tasks to accomplish a goal, decision-making, selective attention and multitasking, and impulse control (Luria, 1980; Shallice, 1982). Different dimensions of executive functions have been described as proceeding through three active and distinct stages of maturation: early childhood (6–8 years), middle childhood (9–12 years), and teenage years (Brocki & Bohlin, 2004). Studies of performance on tasks testing many executive functions showed continued development and improvement through adolescence, in particular inhibitory or impulse control (Leon-Carrion, Garcia-Orza, & Perez-Santamaria, 2004; Luna, Garver, Urban, Lazar, & Sweeney, 2004), how quickly information is processed (Luna et al., 2004), and the size of working memory (Luciana, Conklin, Cooper, & Yarger, 2005).

Possibly because many of these executive functions are still "under construction," particularly those that inhibit impulsive behavior, thinking processes may be more vulnerable to heuristics like the emotional loading of a decision or goal. For example, studies have shown that adolescents make riskier decisions in "hot" (i.e., emotionally laden contexts) more than in "cold" contexts, ignoring important information about the value of an outcome and probabilities of its occurrence (Casey, Jones, & Hare, 2008). In "hot" contexts, teenagers have been found to make decisions that are biased towards acquiring gains and maintaining the "winning, positive" feeling, even when continuing to make this particular choice has clear and negative consequences (Cauffman et al., 2010).

Research findings suggest that emotions are often dysregulated or poorly regulated in maltreated youth (Cicchetti & Toth, 2000). Risks and negative experiences accumulate, possibly triggering fear and anxiety. Emotional dysregulation interferes with good decision-making, and increases the likelihood of making risky decisions that support "good feelings." Understanding when and how executive functions develop, and the role emotions play in decision-making during childhood and adolescence suggests that successful interventions for these children will involve strategies for managing emotions, and improve impulse control.

Moving Toward Adolescence

Youth grow more independent from their parents as they move into their adolescent years, undergoing a significant and obvious hormonal and physical metamorphosis that is represented by changes in cognitive flexibility, identity, and self-consciousness (Rutter & Rutter, 1993). While adolescence has long been recognized as a time of physiological change—the time when hormones rage and children transform into adults—it is only recently that this developmental period has been identified as a period of great neurological change. In 1989, the National Institute of Mental Health (NIMH) began to conduct a longitudinal study of brain development, collecting magnetic resonance images of typically and atypically developing children every 2 years (Giedd, 2008). This large-scale longitudinal pediatric neuroimaging study of participants aged 4 through 20 revealed that although the amount of white matter appeared to increase linearly, as previous cross-sectional studies had shown (e.g., Pfefferbaum et al., 1994), cortical gray matter did not decrease at an equally linear rate, as expected (Giedd et al., 1999). Instead they found concomitant but nonlinear changes in cortical gray matter, with a preadolescent increase followed by a postadolescent decrease (Giedd et al.). Results of later studies suggested that this decrease in gray matter was likely due to increased myelination (which is the primary characteristic separating gray matter from white matter), and synaptic pruning (Sowell, Thompson, Tessner, & Toga, 2001). What does this mean? It means that during the teenage years, important parts of the brain involved in high level thinking and planning is transforming, speeding up and streamlining its neural processes. Researchers believe that a pruned and more myelinated adult brain speeds processing and reaction times to problems, and focuses the activation of the frontal cortex (Blakemore & Choudhury, 2006). In sum, it seems that the teenage brain is not just bigger or faster, but going through a process that makes adolescents structurally different from both children and adults. This section will describe some of the ways in which adolescents are different, both in the way they think, react to social and emotional situations, and the way view the world.

Decision Making

While many studies of the development of executive functions and decision-making show substantive improvements over time, studies have found that in emotion-laden contexts, teenagers are less able to resist impulsive responses than both children and adults (Somerville, Hare, & Casey, 2011). For example, Somerville et al. used a go/no-go task using neutral (calm faces) and emotional cues (happy faces). The ability to resist pushing the "go" button when the neutral face was the "no-go" cue increased linearly with age. However, when the happy face was the "no-go" cue, adolescents performed worse than children and adults, showing less ability to inhibit this dominant response. When examining brain activity during this task from the fMRI, Somerville and colleagues found a significantly greater magnitude of activity in teenagers' ventral striatum—the area that is activated when anticipating a reward—compared to those of children and adults. These studies combine to provide additional evidence that teenagers' brains function differently, not necessarily less efficiently than adults. Not only do teenagers' judgments seem to be more strongly influenced by their emotions, but also the decisions they make are more likely to be oriented towards acquiring immediate gains rather than minimizing loss. Teenagers' preference for acquiring gains contrasts noticeably with adult preferences, who are strongly biased towards avoiding loss rather than acquiring gains (Tversky & Kahneman, 1991).

The Social Context: Decision-Making, Risk-Taking, and Social Cognitions

One of the places teenagers display the deficits in their decision-making is when they are behind the wheel of a car. Research tells us that 15–24 year olds account for 14 % of the population, but nearly 30 % of the costs of motor vehicle injuries (Finkelstein, Corso, & Miller, 2006). Apart from making poorer decisions about the risks and hazards while driving, the presence of other teen passengers increases their risk of accident and injury; and that risk increases with each additional passenger (Simons-Morton, Lerner, & Singer, 2005). One study using driving simulation games, compared driving risks taken when alone and with two peers in study participants ranging from adolescence to adulthood (Gardner & Steinberg, 2005). They found that while adolescents and adults took similar numbers of risks when alone, they performed differently when driving with friends: adolescents took almost three times the number of risks when driving in the presence of their friends as adults. A study repeating Gardner and Steinberg's driving task using fMRI found that when adolescents were in the presence of peers, there was less activity in the brain areas related to cognitive control (e.g., prefrontal cortex) and more activity in the ventral striatum and the orbitofrontal cortex when critical driving decisions had to be made—the same area that processes anticipated rewards (Chein, Albert, O'Brien, Uckert, & Steinberg, 2011). Furthermore, Chien and colleagues found that activity in these brain regions predicted subsequent risk taking.

While research suggests that the presence of peers is likely to increase the emotionality of events and risk-taking, researchers are also considering the possible effects of adolescents' "mentalizing" (i.e., the ability to understand how others' dissimilar mental states would shape different behavior) on their decision-making (e.g., Blakemore & Robbins, 2012). Recent studies using "theory of mind" types of tasks suggest that the ability to understand others' limitations and make judgments based on this understanding is still developing in adolescence, and continues to improve into late teen years (Dumontheil, Apperly, & Blakemore, 2010). Possibly related to adolescents' emerging mentalizing and perspective taking skills is the mounting evidence that adolescents' recognition of others emotions also is not completely developed until late adolescence. Studies investigating age differences in emotional recognition via categorization of facial expressions (e.g., Thomas, De Bellis, Graham, & LaBar, 2007) and using displays of body movement (Ross, Polson, & Grosbras, 2012) found evidence of non-linear improvement in emotional identification during adolescent years, particularly in identifications of anger expressions.

Parenting Adolescents

In western societies, adolescence is generally marked by increased influence of peers and independence from parents. Parents typically have less influence in directly helping to regulate emotions, adopting a more supervisory role, structuring adolescent children's environments to reduce opportunities for risk taking and monitoring physical and psychological well-being. In spite of these shifts in social contexts, research suggests that parenting continues to play a role in supporting positive growth and development, with parents' competence and style relating strongly to adolescents' competence and adjustment (Furstenburg, Cook, Eccles, Elder, & Sameroff, 1999; Steinberg, Blatt-Eisengart, & Cauffman, 2006; Steinberg, Lamborn, Darling, Mounts, & Dornbusch, 1994). More specifically, research has supported *parental monitoring* –defined as the parent's knowledge of their child's whereabouts, activities, and friends (e.g., Fletcher, Steinberg, & Williams-Wheeler, 2004; Jacobson & Crockett, 2000; Patterson & Stouthamer-Loeber, 1984; Pettit, Bates, Dodge, & Meece, 1999) and *parental control-* the extent to which decisions regarding key activities in adolescents' lives were made by parents instead of by adolescents themselves—as reducing the likelihood of children's involvement in risky and delinquent behavior (e.g., Barber, 1996). For example, parental monitoring has been associated with less antisocial behavior (e.g., Patterson & Stouthamer-Loeber; Snyder, Dishion, & Patterson, 1986), substance use (e.g., Steinberg et al., 2006), and improved school performance (Crouter, Macdermid, McHale, & Perry-Jenkins, 1990). The quality of parenting and the family environment has even been found to account for variations in the adjustment of juvenile offenders (Furstenburg et al., 1999; Ikaheimo, Laukkanen, Hakko, & Rasanen, 2013), suggesting that parenting and the family environment have the potential for buffering the development of more serious psychological problems in adolescence.

Maltreatment and Adolescence

While trauma continues to have the same biological effect on the stress response system in older children as it does for younger children, there is clear evidence that certain individual factors mediate the effects of trauma on older children's mental health (Heim et al., 2008). These include early maltreatment (Cicchetti et al., 2010), early attachment relationships, social support, attributional styles, self-esteem, developing cognitions about self and others, and social competence (Cicchetti & Valentino, 2006). One of the most widely documented effects of child maltreatment is an increased risk of internalizing behaviors in middle childhood (Keiley, Howe, Dodge, Bates, & Pettit, 2001; Kim & Cicchetti, 2006) and depression and suicide ideation in adolescence (Dube et al., 2001). Dube and colleagues also found that among a cohort of more than 17,000 primary care clinic patients, having a history of adverse experiences in childhood such as abuse, neglect, domestic violence, and parents' substance abuse doubled to quintupled the likelihood of attempted suicide in adolescence. However, research has not really identified the mechanism that links maltreatment with depression and suicidality in adolescence.

Taken all together, the developmental neurological research described here paints a complex picture of adolescence as a unique developmental period, where the brain transforms, jumping off the ladder of accumulating cognitive skills into a new dimension of functioning. What we know at this point in time is that adolescents can use reasoning skills as well as adults, in situations absent of emotion. When aroused by emotions or the presence of others, however, decisions are likely to be based on perpetuating positive emotion, focusing on opportunities for reward and not minimizing risk. In these situations, behavior is likely to be more impulsive and risky. We know that although emotions are involved in much of adolescents' decision-making, their ability to perceive and understand others' emotions is still developing. This constellation of characteristics may challenge parents and caregivers, and yet their role appears to continue to play an important role in supporting healthy development. Research on the effects of maltreatment on adolescent mental health suggests that early adversity may disrupt adolescents' developing emotional regulation systems (Cicchetti et al., 2010), particularly with respect to their ability to modulate negative emotions. Research on adolescent cognitions reveals the interconnections among emotions, social contexts, and cognitions. The path to psychological wellbeing for adolescents is likely to be similarly complex. Effective interventions should include strategies for managing negative emotions, supporting healthy decision-making and impulse control, and involve parents, helping them to support and monitor their adolescents.

Conclusions

To conclude, we reiterate our belief that there are many paths to more positive functioning for maltreated children, though the paths may be difficult to follow and fraught with distress. If we did not accept and even cling to this premise, it would be difficult to justify spending the time describing and discussing the value of empirically based treatments for maltreated children, much less encourage the reader to read on! After reviewing and describing the elements contributing to positive developmental trajectories, we believe that what determines the most effective intervention for different children will vary by age and developmental stage, though the family environment will likely play a role in their success over the course of development.

Descriptions of healthy development in infancy, childhood, and adolescence support the view that emotional regulation underlies much of psychological wellbeing. However, the interventions that support and facilitate emotional regulation in different developmental stages are likely to be quite different because much of development is described better by multidimensional transformations rather than a linear growth trajectory. For example, we argue that maltreated children's vulnerability to disorganized attachment, and the subsequent negative outcomes associated with this lack of organization (including accompanying risks), suggest that the infant-caregiver relationship is an excellent target for intervention in infants and toddlers. In early childhood, we believe that improving parenting skills is a promising and productive focus for intervention because of its strong influence on children's stress response system, and ability to buffer the effects of stress on children (Dozier et al., 2009). In middle childhood, as executive functions begin to play a bigger role in predicting behavior, we maintain that successful interventions for these children will involve cognitive strategies that help them to regulate their emotions and improve impulse control, thereby reducing their exposure to risk. In adolescence, the connection between emotional regulation, executive functions, and social contexts suggests that in addition to cognitive-based models, which are likely to be essential for improving emotional regulation, decision-making, and impulse control, adolescents may also benefit from efforts to help their parents understand their particular needs, and from activities that involve peers.

In closing, we present the table below, which synopsizes the mental health issues of maltreated infants and toddlers, young children, school age children, and adolescents, describes the targets for change, and lists the empirically-based interventions included in this volume. While this is not an exhaustive list of EBTs for maltreated children, we believe it represents the types of interventions most successful in meeting these children's needs.

Developmental age	Issues addressed by interventions	Targets for change	Intervention
Infants/toddlers	Attachment Emotional regulation Parent–child relationships	Parent self-understanding Parenting behaviors Parent understanding of child Quality of parent–child relationship	Child Parent Psychotherapy (Van Horn & Leiberman) Attachment and Biobehavioral Catch-up (ABC; Dozier, Meade, & Bernard)
Preschooler/early school-age children	Parent–child relationships Emotional regulation Social skills Stress management and coping Externalizing behavior problems	Parenting behaviors Parent understanding of child Child behavior training Child emotional regulation Quality of parent–child relationship	Incredible Years (IY; Webster-Stratton) Multidimensional Treatment Foster Care for Preschoolers (MTFC-P; Fischer & Gilliam) Parent–child Interaction Therapy (PCIT; Urquiza & Timmer) Triple P (Sanders & Pickering)

(continued)

(continued)

Developmental age	Issues addressed by interventions	Targets for change	Intervention
School-age children	Peer relationships Anxiety, depression, PTSD Stress management and coping Parent–child relationships Externalizing behavior problems	Child cognitions Parenting behaviors Child emotional regulation Child behavior training Parent understanding of child	Alternatives for Families: A Cognitive-Behavioral Therapy (AF-CBT; Kolko) Trauma Focused-Cognitive Behavioral Therapy (TF-CBT; Mannarino & Cohen)
Adolescents	Peer relationships Anxiety, depression, PTSD Self-injurious behavior Stress management and coping Externalizing behavior problems Intimate interpersonal relationships parent–child relationships	Child cognitions Child emotional regulation Child behavior training Parenting behaviors Parent understanding of child	Multisystemic Therapy for Child Abuse and Neglect (CAN-MST: Cupit Swenson & Schaeffer) Dialectical Behavior Therapy (Berk & Shelby)

References

Ainsworth, M. D. S., Blehar, M. C., Waters, E., & Wall, S. (1978). *Patterns of attachment: A psychological study of the strange situation*. Hillsdale, NJ: Erlbaum.

Alink, L., Cicchetti, D., Kim, J., & Rogosch, F. (2009). Mediating and moderating processes in the relation between maltreatment and psychopathology: Mother-child relationship quality and emotion regulation. *Journal of Abnormal Psychology, 37*(6), 831–843.

Appleyard, K., Egeland, B., van Dulmen, M. H., & Sroufe, L. A. (2005). When more is not better: The role of cumulative risk in child behavior outcomes. *Journal of Child Psychology and Psychiatry, 46*(3), 235–245.

Bakermans-Kranenburg, M., van IJzendoorn, M., & Juffer, F. (2008). Earlier is better: A meta-analysis of 70 years of intervention improving cognitive development in institutionalized children. *Monographs of the Society for Research in Child Development, 73*(3), 279–293.

Barber, B. K. (1996). Parental psychological control: Revisiting a neglected construct. *Child Development, 67*, 3296–3319.

Beckett, C., Maughan, B., Rutter, M., Castle, J., Colvert, E., Groothues, C., et al. (2006). Do the effects of early severe deprivation on cognition persist into early adolescence? Findings from the English and Romanian Adoptees Study. *Child Development, 77*(3), 696–711.

Belsky, J. (1980). Child maltreatment: An ecological integration. *American Psychologist, 35*(4), 320–335.

Blair, C., Granger, D. A., Kivlighan, K. T., Mills-Koonce, R., Willoughby, M., Greenberg, M. T., et al. (2008). Maternal and child contributions to cortisol response to emotional arousal in young children from low-income, rural communities. *Developmental Psychology, 44*, 1095–1109. doi:10.1037/0012-1649.44.4.1095.

Blakemore, S.-J., & Choudhury, S. (2006). Development of the adolescent brain: Implications for executive function and social cognition. *Journal of Child Psychology and Psychiatry, 47*(3), 296–312.

Blakemore, S.-J., & Robbins, T. (2012). Decision making in the adolescent brain. *Nature Neuroscience, 15*(2), 1184–1191. doi:10.1038/nn.3177.

Booth-LaForce, C., & Oxford, M. (2008). Trajectories of social withdrawal from grades 1 to 6: Prediction from early parenting, attachment, and temperament. *Developmental Psychology, 44*(5), 1298–1313.

Bowlby, J. (1951). *Maternal care and mental health* (World Health Organization (WHO) monograph, serial no. 2). Geneva, Switzerland: WHO.

Bowlby, J. (1973). *Attachment and loss: Vol. 2. Separation: Anxiety and anger.* New York: Basic Books.

Bowlby, J. (1982). *Attachment and loss: Vol. 1. Attachment* (2nd ed.). New York: Basic Books. (Original work published 1969)

Brocki, K. C., & Bohlin, G. (2004). Executive functions in children aged 6 to 13: A dimensional and developmental study. *Developmental Neuropsychology, 26*, 571–593.

Bugental, D. B., Martorell, G. A., & Barraza, V. (2003). The hormonal costs of subtle forms of infant maltreatment. *Hormones and Behavior, 43*, 237–244. doi:10.1016/S0018-506X(02)00008-9.

Carlson, M., & Earls, F. (1997). Psychological and neuroendocrinological sequelae of early social deprivation in institutionalized children in Romania. In M. Carlson & F. Earls (Eds.), *The integrative neurobiology of affiliation* (pp. 419–428). New York: New York Academy of Sciences.

Carlson, V., Cicchetti, D., Barnett, D., & Braunwald, K. (1989). Disorganized/disoriented attachment relationships in maltreated infants. *Developmental Psychology, 25*(4), 525–531.

Casey, B. J., Jones, R. M., & Hare, T. A. (2008). The adolescent brain. *Annals of the New York Academy of Science, 1124*, 111–126.

Cauffman, E., Shulman, E. P., Steinberg, L., Claus, E., Banich, M. T., Graham, S., et al. (2010). Age differences in affective decision making as indexed by performance on the Iowa Gambling Task. *Developmental Psychology, 46*, 193–207.

Chein, J., Albert, D., O'Brien, L., Uckert, K., & Steinberg, L. (2011). Peers increase adolescent risk taking by enhancing activity in the brain's reward circuitry. *Developmental Science, 14*, F1–F10.

Cicchetti, D., & Lynch, M. (1993). Toward an ecological/transactional model of community violence and child maltreatment: Consequences for children's development. *Psychiatry, 56*, 96–118.

Cicchetti, D., & Rogosch, F. A. (1997). The role of self-organization in the promotion of resilience in maltreated children. *Development and Psychopathology, 9*, 799–817.

Cicchetti, D., Rogosch, F. A., Gunnar, M. R., & Toth, S. L. (2010). The differential impacts of early physical and sexual abuse and internalizing problems on daytime cortisol rhythm in school-aged children. *Child Development, 81*(1), 252–269. doi:10.1111/j.1467-8624.2009.01393.

Cicchetti, D., Rogosch, F., Toth, S., & Sturge-Apple, M. (2011). Normalizing the development of cortisol regulation in maltreated infants through preventive interventions. *Development and Psychopathology, 23*, 789–800.

Cicchetti, D., & Toth, S. L. (2000). Developmental processes in maltreated children. In D. Hansen (Ed.), *Nebraska symposium on motivation: Vol. 46. Motivation and maltreatment* (pp. 85–160). Lincoln, NE: University of Nebraska Press.

Cicchetti, D., & Valentino, K. (2006). An ecological transactional perspective on child maltreatment: Failure of the average expectable environment and its influence upon child development. In D. Cicchetti & D. J. Cohen (Eds.), *Developmental psychopathology* (2nd ed., Vol. 3, pp. 129–201). New York: Wiley.

Crouter, A. C., MacDermid, S. M., McHale, S. M., & Perry-Jenkins, M. (1990). Parental monitoring and perceptions of children's school performance and conduct in dual- and single-earner families. *Developmental Psychology, 26*, 649–657.

Cyr, C. A., Euser, E. M., Bakermans-Kranenburg, M. J., & Van Ijzendoorn, M. H. (2010). Attachment insecurity and disorganization in maltreating and high-risk families: A series of meta-analyses. *Development and Psychopathology, 22*, 87–108.

Denham, S. A., Workman, E., Cole, P. M., Weissbrod, C., Kendziora, K. T., & Zahn-Waxler, C. (2000). Prediction of externalizing behavior problems from early to middle childhood: The role of parental socialization and emotional expression. *Development and Psychopathology, 12*, 23–45. doi:10.1017/S0954579400001024.

Downey, G., & Coyne, J. C. (1990). Children of depressed parents: An integrative review. *Psychological Bulletin, 108*, 50–76.

Dozier, M., Lindhiem, O., Lewis, E., Bick, J., & Bernard, K. (2009). Effects of a foster parent training program on young children's attachment behaviors: Preliminary evidence from a randomized clinical trial. *Child and Adolescent Social Work Journal, 26*(4), 321–332.

Dube, S. R., Anda, R. F., Felitti, V. J., Chapman, D. P., Williamson, D. F., & Giles, W. H. (2001). Childhood abuse, household dysfunction, and the risk of attempted suicide throughout the life span: Findings from the adverse childhood experiences study. *Journal of the American Medical Association, 286*, 3089–3096.

Dumontheil, I., Apperly, I. A., & Blakemore, S.-J. (2010). Online usage of theory of mind continues to develop in late adolescence. *Developmental Science, 13*, 331–338.

Ellis, B. J., Boyce, W. T., Belsky, J., Bakermans-Kranenburg, M. J., & Van Ijzendoorn, M. H. (2011). Differential susceptibility to the environment: An evolutionary neurodevelopmental theory. *Development and Psychopathology, 23*, 7–28. doi:10.1017/S0954579410000611.

Ellis, B. J., Jackson, J., & Boyce, W. T. (2006). The stress response system: Universality and adaptive individual differences. *Developmental Review, 26*(2), 175–212.

Felitti, V., Anda, R. F., Nordenberg, D., Williamson, D. F., Spitz, A. M., Edwards, V., et al. (1998). Relationship of childhood abuse and household dysfunction to many of the leading causes of death in adults: The Adverse Childhood Experiences (ACE) Study. *American Journal of Preventive Medicine, 14*(4), 245–258.

Finkelstein, E. A., Corso, P. S., & Miller, T. R., Associates. (2006). *Incidence and economic burden of injuries in the United States*. New York: Oxford University Press.

Fisher, L., Ames, E., Chisholm, K., & Savoie, L. (1997). Problems reported by parents of Romanian orphans adopted to British Columbia. *International Journal of Behavioral Development, 20*(1), 67–82.

Fisher, P. A., Gunnar, M. R., Chamberlain, P., & Reid, J. B. (2000). Preventive intervention for maltreated preschoolers: Impact on children's behavior, neuroendocrine activity, and foster parent functioning. *Journal of the American Academy of Child and Adolescent Psychiatry, 39*, 1356–1364.

Fletcher, A., Steinberg, L., & Williams-Wheeler, M. (2004). Parental influences on adolescent problem behavior: Revisiting Stattin and Kerr. *Child Development, 75*(3), 781–796.

Furstenburg, F. F., Cook, T., Eccles, J., Elder, G., & Sameroff, A. (1999). *Managing to make it: Urban families and adolescent success*. Chicago: University Press.

Gardner, M., & Steinberg, L. (2005). Peer influence on risk taking, risk preference, and risky decision making in adolescence and adulthood: An experimental study. *Developmental Psychology, 41*, 625–635.

Gartstein, M., Bridgett, D., Dishion, T., & Kaufman, N. (2009). Depressed mood and maternal report of child behavior problems: Another look at the depression-distortion hypothesis. *Developmental Psychology, 30*(2), 149–160.

Gershoff, E. T. (2002). Corporal punishment by parents and associated child behaviors and experiences: A meta-analytic and theoretical review. *Psychological Bulletin, 128*, 539–579. doi:10.1037/0033-2909.128.4.539.

Giedd, J. (2008). The teen brain: Insights from neuroimaging. *Journal of Adolescent Health, 42*, 335–343.

Giedd, J., Blumenthal, J., Jeffries, N. O., Castellanos, F. X., Liu, H., Zijdenbos, A., et al. (1999). Brain development during childhood and adolescence: A longitudinal MRI study. *Nature Neuroscience, 2*, 861–863.

Goodman, S., & Gotlib, I. (1999). Risk for psychopathology in the children of depressed mothers: A developmental model for understanding mechanisms of transmission. *Psychological Review, 106*(3), 458–490.

Goodman, G. S., Quas, J. A., Batterman-Faunce, J. M., Riddlesberger, M. M., & Kuhn, J. (1997). Children's reactions to and memory for a stressful event: Influences of age, anatomical dolls, knowledge, and parental attachment. *Applied Developmental Science, 1–2*, 54–75.

Guerra, N. G., Hammons, A. J., & Clutter, M. O. (2011). Culture, families, and children's aggression: Finings from Jamaica, Japan, and Latinos in the United States. In N. G. Guerra, A. J. Hammons, & M. O. Clutter (Eds.), *Socioemotional development in cultural context* (pp. 281–304). New York: Guilford Press.

Guerra, N. G., Huesmann, R., & Spindler, A. (2003). Community violence exposure, social cognition, and aggression among urban elementary school children. *Child Development, 74*(5), 1561–1576.

Gunnar, M., Larson, M., Hertsgaard, L., Harris, M., & Brodersen, L. (1992). The stressfulness of separation among nine-month-old infants: Effects of social context variables and infant temperament. *Child Development, 63*(2), 290–303.

Heim, C., Ehlert, U., & Hellhammer, D. H. (2000). The potential role of hypocortisolism in the pathophysiology of stress-related bodily disorders. *Psychoneuroendocrinology, 25*, 1–35.

Heim, C., Newport, D. J., Mletzko, T., Miller, A. H., & Nemeroff, C. B. (2008). The link between childhood trauma and depression: Insights from HPA axis studies in humans. *Psychoneuroendocrinology, 33*, 693–710.

Herman, J. P., Figueiredo, H., Mueller, N. K., Ulrich-Lai, Y., Ostrander, M., Choi, D., et al. (2003). Central mechanisms of stress integration: Hierarchical circuitry controlling hypothalamo-pituitary-adrenocortical responsiveness. *Frontiers in Neuroendocrinology, 24*, 151–180.

Hill-Soderlund, A. L., Mills-Koonce, W. R., Propper, C., Calkins, S., Granger, D. A., Moore, G. A., et al. (2008). Parasympathetic and sympathetic responses to the strange situation in infants and mothers from avoidant and securely attached dyads. *Developmental Psychobiology, 50*, 361–376. doi:10.1002/dev.20302.

Ikaheimo, O., Laukkanen, M., Hakko, H., & Rasanen, P. (2013). Association of family structure to later criminality: A population-based follow-up study of adolescent psychiatric inpatients in Northern Finland. *Child Psychiatry and Human Development, 44*(2), 233–246.

Jacobson, K. C., & Crockett, L. J. (2000). Parental monitoring and adolescent adjustment: An ecological perspective. *Journal of Research on Adolescence, 10*(1), 65–97.

Juster, R.-P., McEwen, B. S., & Lupien, S. J. (2009). Allostatic load biomarkers of chronic stress and impact on health and cognition. *Neuroscience and Biobehavioral Reviews, 35*, 2–16.

Keiley, M. K., Howe, T. R., Dodge, K. A., Bates, J. E., & Pettit, G. S. (2001). The timing of child physical mal- treatment: A cross-domain growth analysis of impact on adolescent externalizing and internalizing problems. *Development and Psychopathology, 13*, 891–912.

Kim, J., & Cicchetti, D. (2006). Longitudinal trajectories of self-system processes and depressive symptoms among maltreated and nonmaltreated children. *Child Development, 77*, 624–639.

Knudsen, E. I. (2004). Sensitive periods in the development of brain and behavior. *Journal of Cognitive Neuroscience, 16*, 1412–1425.

Leon-Carrion, J., Garcia-Orza, J., & Perez-Santamaria, F. J. (2004). The development of the inhibitory component of the executive functions in children and adolescents. *International Journal of Neuroscience, 114*, 1291–1311.

Luciana, M., Conklin, H. M., Cooper, C. J., & Yarger, R. S. (2005). The development of nonverbal working memory and executive control processes in adolescents. *Child Development, 76*, 697–712.

Luijk, M. P. C. M., Saridjan, N., Tharner, A., van IJzendoorn, M. H., Bakermans-Kranenburg, M. J., Jaddoe, V. W. V., et al. (2010). Attachment, depression, and cortisol: Deviant patterns of insecure-resistant and disorganized infants. *Developmental Psychobiology, 52*, 441–452. doi:10.1002/dev.20446.

Luna, B., Garver, K. E., Urban, T. A., Lazar, N. A., & Sweeney, J. A. (2004). Maturation of cognitive processes from late childhood to adulthood. *Child Development, 75*, 1357–1372.

Lupien, S., Oueliet-Morin, I., Hupbach, A., Tu, M., Buss, C., & Walker, D. (2006). Beyond the stress concept: Allostatic load—A developmental biological and cognitive perspective. In S. Lupien, I. Oueliet-Morin, A. Hupbach, M. Tu, C. Buss, D. Walker, J. Pruessner, & B. McEwen (Eds.), *Developmental psychopathology: Vol. 2. Developmental neuroscience* (2nd ed., pp. 578–628). Hoboken, NJ: Jon Wiley & Sons Inc.

Luria, A. R. (1980). *Higher cortical functions in man* (2nd ed.). Oxford, UK: Basic Books.

Lyons-Ruth, K., Alpern, L., & Repacholi, B. (1993). Disorganized infant attachment classification and maternal psychosocial problems as predictors of hostile-aggressive behavior in preschool children. *Child Development, 64*, 572–585.

Main, M., & Hesse, E. (1990). Parents' unresolved traumatic experiences are related to infant disorganized attachment status: Is frightened and/or frightening parental behavior the linking mechanism? In M. T. Greenberg, D. Cicchetti, & E. M. Cummings (Eds.), *Attachment in the preschool years: Theory, research, and intervention* (pp. 161–182). Chicago: University of Chicago Press.

Main, M., & Solomon, J. (1986). Discovery of an insecure-disorganized/disoriented attachment pattern. In M. Main & J. Solomon (Eds.), *Affective development in infancy* (pp. 95–124). Westport, CT: Alex.

Martorell, G. A., & Bugental, D. B. (2006). Maternal variations in stress reactivity: Implications for harsh parenting practices with very young children. *Journal of Family Psychology, 20–4*, 641–647.

McEwen, B. (2000). Allostasis and allostatic load: Implications for neuro-psychopharmacology. *Neuropsychopharmacology, 22*, 108–124.

McEwen, B., & Stellar, E. (1993). Stress and the individual mechanisms leading to disease. *Journal of the American Medical Association, Archives of Internal Medicine, 153*, 2093–2101.

McLeod, B. D., Weisz, J. R., & Wood, J. J. (2007). Examining the association between parenting and childhood depression: A meta-analysis. *Clinical Psychology Review, 27*, 986–1003. doi:10.1016/ j.cpr.2007.03.001.

McLeod, B. D., Wood, J. J., & Weisz, J. R. (2007). Examining the association between parenting and childhood anxiety: A meta-analysis. *Clinical Psychology Review, 27*, 155–172. doi:10.1016/ j.cpr.2006.09.002.

O'Connor, T. G. (2003). Early experiences and psychological development: Conceptual questions, empirical illustrations, and implications for intervention. *Development and Psychopathology, 15*(3), 671–690.

Patterson, G. R. (1982). *Coercive family process*. Eugene, OR: Castilia.

Patterson, G. R., & Stouthamer-Loeber, M. (1984). The correlation of family management practices and delinquency. *Child Development, 55*, 1299–1307.

Pettit, G., Bates, J., Dodge, K., & Meece, D. (1999). The impact of after-school peer contact on early adolescent externalizing problems is moderated by parental monitoring, perceived neighborhood safety, and prior adjustment. *Child Development, 70*(3), 768–778.

Pfefferbaum, A., Mathalon, D. H., Sullivan, E. V., Rawles, J. M., Zipursky, R. B., & Lim, K. O. (1994). A quantitative magnetic resonance imaging study of changes in brain morphology from infancy to late adulthood. *Archives of Neurology, 51*(9), 874–887.

Pollak, S., Cicchetti, D., Hornung, K., & Reed, A. (2000). Recognizing emotion in faces: The developmental effects of child abuse and neglect. *Developmental Psychology, 36*, 679–688.

Ross, P. D., Polson, L., & Grosbras, M.-H. (2012). Developmental changes in emotion recognition from full-light and point-light displays of body movement. *PLoS One, 7*(9), e44815. doi:10.1371/journal.pone.0044815.

Rubia, K., Russell, T., Overmeyer, S., Brammer, M. J., Bullmore, E. T., Sharma, T., et al. (2001). Mapping motor inhibition: Conjunctive brain activations across different versions of go/no-go and stop tasks. *NeuroImage, 13*, 250–261.

Rutter, M., & Rutter, M. (1993). *Developing minds*. London: Penguin.

Sanchez, M. M., McCormack, K., Grand, A. P., Fulks, R., Graff, A., & Maestripieri, D. (2010). Effects of sex and early maternal abuse on adrenocorticotropin hormone and cortisol responses to the corticotrophin-releasing hormone challenge during the first 3 years of life in group-living rhesus monkeys. *Development and Psychopathology, 22*, 45–53.

Schechter, W., & Willheim, E. (2009). Disturbances of attachment and parental psychopathology in early childhood. *Child and Adolescent Psychiatric Clinics of North America, 18*(3), 665–686.

Shallice, T. (1982). Specific impairments of planning. *Philosophical Transactions of the Royal Society of London. Series B, Biological Sciences, 298*, 199–209.

Simons-Morton, B., Lerner, N., & Singer, J. (2005). The observed effects of teenage passengers on the risky driving behavior of teenage drivers. *Accident Analysis and Prevention, 37*(6), 973–982.

Snyder, J., Dishion, T. J., & Patterson, G. R. (1986). Determinants and consequences of associating with deviant peers during preadolescence and adolescence. *Journal of Early Adolescence, 6*, 29–43.

Somerville, L. H., Hare, T., & Casey, B. J. (2011). Frontostriatal maturation predicts cognitive control failure to appetitive cues in adolescents. *Journal of Cognitive Neuroscience, 23*, 2123–2134.

Sowell, E. R., Thompson, P. M., Tessner, K. D., & Toga, A. W. (2001). Mapping continued brain growth and gray matter density reduction in dorsal frontal cortex: Inverse relationships during postadolescent brain maturation. *Journal of Neuroscience, 21*, 8819–8829.

Sroufe, L. A. (2005). Attachment and development: A prospective study from birth to adulthood. *Attachment & Human Development, 7*(4), 349–367.

Sroufe, L. A., Egeland, B., & Kreutzer, T. (1990). The fate of early experience following developmental change: Longitudinal approaches to individual adaptation in childhood. *Child Development, 61*(5), 1363–1373.

Staub, E. (1996). Cultural-societal roots of violence: The examples of genocidal violence and of contemporary youth violence in the United States. *American Psychologist, 51*(2), 117–132.

Steinberg, L., Blatt-Eisengart, I., & Cauffman, E. (2006). Patterns of competence and adjustment among adolescents from authoritarian, indulgent, and neglectful homes: A replication in a sample of serious juvenile offenders. *Journal of Research on Adolescence, 16*, 47–58.

Steinberg, L., Lamborn, S. D., Darling, N., Mounts, N. S., & Dornbusch, S. M. (1994). Over-time changes in adjustment and competence among adolescents from authoritative, authoritative, indulgent, and neglectful families. *Child Development, 65*, 754–770.

Thomas, L., De Bellis, M., Graham, R., & LaBar, K. (2007). Development of emotional facial recognition in late childhood and adolescence. *Developmental Science, 10*(5), 547–548.

Tversky, A., & Kahneman, D. (1991). Loss aversion in riskless choice: a reference dependent model. *Quarterly Journal of Economics, 106*(4), 1039–1061.

U.S. Department of Health & Human Services (USDHHS), Administration for Children, Youth and Families, & Children's Bureau. (2011). *Child maltreatment 2010.* Available from http://www.acf.hhs.gov/programs/cb/stats_research/index.htm#can. Accessed 23 Oct 2012.

Van IJzendoorn, M., Bakermans-Kranenburg, M., & Juffer, F. (2007). Plasticity of growth in height, weight, and head circumference: Meta-analytic evidence of massive catch-up after international adoption. *Journal of Developmental and Behavioral Pediatrics, 28*(4), 334–343.

Yehuda, R., Cai, G., Golier, J. A., Sarapas, C., Galea, S., Ising, M., et al. (2009). Gene expression patterns associated with posttraumatic stress disorder following exposure to the World Trade Center attacks. *Biological Psychiatry, 66*(7), 708–711.

Zeanah, C., Smyke, A., Koga, S., & Carlson, E. (2005). Attachment in institutionalized and community children in Romania. *Child Development, 76*(5), 1015–1028.

Zhang, L. X., Levine, S., Dent, G., Zhan, Y., Xing, G., Okimoto, D., et al. (2002). Maternal deprivation increases cell death in the infant rat brain. *Brain Research. Developmental Brain Research, 133*(1), 1–11.

Part II
Interventions for Infants and Toddlers

There is a strong body of research supporting the value of early positive and responsive caregiving for infants and toddlers, and the value of emotional regulation for development. Maltreated children's vulnerability to disorganized attachment, and the subsequent negative outcomes associated with this lack of organization (including accompanying risks), suggest that the ingredients of attachment in the infant-caregiver relationship would be excellent targets for early intervention. We present two evidence-based interventions that focus specifically on these target areas and have been proven effective for traumatized infants and toddlers. In Chap. 4, Dozier and colleagues describes Attachment and Biobehavioral Catchup (ABC); and in Chap. 5, van Horn and Reyes present Child-parent Psychotherapy (CPP).

Chapter 4
Attachment and Biobehavioral Catch-Up: An Intervention for Parents at Risk of Maltreating Their Infants and Toddlers

Mary Dozier, Elizabeth Meade, and Kristin Bernard

When young children are abused or neglected, they have difficulty regulating behavior, physiology, and emotions. The parents of these children especially need to provide nurturing, synchronous, and non-frightening care. It is critical that parents behave in nurturing ways so that children develop secure, organized attachments, that they behave in contingent responsive ways to enhance the development of adequate regulatory capabilities, and that they avoid frightening behavior which undermines children's ability to develop organized attachments and regulatory capabilities. Attachment and Biobehavioral Catch-up (ABC) was developed to target these three issues.

Theoretical Background

Attachment Theory

According to attachment theory, infants and young children develop attachments to parents or other caregivers such that children seek proximity to attachment figures under conditions of threat. From an evolutionary perspective, chances of survival are enhanced if children seek out caregivers under threatening circumstances. By the time infants are able to move away from the caregiver, they develop the felt need to maintain proximity under threatening circumstances (e.g., unknown environment, presence of stranger, darkness; Bowlby, 1969/1982). The reliance on the

M. Dozier, Ph.D. (✉) • E. Meade
Department of Psychology, University of Delaware, Newark, DE, USA
e-mail: mdozier@psych.udel.edu; emeade@psych.udel.edu

K. Bernard, Ph.D.
Department of Psychology, Stony Brook University, Stony Brook, NY, USA
e-mail: Kristin.Bernard@stonybrook.edu

S. Timmer and A. Urquiza (eds.), *Evidence-Based Approaches for the Treatment of Maltreated Children*, Child Maltreatment 3, DOI 10.1007/978-94-007-7404-9_4, © Springer Science+Business Media Dordrecht 2014

caregiver is nearly universal, with children developing attachments to parents regardless of whether parents are nurturing or not nurturing, synchronous or not synchronous (van IJzendoorn, Bakermans-Kranenburg, & Sagi-Schwartz, 2006). Indeed, even when parents are abusive or neglecting, children typically develop attachments (Weinfield, Sroufe, Egeland, & Carlson, 2008). The exception is when children do not have a caregiver, or when caregivers are essentially staff, as seen in impersonal institutional settings. In such settings, children sometimes fail to develop a primary attachment (Zeanah, Smyke, Koga, & Carlson, 2005). Again, though, such conditions are rare.

What differentiates children with varying caregiving histories is the quality and organization of their attachment to their primary caregivers. Children with organized attachments (including secure, avoidant, and resistant attachments) have a coherent strategy for engaging the parent when distressed, whereas children with disorganized attachments lack such a strategy (Main & Solomon, 1990). Attachments are organized around the way that parents typically respond when their child is distressed. When parents are nurturing, children often develop secure attachments. Such children seek out their parents directly when distressed, confident in their parents' availability (Ainsworth, Blehar, Waters, & Wall, 1978). When parents reject children's bids for reassurance, children often develop avoidant attachments, turning away from their parents when distressed. As with other organized attachments, children's avoidant strategies have been described as well-suited to their maintaining optimal proximity to the caregiver (Main & Hesse, 1990). That is, when parents are uncomfortable with children's bids for reassurance, turning away from the parent when distressed represents an effective strategy for avoiding rejection. When parents are inconsistent in availability, children often develop resistant attachments, showing a combination of proximity-seeking and resistance. As with avoidant strategies, resistant attachments can be seen to maximize proximity. That is, when parents are inconsistent, frequent bids for reassurance maximize the likelihood that parents will respond. Thus, although perhaps appearing non-optimal, these avoidant and resistant attachments are well-suited to parents' availability, and represent organized strategies (De Wolff & van IJzendoorn, 1997; van IJzendoorn, 1995). Differences among these organized attachments, whether secure, avoidant, or resistant, are only weakly predictive of later problematic outcomes (Fearon, Bakermans-Kranenburg, van IJzendoorn, Lapsley, & Roisman, 2010).

On the other hand, disorganized attachments are predictive of later problematic outcomes. Children often develop disorganized attachments when parents are threatening or frightening (Main & Hesse, 1990; Schuengel, Bakermans-Kranenburg, & van IJzendoorn, 1999; True, Pisani, & Oumar, 2001). Disorganized attachments represent a breakdown or lack of strategy for interacting with the parent when the child is distressed (Main & Solomon, 1990). Whereas avoidant and resistant attachments are only weakly associated with long-term problematic outcomes, disorganized attachment predicts a host of problematic outcomes, with the most robust effects seen for externalizing symptoms (Fearon et al., 2010; Lyons-Ruth, Easterbrooks, & Cibelli, 1997).

Disorganized and insecure attachments are much more common among maltreated children than among low-risk children (Cyr, Euser, Bakermans-Kranenburg, & van

IJzendoorn, 2010). In research in our lab, we have also found that when maltreated children enter foster care, they often behave in ways that push caregivers away (Stovall & Dozier, 2000; Stovall-McClough & Dozier, 2004). More specifically, such children often act as if they do not need their caregivers or are unsoothable. These behaviors that make it less likely that caregivers will provide nurturing care subsequently (Stovall-McClough & Dozier).

Caregivers may struggle to provide nurturance for other reasons as well. Parent "state of mind with regard to attachment" is the strongest predictor of attachment quality (Dozier, Stovall, Albus, & Bates, 2001; van IJzendoorn, 1995). State of mind refers to how adults process their own attachment-related experiences, and is assessed through the Adult Attachment Interview (Main & Goldwyn, 1998). Caregivers with "autonomous" states of mind are open and reflective when describing attachment-related memories. Caregivers with "nonautonomous" states of mind may dismiss the importance of or get angrily caught up in attachment-related issues. Attachment state of mind is moderately associated with parental sensitivity (van IJzendoorn), with autonomous parents typically responding more sensitively to children's signals than non-autonomous parents. Thus, caregivers' conceptualizations of their attachment-related histories may make it difficult to provide the nurturance that maltreated children especially need. Maltreating parents are much more likely than other parents to have had challenging experiences as children themselves and are less likely than other parents to have autonomous states of mind (Bailey, Moran, & Pederson, 2007; Hesse & Main, 2000). Additionally, maltreating parents often face a number of ongoing stressors, such as poverty, psychopathology, and lack of social support, which may interfere further with providing sensitive care (Cicchetti, Rogosch, & Toth, 2006; Lyons-Ruth, Connell, Zoll, & Stahl, 1987). Foster parents, on the other hand, may face challenges with feeling "committed" to a child who is not their own, and sometimes receive messages from agencies that it is better not to become emotionally invested in a relationship that may be temporary (Dozier & Lindhiem, 2006). Importantly, maltreated children and their caregivers both bring issues to the relationship that may make an organized and secure attachment less likely.

Stress Neurobiology

In early infancy, children are dependent on caregivers for help in regulating many functions. With time and with many successful experiences at co-regulation, children gradually are able to take over these regulatory functions themselves (Feldman, 2007; Hofer, 1994, 2006; Winberg, 2005). But, when parents fail in their role as co-regulators, children often have difficulty developing their regulatory capabilities. Neglect and abuse have been associated with perturbations in the regulation of behavior and physiology. These perturbations have been seen among non-human primates and rodents through experimental studies, and among human infants and young children living under adverse conditions (Gunnar, Fisher, & The Early Experience, Stress, and Prevention Network, 2006).

The Hypothalamic-Pituitary-Adrenal (HPA) axis matures in the early post-natal period in many mammals, and is sensitive to environmental input. An end product of the HPA system is cortisol (cortisol in humans, corticosterone in rodents). Diurnal creatures such as humans show high morning values of cortisol with the level decreasing across the day to near zero values at night. These high morning values help ensure that members of the species are awake at the same time of the day as one another, with higher levels providing more glucose for metabolism.

In a study of foster children's morning cortisol production, Bruce, Fisher, Pears, and Levine (2009) found that unlike a low-income, non-maltreated comparison group, foster children were more likely to have had low morning levels of cortisol, particularly among children with a history of neglect. Consistent with this work, we also have found that adversity is associated with disruptions to this daily pattern in cortisol production (Bruce et al., 2009; Fisher, Stoolmiller, Gunnar, & Burraston, 2007; Fisher, Van Ryzin, & Gunnar, 2011). In findings from our lab and Philip Fisher's lab at Oregon Social Learning Center, children who have experienced adversity have shown flatter slopes of cortisol production across the day relative to children living under low-risk conditions (Fisher, Gunnar, Dozier, Bruce, & Pears, 2006). Bernard, Butzin-Dozier, Rittenhouse, and Dozier (2010) found that children living with high-risk parents showed the flattest slopes with lowest morning values of cortisol, and that children in foster care showed intermediate values, with low-risk children showing the steepest slopes and highest wake-up values (Bernard et al., 2010).

A stress neurobiology perspective dovetails with an attachment perspective. The reason that high-risk parenting is thought to be associated with dysregulation of the neuroendocrine system is that the parent is failing to provide necessary input to the child (in the case of neglect), or is providing problematic input (in the case of frightening behavior).

Attachment and Biobehavioral Catch-Up

Overview of Intervention

The ABC Intervention targets three issues, as suggested by attachment and stress neurobiology theory and findings. First, children need parents to behave in nurturing ways when they are distressed; second, children need parents to behave in synchronous ways when they are not distressed; and third, children need their parents to avoid frightening behavior at all times.

First, young children of maltreating or high-risk parents especially need nurturing care. Although children from low-risk environments can usually organize attachment around the availability of non-nurturing caregivers, high-risk children have greater difficulty doing so (Cyr et al., 2010; Dozier et al., 2001). Therefore, the first objective of the Attachment and Biobehavioral Catch-up intervention is to help parents behave in nurturing ways when their children are distressed.

Second, such children need a responsive environment if they are to develop adequate regulatory capabilities. We operationalize synchrony as parents following their children's lead. In our work, we observed that some caregivers learned to interact synchronously with children, but their interactions seemed rote and emotionless. For this reason, we encourage parents to delight in their children, showing genuine, unconditional positive affect and positive regard. Our research suggests that delight may be one way that caregiver commitment is communicated to children (Bernard & Dozier, 2011). The second objective of the intervention is therefore to help parents learn to behave in more synchronous and delighted ways with their young children.

Third, neglecting parents are at elevated risk for interacting with children in ways that could be frightening and intrusive, behaviors that have been shown to interfere with children's abilities to organize their behavior and physiology (e.g., Hane & Fox, 2006; van IJzendoorn, Schuengel, & Bakermans-Kranenburg, 1999). Therefore, the third intervention component helps parents recognize how their behavior may be frightening to a child, and learn alternative strategies to using frightening or intrusive parenting behaviors.

Description of Intervention

The ABC intervention is a 10-session program that is conducted in families' homes by a "parent coach" with parents and children present. We consider it critical that the intervention take place in the environment in which parents live their lives, increasing the likelihood that parents will generalize the skills acquired. Sessions are videotaped for the purposes of supervision and video feedback to parents. Sessions include manual-guided discussion of intervention content, review of parent homework, activities that allow parents to practice targeted behavior, and video feedback. Although the intervention is manualized, parent coaches' "In the Moment" comments, described in more detail below, are considered the most critical aspect of the program.

The ABC intervention has been used with both foster parents and maltreating birth parents referred by Child Protective Services as part of a foster care diversion program. As a preventative intervention for children who have experienced maltreatment, we do not screen out parents or children, and provide services broadly. The intervention is best suited to parents of children who are between about 6 and 24 months of age. Although it is possible to intervene with infants between the ages of birth and 6 months of age, the intervention is likely more powerful with children in the preferred age range because there are more opportunities for practice on intervention targets, that is, the parent behaviors targeted by the intervention. When the intervention is conducted with newborns and young infants, frequent napping and fewer spontaneous behaviors (such as vocalizing, reaching for objects, etc.) give parents fewer opportunities to respond to their child and thus practice the intervention targets. We are currently testing the efficacy of an intervention for children older than 24 months, but it includes some key features not discussed here.

"In the Moment" Comments

Parent coaches use "In the Moment" comments to provide feedback to parents regarding their behaviors that relate to intervention targets. These comments focus attention on parents' opportunities for behaving in nurturing and synchronous ways during the sessions, and help them recognize and practice the key targeted behaviors. Parent coaches are expected to make "In the Moment" comments about once per minute on average. Parent coaches are expected to pause or interrupt themselves during discussions of manual content to bring the focus of the session back to the parent–child interaction. Manual content often takes a back seat to "In the Moment" comments. Early on in intervention, when parents may not yet exhibit many synchronous or nurturing behaviors, parent coaches make "In the Moment" comments that shape the parent's behavior by focusing on the positive aspects of an overall negative behavior. Parent coaches may also scaffold parent behavior by providing suggestions for how the parent can respond to the child as an interaction unfolds. When parents engage in synchronous and nurturing interactions, parent coaches make supportive comments that describe parents' behaviors, link behaviors to intervention targets, and describe the effects of their behaviors on children. For example, the following illustrates a comment that meets all three criteria: (in response to parent taking a toy that child handed her) "He handed you that toy and you took it right from him (i.e., description). That's a great example of you following his lead (i.e., target). That lets him know he has an effect on the world (i.e., effect on child)." When parent coaches have developed sufficient rapport with the parent, they begin to make gentle corrections in response to the parent's behavior. As the parent develops greater skill and insight into the intervention target behaviors, the parent coach can also encourage the parent to reflect upon behavior, with "In the Moment" comments such as, "Are you following or leading right now?"

We train parent coaches to evaluate their own "In the Moment" comments by coding 5-min clips of their videotaped sessions. Parent coaches video-record all of their sessions by mounting a small camera on a tripod. Parent coaches identify specific behaviors related to the three intervention targets (i.e., nurturance, synchrony, frightening behavior) that the parent displays within the 5-min clip. Then, the parent coaches identify how they responded to the parent's behavior, specifically whether or not they followed the behavior with an "In the Moment" comment. For each "In the Moment" comment, the parent coach rates whether the comment appropriately matched the parent's behavior (i.e., was the comment "on target"), as well as the quality of the comment. As mentioned previously, high quality comments describe the parent's behavior, label the intervention target, and link the behavior to its effects on the child. We have found that this process of self-supervision improves the quality and the frequency of parent coaches' comments. We think "In the Moment" comments are important for a number of reasons, including making the intervention content alive for parents, giving parents practice with the behaviors while receiving feedback from the parent coach, and helping parents see that the behaviors are valued. The number of "In the Moment" comments that parent coaches make is associated with increases in parental sensitivity (Meade & Dozier, 2012).

Client Assessment

We use a standardized play assessment prior to and following the intervention to allow the parent coach to assess parent synchrony. We also recommend using the Strange Situation post-intervention to assess attachment/nurturing behavior. Additionally, parents' behavior is coded in two ways following each session: on standardized 5-point scales, and through "In the Moment" coding of video clips of sessions. Throughout all sessions, parent coaches evaluate parents' strengths and weaknesses with regard to intervention targets. Because intervention sessions are conducted in families' homes with children and parents present, information is continuously available to evaluate parents' strengths with regard to nurturance, following the lead, delight, and frightening behaviors. Following each session, parent coaches rate parents' strength in each target behavior using 5-point scales. Parent coaches also update their plans for addressing each target behavior weekly using a standardized rating tool. The plan to address parent weaknesses becomes increasingly urgent in later sessions, as the last session with the family approaches. Because sessions 9 and 10 do not introduce any new intervention content, parent coaches are able to focus intently on their plan. Our planning tool and a sample target behavior scale are shown below:

Scale for Rating Parent Nurturance

1. Not at all nurturing
2. An inkling of nurturance
3. Some mixture of nurturing and not nurturing, or ambiguous
4. Very nurturing, but may cut off too early, or not nurture every opportunity, or be fully nurturing.
5. Very nurturing. This parent shows nurturing behavior at virtually every opportunity. This is seen when child falls, asks for help, asks for closeness (e.g., leans in)

Planning Tool for Parent Coaches

For each of the target behaviors (nurturance, following the lead, delight, and frightening behavior), indicate what needs to happen in the next session:

1. Already strong/need to reinforce
2. Time to work on now, directly
3. Late, missed it, need remedial work
4. Can work on, but only indirectly
5. Wait until further in

In addition to the scales for rating parent behavior, parent coaches' "In the Moment" coding of 5-min video clips of sessions also includes assessment of parent behavior. Described in more detail above, the "In the Moment" coding system requires parent coaches to record and code each parent behavior that relates to intervention targets. As a counterpart to the global ratings, this process encourages parent coaches to objectively assess parent behaviors in greater detail and specificity. This information is used in treatment planning and tracked from session to session.

Description of Sessions

Sessions 1 and 2 emphasize the importance of nurturing care for children who have experienced adversity. In session 1, the parent coach discusses how children's previous experiences with caregivers may lead them to be difficult to soothe or to act as if they do not need the parent. As homework, parents are asked to complete a log of how their child behaves when hurt, frightened, or upset.

In session 2, the homework is reviewed, discussing the ways the child tends to behave when distressed, and the parent's responses to the child in these situations. Video clips of children who behave in secure, avoidant, and resistant ways are used to illustrate how much easier it is to provide nurturance to a child who directly seeks out comfort and is easy to soothe. Parents are helped to recognize how important it is for children to have confidence that their parents will reassure them when they are distressed. They are encouraged to respond in nurturing ways when their child is distressed, overriding the reactions and feelings that the child's avoidant, resistant or disorganized behavior may elicit initially.

Sessions 3 and 4 emphasize the importance of synchronous, or contingently responsive parenting behaviors. In session 3, parent coaches talk about this with parents as "following the child's lead." Parents are asked to engage in two activities focused on following the child's lead: playing with a book with pull-out shapes and playing with blocks. Prior to the activities, parents are shown video clips of other parents playing with these toys, and the differences between "following" and "leading" in play are emphasized. The parent coach then supports the parent as she engages with her child in the activities, pointing out times when the parent follows the lead, and making suggestions for other ways she might respond to the child. Video feedback can be provided in session 3, directly after the activities, or in session 4, when the parent coach has had the opportunity to review the video and choose short clips (e.g., 10 s) of times when the parent engaged in synchronous interaction and times when the parent did not.

In session 4, parents are asked to follow their child's lead in a pudding making activity. This activity is particularly challenging for parents because it is hard for them not to "take charge." Again, prior to the activity, parent coaches show video clips of other parents interacting synchronously and non-synchronously while making pudding with their children. During the activity, parent coaches use "In the Moment" comments to support parents in following their children's lead. Later, video feedback is used to further reinforce parents' understanding of interactional synchrony.

In session 5, the concept that some parental behavior can have a negative effect on children is introduced. This discussion begins with a description and illustration of the effects of parents' intrusive behavior on children. Activities with puppets and noisy toys are used because they elicit intrusive and/or frightening behavior. As in the sessions focused on synchrony, the parent coach supports the parent in the process of reading and responding to the child's signals for engagement and disengagement through the use of "In the Moment" comments.

Session 6 introduces the idea that parents can frighten their children with their behavior. Parents are asked to consider experiences of being frightened themselves as children, and then to consider times when their behavior might frighten their children. The parent coach discusses how challenging it is to be aware that a behavior is frightening or to recognize the consequences of frightening behavior. Videos of the parent in instances when they were and were not frightening are presented if applicable.

Sessions 7 and 8 ask parents to think about experiences from their past that affect their current parenting. The objective of these sessions is helping parents to become aware of influences that drive their parenting behavior. In making parents aware and conscious of such influences, their behavior becomes less automatic. They can then "over-ride" these influences and behave in nurturing or responsive ways.

In session 7, we introduce the topic as "voices from the past." The parent coach approaches this session with a clear conceptualization of the critical issues on which the parent needs to work. If the primary issue is nurturance, for example, voices from the past will be approached with the objective of: identifying attachment experiences relevant to nurturing behaviors; recognizing times when these experiences affect current feelings about whether the parent should provide nurturance; and over-riding these initial responses, providing nurturance despite the "voices from the past." The parent coach guides the parent in recognizing voices from the past by providing examples of other parents' voices from the past, and presenting video clips of times when a voice from the past might have prevented the parent from responding in a nurturing or synchronous way.

In session 8, the topic of "voices from the past" is continued, with an emphasis on helping parents develop a plan to override their automatic way of responding, in order to respond in a way that supports the needs of their children. Parents are encouraged to begin to recognize the times when a voice from the past influences their behavior, and to consciously choose to respond in a different way.

Given the topic of sessions 7 and 8, it is tempting for parent coaches to direct attention to the parent, rather than the parent's behaviors toward the child. However, it is critical that the emphasis on "In the Moment" comments is maintained. Furthermore, it can be powerful to link the discussion about "voices from the past" to what is occurring between the parent and child during the session. For example, a parent might be soothing her crying child as she is describing how her mother would ignore her distress or respond by telling her she was spoiled. In this case, a parent coach might point out the parent's strengths in recognizing her voices from the past and in making active efforts to behave differently (commenting specifically on her ability to be nurturing in the moment).

Sessions 9 and 10 serve to consolidate intervention gains. The primary objective of these sessions is to continue the emphasis on parents nurturing their children, following their children's lead with delight, and behaving in non-frightening ways. In session 10, parent coaches show videos that highlight the progress parents have made in each of the three areas, and celebrate their effort and gains.

Overview of ABC Intervention Focus Areas by Session

Session sequence	Session title	Session content
Sessions 1–2	Providing nurturance to the child	Helps parents understand that the child needs them to be nurturing when distressed
Sessions 3–5	Following the child's lead with delight	Emphasizes the importance of following the child's lead in interactions. Helps parents become attuned and responsive to the child's signals for engagement and disengagement
Session 6	Frightening behavior	Helps parents understand that frightening behavior is problematic for the child and helps parents develop alternative ways of interacting
Sessions 7–8	Over-riding parents' own issues	Parents are helped to develop strategies so they can override automatic ways of responding, providing nurturing, sensitive care even if it does not come naturally
Sessions 9–10	Consolidating	Consolidates parents' gains, provides practice with behaviors still in need of improvement

Evidence Base for the ABC Intervention

The efficacy of the ABC intervention has been assessed in randomized clinical trials with both foster parents and CPS-referred birth parents. The CPS-referred parents were involved in a foster care diversion project. In both sets of studies, children were randomly assigned to receive the ABC intervention or a control intervention. We describe below the results of investigations into the relationship between participation in the ABC Intervention and children's attachment style, emotional regulation, and neurological processes reflected by cortisol levels.

Attachment was assessed through the Strange Situation at post-intervention to determine whether children participating in ABC compared to a control intervention were more likely to develop an organized attachment. The Strange Situation is a laboratory assessment in which parent and child are separated and reunited twice over an approximately 24-min period (Ainsworth et al., 1978), and is considered the "gold-standard" for assessing young children's attachment quality. The reunion behavior of the child is used to classify children as having a secure, avoidant, resistant, or disorganized attachment. As described earlier, disorganized attachment is of greatest concern because of its association with long-term problematic outcomes (Fearon et al., 2010). In the CPS-involved birth parent sample, children who were randomly assigned to the ABC intervention showed lower rates of disorganized attachment than children assigned to the control intervention (Bernard et al., 2012). Specifically, when children's attachments to their high-risk birth parents were assessed, 32 % of children in the ABC intervention group had disorganized attachments, in contrast with 57 % in the control intervention group.

We assessed emotion expression in challenging tasks through the Tool Task (Matas, Arend, & Sroufe, 1978). When children in the CPS-referred birth parent sample were about 2-years-old, they were presented with several tasks that were too difficult for them to master alone. Children from the ABC intervention group expressed less negative affect, and less anger toward their mothers relative to children in the control group when engaged in these challenging and frustrating tasks (Lind, Bernard, Wallin, & Dozier, 2012).

Children's diurnal cortisol was assessed by asking parents to take salivary samples at wake-up and bedtime over 2 days. Children whose birth parents received the ABC intervention showed more normative cortisol production than those whose parents received the control intervention (Dozier, Bernard, Bick, & Gordon, 2012). Children whose parents received the ABC intervention showed a steeper slope and higher wake-up values relative to children in the control group. A non-normative cortisol pattern across the day reflects a disruption to a basic biological process. We consider the intervention's ability to restore this normative pattern by improving parenting responsiveness remarkable.

In addition to physiological measures of children's regulation, ABC has also been shown to improve children's executive function, a capacity that enables behavioral self-regulation (Barkley, 2001). Specifically, foster children in the ABC group showed more advanced executive functioning on an executive function task in which they were asked to shift rules (the Dimensional Change Card Sort, Zelazo, 2006) relative to children in the control group (Lewis-Morrarty, Dozier, Bernard, Terraciano, & Moore, 2012). That is, when asked to sort cards according to a particular dimension, or rule, children in all groups performed well. However, after being asked to change the rule by which they were sorting, children from the ABC intervention group showed significantly better performance than children in the control group. Being able to switch dimensions is associated with other executive functions, such as planning and inhibitory control. Deficits in executive functions are associated with disorders such as ADHD (Mulas et al., 2006).

These findings support the efficacy of the ABC intervention in enhancing attachment quality, cortisol production, emotion expression, and inhibitory control among children living with high risk birth parents and with foster parents. Given that the ABC intervention is relatively short-term, it is impressive that effects emerge across domains of functioning and in diverse samples of children. We expect that both the targeted approach developed based on research and the explicit focus on specific parent behaviors during sessions support its effectiveness.

ABC Case Study

Deanna was a 23-year-old mother of 3 children. She had been investigated by Child Protective Services (CPS) when neighbors complained that drug dealing was taking place in her home. She was referred by CPS to the ABC parenting intervention as part of a foster care diversion program, but her participation was not mandatory.

Deanna's children were 18 months, 3, and 4 years old. She struggled with substance use and unstable living arrangements. She moved in and out of her mother's house from time to time. She had recently moved back in with her mother after the CPS complaint and before our intervention began. She lived with her boyfriend for several sessions of the intervention. However, he abused alcohol and illegal drugs, so the arrangement did not last long.

We invited Deanna, her mother, and the three children (and anyone else in the home) to participate in the intervention sessions. There were times when as many as 8–10 members of the family were involved in sessions.

Based on our observations in the first of the ten sessions, Deanna was staunchly not nurturing, not synchronous, and often engaged in frightening behaviors. We note again that these behaviors are observed in the context of the intervention rather than through an assessment process outside of the context of the intervention. For example, with regard to nurturing behaviors, when Deanna's mother left the home during the second intervention session and the 18-month-old Sam began crying uncontrollably, she mocked him, saying that he should not be acting like a baby. When first asked to follow his lead while playing with blocks, she immediately took control, asking questions, correcting, and directing any play. With regard to frightening behavior, she quickly resorted to an angry, threatening expression when Sam engaged in even mildly negative (but developmentally appropriate) behavior, and was more overtly frightening with the older children once yelling, "Just because she [the parent coach] is here don't mean nothing. She's going to videotape the real me!"

Sessions 1 and 2

An initial challenge with Deanna was to gain her trust while introducing the changes we wanted to see across all domains. It can be very threatening to have an "expert" provide feedback regarding parenting. Therefore, the parent coach was very careful to provide supportive feedback almost immediately after walking in the door. Even though Deanna was often not nurturing and not synchronous, the parent coach commented on the small behaviors seen that could be commented on in a positive way. For example, when Sam held out a toy to Deanna and she took it absentmindedly, the parent coach commented, "He held that toy out to you and you took it right from him. We'll be talking about how important that is in later sessions, but I just want to mention now what a great example that is of following his lead." On another occasion, Sam cried for an extended time after his grandmother left and kicked at Deanna multiple times. Her response could be described as hostile overall, but there was a moment in which Sam leaned against her and she briefly put her hand on his back. The parent coach commented, "Even though your job is hard because he's not showing you clearly that he needs you, reaching out to touch him like that is so important. We'll be talking about how critical it is to provide that nurturance just like that."

Sessions 3–5

In session 3, Deanna was given the task of following Sam's lead while reading a book with him. She immediately started asking him what was on each page, and corrected him when he said the wrong thing. At her first opportunity, the parent coach ignored Deanna's critical tone of voice and said, "He said 'dog' and then you said 'dog' (when the picture was actually of a cow). That's great! It doesn't matter if it's a dog or not, does it?" Deanna beamed, and started following Sam's lead. She continued to need support nearly continuously, but when supported, her behaviors with Sam were markedly different than they had been. The parent coach had many opportunities to make positive "In the Moment" comments as a result. When Deanna started taking the lead, the parent coach was able to gently remind her by asking, "Who is leading now?" without eliciting anger or defensiveness. Deanna may have felt more comfortable with the parent coach after receiving many positive comments, which prevented her from becoming defensive to the gentle reminders.

Sam became upset several times during sessions 3 through 5, and the parent coach used these times to help Deanna recognize the importance of providing him nurturing care. Deanna's initial responses conveyed that Sam needed to be a big boy, or that he was not really upset or hurt. Gradually, with positive feedback from the parent coach for each nurturing behavior, she started offering more nurturing care.

Session 6

In session 6, Deanna recalled times when her mother had threatened her sisters and her, and acknowledged that she had felt very scared at such times. She was surprisingly open and non-defensive in her recollection of these memories. She described acting in similar ways with Sam and his siblings. Nonetheless, she resisted thinking that Sam was afraid of her, and downplayed that it was a problem. Although session 6 involved Deanna thinking about times from her own past that were difficult, the parent coach continued to make frequent "In the Moment" comments regarding following the lead and nurturance as Deanna interacted spontaneously with Sam. We consider it essential to keep the focus on the parent's behaviors with her child even as she thinks about her own difficult experiences.

Sessions 7 and 8

Approaching session 7, the parent coach was aware that Deanna needed to work on nurturing and synchronous behavior. Given that she appeared to be struggling with being nurturing toward Sam, this was the primary focus of the session. She had made progress in the treatment program, but it seemed critical to help her become more aware of her voices from the past if she were to maintain the gains beyond the ten sessions. The parent coach first showed a video from session 5 in which Deanna responded in a nurturing way when Sam was upset. The parent coach pointed out how nurturing Deanna was, and how different it was from the way she had talked about her mother responding to her. They looked at this video several times, considering how impressive it was to provide nurturing care even though Deanna's voices from the past suggested to her that she would just spoil Sam. The parent coach then showed a clip from session 2 when Deanna had not initially been nurturing when Sam was upset over his grandmother's departure. Deanna was helped to realize that her automatic responses (to behave in non-nurturing ways) were guided by her voices from the past.

Throughout the sessions, the parent coach made frequent "In the Moment" comments and linked the comments to voices from the past when possible. For example, Sam pinched his finger in a toy, fussed, and looked up at Deanna. Deanna quickly asked, "Hey booty, did that hurt?" The parent coach said, "Oh my gosh, listen to you. Even though your voice from the past tells you that he doesn't need you to respond, look what you do. You're there for him when he needs you. It's so impressive that you can over-ride that voice from the past."

Sessions 9 and 10

In the final two sessions, the parent coach worked to solidify the gains that Deanna had made throughout the sessions. She presented videos showing changes that were evident in Deanna's behavior, such as responding in more nurturing ways and following her child's lead. Deanna even noticed and pointed out examples from the video clips when she was not nurturing or took the lead during play. Her increasing awareness of these problematic behaviors that were previously automatic allowed her to interrupt herself in the moment, and provide Sam with more appropriate responses. When showing later videos of Deanna behaving in sensitive and synchronous ways, the parent coach reminded Deanna of how these particular behaviors would affect Sam – such as strengthening his trust in her, enhancing his ability to regulate his behavior and physiology, and supporting his sense of competence and self-esteem.

This intervention has been developed as a 10-session program with annual booster sessions that review progress and challenges. If parents are able to complete all ten sessions of the initial intervention, no additional sessions are provided until the annual booster sessions, even when parents have not fully reached treatment goals. Deanna had made significant progress toward all targets by the end of the ten sessions.

Conclusion

The ABC Intervention was designed to enhance parenting among parents of high-risk children who have faced early adversity. The three objectives of increasing nurturance, increasing parent–child synchrony, and reducing frightening behavior are primarily targeted by providing specific, positive feedback to parents about their behavior during the sessions. We have several ways to assess progress related to intervention targets. First, parent coaches assess parents' strength in each intervention target behavior following every session. Second, we code parents' behavior during a 5-min period each session. Third, we encourage agencies to use a standardized play assessment prior to and following the intervention to allow assessment of synchronous interactions, and to assess attachment/nurturing behavior through the Strange Situation post-intervention. The intervention has a strong evidence-base with support from two randomized clinical trials showing effects on children's attachment organization, physiological regulation, and executive functioning. We consider the ABC intervention to be especially appropriate for parents involved with the child welfare system at risk for maltreating their young children. Furthermore, ABC's short duration, targeted and supportive approach, and implementation in parents' homes are expected to bolster parents' engagement and ability to make lasting behavioral changes.

References

Ainsworth, M. D. S., Blehar, M. C., Waters, E., & Wall, S. (1978). *Patterns of attachment: A psychological study of the strange situation*. Hillsdale, NJ: Erlbaum.

Bailey, H. N., Moran, G., & Pederson, D. R. (2007). Childhood maltreatment, complex trauma symptoms, and unresolved attachment in a at-risk sample of adolescent mothers. *Attachment & Human Development, 9*, 139–161.

Barkley, R. A. (2001). The executive functions and self-regulation: An evolutionary neuropsychological perspective. *Neuropsychology Review, 11*, 1–29.

Bernard, K., Butzin-Dozier, Z., Rittenhouse, J., & Dozier, M. (2010). Young children living with neglecting birth parents show more blunted daytime patterns of cortisol production than children in foster care and comparison children. *Archives of Pediatrics & Adolescent Medicine, 164*, 438–443.

Bernard, K., & Dozier, M. (2011). This is my baby: Foster parents' feelings of commitment and displays of delight. *Infant Mental Health Journal, 32*, 251–262.

Bernard, K., Dozier, M., Bick, J., Lewis-Morrarty, E., Lindhiem, O., & Carlson, E. (2012). Enhancing attachment organization among maltreated infants: Results of a randomized clinical trial. *Child Development, 83*, 623–636.

Bowlby, J. (1969/1982). *Attachment and loss* (Vol. 1). London: Hogarth Press.

Bruce, J., Fisher, P. A., Pears, K. C., & Levine, S. (2009). Morning cortisol levels in preschool-aged foster children: Differential effects of maltreatment type. *Developmental Psychobiology, 51*, 14–23. doi:10.1002/dev.20333.

Cicchetti, D., Rogosch, F. A., & Toth, S. L. (2006). Fostering secure attachments in infants in maltreating families through preventive interventions. *Development and Psychopathology, 18*, 623–649. doi:10.1017/S0954579406060329.

Cyr, C., Euser, E. M., Bakermans-Kranenburg, M. J., & van IJzendoorn, M. H. (2010). Attachment security and disorganization in maltreating and high-risk families: A series of meta-analyses. *Development and Psychopathology, 22*, 87–108. doi:10.1017/S0954579409990289.

De Wolff, M., & van IJzendoorn, M. H. (1997). Sensitivity and infant attachment: A meta-analysis on parental antecedents of infant attachment. *Child Development, 68*, 571–591. doi:10.2307/1132107.

Dozier, M., Bernard, K., Bick, J., & Gordon, M. K. (2012). *Normalizing the diurnal production of cortisol: The effects of an early intervention for high-risk children*. Unpublished manuscript, University of Delaware, Newark, DE.

Dozier, M., & Lindhiem, O. (2006). This is my child: Differences among foster parents in commitment to their children. *Child Maltreatment, 11*, 338–345. doi:10.1016/j.chiabu.2006.12.003.

Dozier, M., Stovall, K. C., Albus, K. E., & Bates, B. (2001). Attachment for infants in foster care: The role of caregiver state of mind. *Child Development, 72*, 1467–1477. doi:10.1111/1467-8624.00360.

Fearon, R. P., Bakermans-Kranenburg, M. J., van IJzendoorn, M. H., Lapsley, A. M., & Roisman, G. I. (2010). The significance of insecure attachment and disorganization in the development of children's externalizing behavior: A meta-analytic study. *Child Development, 81*, 435–456. doi:10.1111/j.1467-8624.2009.01405.x.

Feldman, R. (2007). Parent-infant synchrony and the construction of shared timing: Physiological precursors, developmental outcomes, and risk conditions. *Journal of Child Psychology and Psychiatry, 48*, 329–354. doi:10.1111/j.1469-7610.2006.01701.x.

Fisher, P., Gunnar, M. R., Dozier, M., Bruce, J., & Pears, K. (2006). Effects of therapeutic interventions for foster children on behavior problems, caregiver attachment, and stress regulatory neural systems. *Annals of the New York Academy of Sciences, 1094*, 215–225. doi:10.1196/annals.1376.023.

Fisher, P. A., Stoolmiller, M., Gunnar, M. R., & Burraston, B. O. (2007). Effects of a therapeutic intervention for foster preschoolers on diurnal cortisol activity. *Psychoneuroendocrinology, 32*, 892–905. doi:10.1016/j.psyneuen.2007.06.008.

Fisher, P. A., Van Ryzin, M. J., & Gunnar, M. R. (2011). Mitigating HPA axis dysregulation associated with placement changes in foster care. *Psychoneuroendocrinology, 36*, 531–539. doi:10.1016/j.psyneuen.2010.08.007.

Gunnar, M. R., Fisher, P. A., & The Early Experience, Stress, and Prevention Network. (2006). Bringing basic research on early experience and stress neurobiology to bear on preventive interventions for neglected and maltreated children. *Development and Psychopathology, 18*, 651–677. doi:10.1017/S0954579406040330.

Hane, A. A., & Fox, N. A. (2006). Ordinary variations in maternal caregiving influence human infants' stress reactivity. *Psychological Science, 17*, 550–556. doi:10.1111/j.1467-9280.2006.01742.x.

Hesse, E., & Main, M. (2000). Disorganized infant, child and adult attachment: Collapse in behavioral and attentional strategies. *Journal of the American Psychoanalytic Association, 48*, 1097–1127.

Hofer, M. (1994). Hidden regulators in attachment, separation, and loss. *Monographs of the Society for Research in Child Development, 59*, 192–207. doi:10.2307/1166146.

Hofer, M. (2006). Psychobiological roots of early attachment. *Current Directions in Psychological Science, 15*, 84–88. doi:10.1111/j.0963-7214.2006.00412.x.

van IJzendoorn, M. H. (1995). Adult attachment representations, parental responsiveness, and infant attachment: A meta-analysis of the predictive validity of the Adult Attachment Interview. *Psychological Bulletin, 117*, 387–403. doi:10.1037/0033-2909.117.3.387.

van IJzendoorn, M. H., Bakermans-Kranenburg, M. J., & Sagi-Schwartz, A. (2006). Attachment across diverse sociocultural contexts: The limits of universality. In K. Rubin (Ed.), *Parental beliefs, parenting, and child development in cross-cultural perspective* (pp. 107–142). Hove, England: Psychology Press.

van IJzendoorn, M. H., Schuengel, C., & Bakermans-Kranenburg, M. J. (1999). Disorganized attachment in early childhood: Meta-analysis of precursors, concomitants, and sequelae. *Development and Psychopathology, 11*, 225–249. doi:10.1017/S0954579499002035.

Lewis-Morrarty, E., Dozier, M., Bernard, K., Terraciano, S., & Moore, S. (2012). Cognitive flexibility and theory of mind outcomes among foster children: Preschool follow-up results of a randomized clinical trial. *Journal of Adolescent Health, 52*, S17–S22. doi:10.1016/j.jadohealth.2012.05.005.

Lind, T., Bernard, K., Wallin, A., & Dozier, M. (2012). *The effects of an attachment-based intervention on children's expression of negative affect in a challenging task*. Unpublished manuscript, University of Delaware, Newark, DE.

Lyons-Ruth, K., Connell, D. B., Zoll, D., & Stahl, J. (1987). Infants at social risk: Relations among infant maltreatment, maternal behavior, and infant attachment behavior. *Developmental Psychology, 23*, 223–232. doi:10.1037/0012-1649.23.2.223.

Lyons-Ruth, K., Easterbrooks, M. A., & Cibelli, C. D. (1997). Infant attachment strategies, infant mental lag, and maternal depressive symptoms: Predictors of internalizing and externalizing problems at age 7. *Developmental Psychology, 33*, 681–692. doi:10.1037/0012-1649.33.4.681.

Main, M., & Goldwyn, R. (1998). *Adult attachment classification system*. London: University College.

Main, M., & Hesse, E. (1990). Parents' unresolved traumatic experiences are related to infant disorganized attachment status: Is frightened and/or frightening parental behavior the linking mechanism? In M. T. Greenberg, D. Cicchetti, & E. Cummings (Eds.), *Attachment in the preschool years: Theory, research, and intervention* (pp. 161–182). Chicago: University of Chicago Press.

Main, M., & Solomon, J. (1990). Procedures for identifying infants as disorganized/disoriented during the Ainsworth strange situation. In M. T. Greenberg, D. Cicchetti, & E. Cummings (Eds.), *Attachment in the preschool years: Theory, research, and intervention* (pp. 161–182). Chicago: University of Chicago Press.

Matas, L., Arend, R. A., & Sroufe, L. A. (1978). Continuity of adaptation in the second year: The relationship between quality of attachment and later competence. *Child Development, 49*, 547–556. doi:10.2307/1128221.

Meade, E., & Dozier, M. (2012). *"In the moment" commenting: A fidelity measurement and active ingredient in a parent training program*. Unpublished manuscript, University of Delaware, Newark, DE.

Mulas, F., Capilla, A., Fernández, S., Etchepareborda, M. C., Campo, P., Maestú, F., et al. (2006). Shifting-related brain magnetic activity in attention-deficit/hyperactivity disorder. *Biological Psychiatry, 59*, 373–379. doi:10.1016/j.biopsych.2005.06.031.

Schuengel, C., Bakermans-Kranenburg, M. J., & Van IJzendoorn, M. H. (1999). Frightening maternal behavior linking unresolved loss and disorganized infant attachment. *Journal of Consulting and Clinical Psychology, 67*, 54–63. doi:10.1037/0022-006X.67.1.54.

Stovall, K. C., & Dozier, M. (2000). The development of attachment in new relationships: Single subject analyses for 10 foster infants. *Development and Psychopathology, 12*, 133–156.

Stovall-McClough, K. C., & Dozier, M. (2004). Forming attachments in foster care: Infant attachment behaviors during the first 2 months of placement. *Development and Psychopathology, 16*, 253–271. doi:10.10170S0954579404044505.

True, M. M., Pisani, L., & Oumar, F. (2001). Infant-mother attachment among the Dogon of Mali. *Child Development, 72*, 1451–1466. doi:10.1111/1467-8624.00359.

Weinfield, N. S., Sroufe, L. A., Egeland, B., & Carlson, E. (2008). Individual differences in infant-caregiver attachment: Conceptual and empirical aspects of security. In J. Cassidy & P. R. Shaver (Eds.), *Handbook of attachment: Theory, research, and clinical applications* (pp. 78–101). New York: Guildford.

Winberg, J. (2005). Mother and newborn baby: Mutual regulation of physiology and behavior – A selective review. *Developmental Psychobiology, 47*, 217–229. doi:10.1002/dev.20094.

Zeanah, C. H., Smyke, A. T., Koga, S. F., & Carlson, E. (2005). Attachment in institutionalized and community children in Romania. *Child Development, 76*, 1015–1028. doi:10.1111/j.1467-8624.2005.00894.x.

Zelazo, P. D. (2006). The Dimensional Change Card Sort (DCCS): A method of assessing executive function in children. *Nature Protocols, 1*, 297–301.

Chapter 5
Child-Parent Psychotherapy with Infants and Very Young Children

Patricia Van Horn and Vilma Reyes

Child-parent Psychotherapy (CPP) for traumatized infants and young children is based on the principles that (1) relationships are central to young children's healthy development, and (2) infants and young children organize their responses to threat and danger, and therefore to trauma, around their attachment relationships. As they develop, infants internalize the caregiving patterns of their earliest attachment figures and, over time, become increasingly able to soothe themselves by bringing caregiving patterns to mind in the attachment figure's absence (Bowlby, 1969/1982). These earliest relational experiences also provide templates from which the developing young child predicts how others will behave and how others will respond to the child's behavior, shaping the child's earliest understanding of relationships. Finally, secure early relationships with caregivers give infants and toddlers a secure base from which to explore the world and to take on the mental and emotional challenges it presents (Bowlby). Thus, secure relationships lay the foundations for resilience by shaping young children's capacities in three critical domains: (1) early self-soothing leading, later, to regulating strong emotions, (2) understanding and forming sustaining relationships, and (3) developing the ability to process information about the world, using that information to solve problems (Lieberman & Van Horn, 2005, 2008).

When interpersonal trauma occurs in the lives of infants and very young children, it can be profoundly disruptive of their development in all of these domains for the very reason it has the potential to damage or destroy trust in relationships. Freud (1920/1955) originally proposed the concept that young children rely on their caregivers to provide a protective shield, fending off traumatic stimuli, both internal and external, that flood the child and overwhelm his or her nascent capacity to cope; Bowlby (1969/1982) expanded this idea further, proposing that an infant's expectation of protection and the mother's role in providing protection from danger and

P. Van Horn, Ph.D. (✉) • V. Reyes, Psy.D.
Department of Psychiatry, University of California, San Francisco, CA, USA
e-mail: patricia.vanhorn@ucsf.edu; vilma.reyes@ucsf.edu

S. Timmer and A. Urquiza (eds.), *Evidence-Based Approaches for the Treatment of Maltreated Children*, Child Maltreatment 3, DOI 10.1007/978-94-007-7404-9_5,
© Springer Science+Business Media Dordrecht 2014

generating a sense of security in the infant in spite of threat were biologically determined. Following these early theorists, contemporary trauma experts posit that infants and young children have the developmentally appropriate expectation that those who care for them will sense oncoming danger, appraise the level of risk it presents, and provide protection from injury and from overwhelming fear and terror (Marans & Adelman, 1997; Pynoos, Steinberg, & Piacentini, 1999). When young children experience the overwhelming sights, sounds, and internal sensations that make up a traumatic experience, their expectation of protection is betrayed. Their trust in their caregivers, the *sine qua non* of children's healthy development, is shattered, at least for the space of the traumatic moment. The younger the child is when such an experience occurs, the more profoundly will his or her development be placed at risk, because early development provides the foundations upon which the child bases later capacities.

We distinguish in this chapter between trauma, an experience that overwhelms the capacity of the individual (regardless of age) to cope, leading to feelings of helplessness and terror, and developmentally costly stress, which certainly affects development but without leading to the existential crisis that psychologists have described in traumatized adults. Janoff-Bulman (1992) describes certain assumptions about themselves and the world that all humans develop as children if their development proceeds unaffected by trauma: these assumptions are that the world is fundamentally benevolent, that life has meaning, and that the self has value. Trauma shatters these assumptions, leading to a new set of beliefs: that the world is a dangerous, meaningless place, and that the self is not worthy of protection but is, in fact, beset by risk from all quarters. When trauma shatters young children's trust in their caregivers, it places at risk their nascent regulatory, relational, and cognitive capacities. If young children are to be restored to positive and hopeful developmental trajectories after trauma it is essential that the ruptures in their relationships with those who care for them be mended. For this reason, CPP focuses on strengthening the caregiving relationship after trauma as the most economical means of protecting children's development and mental health.

CPP has been described fully elsewhere (Lieberman, 1992, 2004; Lieberman & Van Horn, 2005, 2008, 2009), and so here we will describe it briefly, ending with a short discussion of the evidence that supports it. We will next then examine the special challenges of using CPP, which has at its heart making the trauma explicit, and developing a joint narrative between child and caregiver in order to place the trauma in perspective. We will use a case treated by one of us (VR) as an illustration of CPP treatment with pre-verbal children.

Theoretical Underpinnings of CPP

CPP emerged from a tradition of relationship-based therapy developed to address situations in which infants or young children suffered abusive or neglectful caregiving, or in which the parents had suffered traumas in their own early caregiving that they reenacted with their children, putting the children's development at risk (Fraiberg, 1980; Lieberman, Silverman, & Pawl, 2000). The relationship-based therapies focus on the inter-generational transmission of trauma and psychopathology and on translating the parent's and child's feelings and experiences to one another as a means of achieving enhanced emotional reciprocity in the dyad. Interventions are directed at the parent-child relationship itself, particularly addressing the child's sense of the parent as being unable to provide safety and protection, the parent's distorted negative attributions of the child, and the mutual traumatic expectations that the parent and child have of one another.

CPP (Lieberman & Van Horn, 2005, 2008) is psychodynamic with attachment theory as posited by Bowlby (1969/1982). As it moved from a modality for the treatment of a range of relationship difficulties that can beset infancy and early childhood, to use with trauma-specific populations, CPP kept the intervention foci described above, but added other components common to all trauma treatments (Marmar, Foy, Kagan, & Pynoos, 1993). These include helping the traumatized individual achieve and maintain regular levels of affective arousal, re-establishing trust in bodily sensations and emotional cues, and restoring the capacity to respond realistically to threat. It is critical to note that in many dyads in which young children have suffered traumas, their caregivers have as well (Ghosh Ippen, Harris, Van Horn, & Lieberman, 2011); requiring the CPP therapist to attend to caregivers' as well as children's traumatic reminders and expectations, and to the dysregulation in affect and cognition that accompanies them, if the intervention is to be effective. CPP uses relationship-focused strategies to aid coping with traumatic reminders and traumatic expectations, and play or other media to allow co-creation of a coherent narrative of the traumatic experiences. While CPP is sufficiently flexible to allow the incorporation of interventions based in behavioral and social learning theories when these are deemed the most effective ways to address the clinical problem at hand, it does not strive to accomplish behavior change as an end in itself. It seeks to understand the meaning behind children's and parents' behaviors (particularly where the meaning is based in developmentally salient anxieties or traumatic experiences) and to translate these meanings for the parent and the child so that they can better understand one another's views of the world and motivations.

Openings for potential interventions or clinical ports of entry are not selected *a priori* according to theory in CPP, but are selected by the clinician as material presents itself, allowing the clinician to select interventions that he or she believes will most effectively advance the goals of helping the parent and child hold realistic, flexible, and reciprocal views of one another and returning the child to a healthy developmental trajectory. Ports of entry include the caregiver or the child's individual behavior, the interactive exchanges between caregiver and child, the mental representations of each other and of the absent parent, the child's play, and the child or caregiver's perceptions of the therapeutic relationship. There are also systemic ports of entry such as offering concrete assistance by consulting with other providers, teachers, case managers, lawyers, etc. The order of interventions is not dictated, but clinicians are advised to begin with simple interventions, often based in developmental guidance and advocating for safety, and then choosing more complex interventions such as addressing resistance, mistrust, generational transmission of trauma or psychological obstacles (Lieberman & Van Horn, 2005).

CPP uses a variety of treatment modalities including (a) supporting the child's developmental momentum through play, physical contact and language; (b) offering unstructured, reflective, developmental guidance that is consistent with the family's cultural beliefs about the roles of parents and children; (c) modeling appropriate protective behavior if the parent does not respond to threat observed by the clinician; (d) interpreting feelings and actions; (e) providing emotional support and empathic communication; and (f) offering crisis intervention, case management, and concrete assistance with problems of daily living. As CPP clinicians weave these modalities into unified treatments, they pay special attention to themes of trauma, in the present, in the parents' or children's pasts, or in their larger cultural group (Klatzkin, Lieberman, & Van Horn, 2013) in order to help parents and children understand the impact of the trauma on their beliefs and feelings about one another and other important people, and to help them form more balanced views of themselves and others. To facilitate this quest for balance, clinicians engage in an active search for beneficent memories from the parents' care-receiving pasts that may guide and sustain them as they care for their children (Lieberman, Padrón, Van Horn, & Harris, 2004).

Beginning Treatment in CPP

Although CPP is a generally flexible modality, the beginning of a CPP treatment is highly structured for several reasons. First, it is critical that the clinician begin to form a strong alliance with the parent, by meeting alone with the parent at least one time and an average of five times before the joint parent-child sessions begin. In addition to alliance building, meetings with the caregiver serve several purposes. The clinician should use them to perform a good clinical assessment, with or without the use of formal instruments. At a minimum, the clinician can learn the parent's concerns about the child, the details of the traumatic experience (critical for guiding hypotheses about potential traumatic reminders), and the parent's understanding of it and how the child's functioning changed after the traumatic experience, and whether there has been any spontaneous recovery of pre-trauma functioning. The child's behavioral functioning can be assessed using instruments such as the Child Behavior Checklist (CBCL), or the Devereux Early Childhood Initiative (DECA-I/T). The child's trauma symptoms can be assessed using the Trauma Symptom Checklist for Young Children (TSCYC). The child's developmental functioning can be assessed using the Ages and Stages Questionnaire (ASQ). The clinician also uses these meetings to assess the parent's trauma history and his/her capacity for affect regulation and to offer psycho-education about the impact of trauma on both the parent and the child. The assessment of the parent's trauma history can be done using the Life Stressors Checklist-R. Knowing the parent's trauma history allows the clinician to offer support if the parent experiences traumatic reminders of their own history. It can also open a port of entry to discuss the intergenerational transmission of trauma and work together to break the cycle of violence. The parent's ability to regulate their affect is assessed using clinical observation (e.g., does the parent become flooded when discussing trauma material; does the parent have workable strategies for self-calming; how much support does she need to return to baseline), and helps inform the pace of treatment and the amount of support the parent may need via collateral sessions to help him/her process the treatment sessions. The clinician also observes the child and caregiver in free play to assess for the quality of their relationship.

In this assessment phase, the clinician also helps the parent make the link between child's symptoms and his or her trauma history, and encourages understanding of the child's behavior as a normal response to trauma. The clinician informs the parent about trauma reminders and help them identify and prepare for potential trauma reminders for their child and themselves. The role of play in treatment as a way to express and process trauma is explained and distinguished from the way caregivers may typically interact with their children in their family culture. The clinician and parent agree on a set of toys that will be presented to child, including toys related to the child's traumatic experience and toys to help the child and caregiver regulate. The assessment phase ends with a feedback session where the clinician summarizes the results from the screening instruments, and along with the parent decide what the treatment goals will be and how the treatment will be introduced to the child. Parents are encouraged to use the agreed on presentation to prepare children for the first treatment session, but the presentation is also repeated in the session to make clear that there is a shared awareness among the child, parent, and clinician about the nature of the problems the child is facing.

Treatment Phase

The length of the treatment phase is dependent on the family's needs. It is critical that in the first parent-child session, and thereafter as necessary, the parent and therapist work together to use words to tell the child that the trauma is the reason the child is coming to therapy. If the child is experiencing post-traumatic symptoms or behavioral problems, these can be woven into the explanation for treatment as well. For example, a child may be told, "You saw your daddy hit your mom and make her face bleed. You cried and told him to stop. That is so scary for kids, and your mom is worried that you are still scared about what you saw. She says that you have bad dreams and that sometimes you get so mad that you hit other people. My job is to help your mom help you understand what happened and help you feel better." In short, the therapist brings the discussion of the traumatic experience into the treatment session at the beginning of treatment, and ties the trauma, in a cause and effect manner, to symptoms that the child is experiencing. Thereafter, the clinician generally does not guide the child to play specifically about the trauma, but stays alert to play or talk about the trauma that the child may bring to the session. The clinician tracks the child's response to introduction to treatment and supports the parent in their understanding of child's reaction. The clinician may provide psychoeducation about typical responses to trauma and offer a benevolent explanation of reactions in the child or caregiver. For example, the clinician may help a parent understand child's avoidant behavior such as wanting to leave, or a triggered emotional response such as becoming overly active or clingy.

CPP's format allows children to bring up trauma material in their own time. For some children, trauma play may emerge in the first session. For others, a period of organizing play may come before active play about the trauma. For others, trauma material may come and go in children's play as they work through both the trauma and through developmental concerns that may not be trauma related (e.g., exploring the wish for and the fear of increased autonomy). Consistent with the overall goal of supporting a satisfying and reciprocal parent-child relationship, and returning the child to a positive developmental trajectory, CPP encourages the therapist to follow the child's lead in play, and to support the parent in following the child's lead as well.

Although CPP is flexible, it, like most trauma treatments, often proceeds in stages. Early CPP sessions may focus on establishing physical and psychological safety for both parent and child. Interventions during this period may include safety planning, help finding safe housing or legal assistance, and help stabilizing the child's preschool or day care placement. It may also include psycho-education about trauma or helping both parent and child learn ways to relax and calm themselves when they are emotionally activated either by trauma reminders or by the daily stresses of their lives. In later stages of the treatment there is likely to be a greater focus on creating a trauma narrative where the parent acknowledges what the child has witnessed and remembers and a coherent story that validates both the parent and the child's experience is co-created. The clinician encourages the parent to restore his/her capacity to be a protective shield for the child and this narrative often includes the parent's intention to keep child safe in the future. The clinician will also focus on undoing the distorted expectations that parents and children may have formed about each other as a result of the trauma. This may involve helping the parent identify negative views/representations of the child or vice versa, making a connection to the ways in which this impacts their relationship and thinking of new, more positive ways to relate to each other in the here and now. The clinician remains alert at all stages of the treatment for cues that the trauma is shaping the child's or caregiver's thoughts and feelings, and uses psychoeducation or interpretation, as appropriate to assist with coping and/or correct distortions. Other CPP objectives in the treatment phase are to strengthen the dyadic affect regulation capacities by supporting and labeling the parent and child's emotional experiences, fostering their abilities to regulate affect and providing developmental guidance around emotional reactions and typical early childhood fears. CPP also strengthens the dyadic body-based regulation by helping the parent and child increase awareness of their physiological responses and body-based trauma reminders, and to learn body-based regulation techniques. Another objective in treatment is to normalize the traumatic response and support the child in returning to a normal developmental trajectory by supporting adaptive behavior, positive identity development and age appropriate healthy play.

A follow up assessment is conducted after 20 treatment sessions to decide if needs persist, and if treatment will continue or if a termination will be planned. This is also an opportunity to re-assess and possibly re-establish treatment goals.

The Termination Phase

The timing of termination is negotiated when clinician and parent determine that treatment goals have been met. Often, treatment ends when the parent has an increased understanding of the impact of trauma, can place the traumatic experience in perspective, is capable of keeping themselves and child safe and has an increased ability to respond to their child's needs. When the parent can confidently assume the role of the child's guide through the trauma and can continue the healing in their relationship independently of the clinician's help, it is a good sign of termination readiness. The treatment phase is integral to trauma treatment and the clinician allows for at least 2 months to process and plan for this with the caregiver. CPP clinician acknowledges how goodbyes can be traumatic reminders for many parents and children and aim to provide a corrective emotional experience. The clinician strives to give the dyad a sense of agency by empowering them to be part of the process, providing predictability and supporting them in the feelings that may arise. The family's story and the themes of the treatment are summarized, highlighting a sense of hope in the future. The clinician helps the caregiver anticipate and plan for trauma reminders in the future, and be able to recognize if child's symptoms are significant enough to warrant a return to treatment.

Evidence for the Efficacy of CPP

Early trials of CPP as an intervention focused on relational stress leading to developmental risk demonstrated its efficacy with high-risk samples. These studies, conducted by two different research groups, found superior outcomes for CPP with anxiously attached toddlers of immigrant mothers (Lieberman, Weston, & Pawl, 1991) and toddlers of depressed mothers (Cicchetti, Toth, & Rogosch, 1999). More recently, and after CPP was adapted to include trauma-related goals, randomized trials from two different research groups provided evidence for the efficacy of CPP with traumatized children between the ages of 12 months and 5 years. It has been shown to significantly reduce both PTSD symptoms and behavior problems in preschool children exposed to physical violence between their parents (Lieberman, Van Horn, & Ghosh Ippen, 2005); these improvements have not only persisted for 6 months after the conclusion of treatment, but both children and parents receiving CPP have continued to improve in their functioning during the months after treatment when compared to a control group parents and children who received case management plus treatment as usual in the community (generally individual treatment for parent, child, or both) (Lieberman, Ghosh Ippen, & Van Horn, 2006).

In a sample of maltreated toddlers, toddlers treated using CPP demonstrated improved rates of secure attachment compared to a control group of children who received treatment as usual (Cicchetti, Rogosch, & Toth, 2006; Toth, Rogosch, & Cicchetti, 2006). In a study involving maltreated preschoolers, CPP significantly improved the number of children's positive representations of their mothers compared to a control group of children who received treatment as usual (Toth, Maugham, Manly, Spagnola, & Cicchetti, 2002).

CPP with Infants and Very Young Children

Clinicians must make adaptations based on developmental needs and limitations when they offer CPP to preverbal children. Most obviously, because infants and toddlers have less capacity for symbolic representation of feelings and ideas, play holds a less prominent position in interventions with very young children. Instead, the clinician works more actively with the caregiver, engaging her as an active partner in helping restore the child to a positive developmental trajectory. Clinicians focus on helping caregivers see traumatic experiences as a causative force behind their infant or toddler's behavior. They offer developmental guidance to help caregivers give the extra reassurance and soothing that a traumatized infant needs to begin to feel sufficiently secure to learn to soothe him or herself. Clinicians also help caregivers notice how even preverbal children respond to language and tone of voice, and help find words to say that allow children to begin to organize and master their experiences rather than being helpless captives of them. As the case that follows illustrates, these tasks are especially challenging when the caregiver is also severely traumatized and does not notice her baby's bids for help either because she is struggling to keep her own strong affects under control or because she sees the baby as a potential threat in an all too dangerous world.

The Case of Ms. Santiago and Luis

Ms. Santiago, an immigrant from a Central American country, was 33 years old when she brought her son Luis, slightly over two, for treatment. Her initial concerns were related to Luis' behavior. She reported that he was aggressive with her and with other adults and children. By his second birthday, Luis had been expelled from two childcare centers because of his intense emotional outbursts. One center called Ms. Santiago before the end of Luis' first day there and asked her to come get him and not to bring him back. The center staff felt that his screaming and aggression were more than they could manage. Ms. Santiago said that other potential babysitters had similar reactions to Luis, refusing to care for him after spending less than a day with him. Ms. Santiago was desperate to find someone who could help her with her son. She angrily described Luis as defiant, stubborn, and determined to make her miserable.

Trauma History

In her initial meetings with the clinician, Ms. Santiago reported frequent verbal conflicts between Luis' father and herself that began shortly after Luis' birth. She said that she left Luis' father soon after Luis' first birthday, and that since then Luis had rare and inconsistent visits from his father. Within weeks of the separation, Ms. Santiago became involved in a new relationship, one marked by severe physical and sexual violence. Between Luis' first and second birthdays, he and his mother lived in constant transition. Ms. Santiago typically took Luis with her and left after an incident of violence. For weeks at a time, she would support herself and Luis by prostituting, these encounters sometimes also resulting in violence. She and Luis slept on the streets, in churches, or in emergency shelters. During these times, Ms. Santiago used substances daily. When her situation became intolerable, she would return to her boyfriend and stay until his violence again sent her and Luis to the streets. Shortly before Luis turned two, he was present when Ms. Santiago's boyfriend attempted to rape her. As she screamed for help, Luis intervened, trying to place his body between his mother and her boyfriend. The boyfriend hit Luis and threw him across the room. Neighbors called the police and Ms. Santiago and Luis were both taken for medical care. Although Luis' examination revealed no traumatic brain injury, the hospital called child protective services. A case was opened, and Ms. Santiago and Luis were placed in a family shelter. The CPS social worker was able to contact Luis' father, and Luis began spending two nights a week in his father's home. Although Luis' father was willing to have limited involvement in his care, he refused to become involved in his therapy, telling the clinician, "I had nothing to do with all that my son has suffered."

Although the problem that brought the family to treatment was Luis' behavior, it was apparent that Ms. Santiago also had serious difficulties. In addition to the trauma of the recent years, Ms. Santiago reported significant childhood maltreatment. Her mother abandoned her before she was 7 years old, and placed her in the care of relatives who demeaned and beat her. She reported being raped by an uncle when she was nine, and said that her relatives did not believe her and did nothing to protect her. As a result of her experiences, Ms. Santiago was depressed and hypervigilant, with a number of psychosomatic symptoms including headaches and nausea. She reported frequent flashbacks, especially to her experiences of rape and prostitution as an adult and she had apparent dissociative episodes during every assessment session in response to being asked about her experiences. When these occurred, the clinician helped Ms. Santiago focus on the present, grounding her in the room, offering her sips of water, and helping her breathe slowly and deeply. Though Ms. Santiago responded to these techniques in the moment, she was unable to reflect on the function that dissociation played in protecting her from feeling the impact of her experiences.

Thus, the first obstacle to treatment became apparent in the course of the assessment. In spite of her own obvious symptoms and Luis' severe behavioral dysregulation, Ms. Santiago consistently minimized the importance of the traumatic experiences that they had both endured. She insisted that Luis was asleep during most of the violent incidents and didn't know about them. The clinician gently noted that she could see that it was very difficult for Ms. Santiago to think about and talk about all of the things that had happened to her, and difficult for her to know how much Luis had suffered. Ms. Santiago ultimately agreed to words that the clinician could tell Luis why he was coming for therapy. "You got so hurt by mommy's friend. The police came and you had to go to the hospital. You were hurt and scared, and that made you so angry that now you want to hit everyone. You will come here to play, and your mommy and I will help you feel better, so you don't have to hit." Though Ms. Santiago agreed that these words could be spoken, it was clear that she did not believe them. In spite of the clinician's best efforts at psychoeducation about the impact of trauma, Ms. Santiago continued to interpret Luis' behavior as stubbornness and defiance aimed at her. Nonetheless, the clinician believed that it was critically important to establish this trauma frame for the treatment, most immediately to begin to help Luis construct an integrated narrative of his life, but also to hold the hope that Ms. Santiago would be able to see Luis in this light rather than through her more distorted negative attributions.

Planning Treatment

Ms. Santiago's and Luis' physical safety was assured as treatment began. They were securely housed in a residential treatment facility where they would be able to stay for up to 2 years. Ms. Santiago's substance use was addressed and she had been able to stay clean during the weeks leading up to the assessment and throughout an assessment period that proceeded as described above. Nevertheless, there were significant challenges to emotional safety. Both Luis and his mother were highly symptomatic and Ms. Santiago's reluctance to discuss her experiences or to identify them as causally related to her or Luis's problems meant that direct intervention would be a challenge. The clinician was aware that Ms. Santiago's recovery from substance abuse was new and fragile, and that she would need to develop strategies for managing her affect when recalling traumatic events or when confronted by Luis' distressing behaviors to diminish the likelihood of relapse. Substance use had long been Ms. Santiago's strategy for blunting her strong negative feelings, and the clinician wanted to offer her more adaptive ways to cope. Finally, Ms. Santiago's negative attributions regarding Luis' behavior seemed fixed and almost unalterable. The clinician was concerned that Ms. Santiago's own history of severe trauma left her expecting to be victimized by everyone she met, including her own 2-year-old son. If this were indeed the case, Ms. Santiago might be unable to see Luis as struggling to communicate distress through his behavior. If she continued to respond to him as persecutory rather than hurt and distressed, it would be difficult for her to offer him the reassurance he needed in order to feel safe with her and to use her care as a model for self-soothing.

Before the first child-parent session, the clinician met with Ms. Santiago to discuss goals for treatment. Ms. Santiago was interested in behavioral change for Luis. She wanted him to be less aggressive and less defiant, and continued to minimize the impact of trauma in a way that made it difficult to set trauma-related goals. She was also unwilling to think about her substance abuse as a response to trauma and the wish to blunt the feelings of sadness, anger, and fear aroused by trauma. She assured the clinician that she would have no trouble maintaining her sobriety, saying, "I'm all through with that. I know Luis needs me. I won't go back to that." Ms. Santiago did, however, agree with the clinician that Luis' behavior made her very upset and distressed, and she was willing to set a goal of learning ways to keep her own feelings under control at these times so that she would be more effective in teaching Luis different ways to behave when he was angry.

Meeting Luis: Initial Sessions

Ms. Santiago brought Luis to the first therapy session in his stroller, and he remained there for the entire session. He showed no interest in the toys that the clinician made available. In fact he seemed disconnected from the present moment and disinterested in any external stimuli, including the clinician and his mother. Sometimes he sat silently. When the clinician spoke to him, he seemed not to notice or hear her. At other times he screamed in a loud, high-pitched, wordless wail that went on for several minutes. At these times Ms. Santiago tried frantically to calm him. Initially, she would offer him a bottle, which he generally struck from her hand, making the bottle fly across the room. She attempted to talk to him, using face-paced, high-pitched speech and placing her face only inches from his. Luis continued screaming, arching his back and turning his face away. Seeming not to notice, Ms. Santiago kept talking to him, but increased the level of stimulation, rattling her keys in front of Luis' face or trying to interest him in pictures on her cell phone screen. After several frantic attempts to calm him, none of which succeeded, Ms. Santiago laughed nervously and said, "You see why no one wants to care for him. He's impossible. He doesn't care about anyone." As Luis continued to scream, Ms. Santiago began to tremble visibly and appeared to dissociate, staring at the wall. The clinician responded to Ms. Santiago, speaking softly to her, agreeing that it was very difficult to listen to such distressed screaming from a child. She said repeatedly and softly, "You're both safe here. I won't let anything happen to you here. You're safe here." As she spoke, she reached for the wheel of Luis' stroller and rolled it back and forth slowing, matching the rhythm of her voice. Luis was calmed by this and stopped screaming. Continuing to move the stroller back and forth, but being careful not to look directly into Luis' face for fear of over-stimulating him, the clinician asked Ms. Santiago, "What do you think happened? Do you know why he screamed?" Ms. Santiago had no response. Nor could she respond to the clinician's questions about what might have helped Luis to calm. She seemed appreciative of the clinician's observations about how difficult it had been for her, Ms. Santiago, to listen to the screaming and how hard she had tried to help Luis stop. She said, "I try everything. Nothing works." The clinician noticed that something had helped him stop and pointed out what she was doing with the stroller. She invited Ms. Santiago to take the other wheel and help her rock Luis slowly back and forth. Ms. Santiago took the wheel nearest her and began to roll the stroller. As she got into a rhythm, the clinician moved her own hand away. After a moment, the clinician observed, "You're rocking him by yourself and he is still calm. Maybe he likes that slow, steady movement."

The second and third sessions looked much like the first one except that the clinician urged Ms. Santiago to try rocking the stroller earlier in the process. As Luis reliably calmed in response to being rocked in this way, the clinician asked Ms. Santiago to describe how she felt as she moved the stroller slowly back and forth. She replied that she felt calmer, too. As Ms. Santiago rolled the stroller back and forth, rocking her body in rhythm with it, she and Luis looked at each other silently. The clinician said, "That movement seems to help you both. It reminds me of a mother sitting in a big rocking chair and rocking her baby. The same feeling."

Ms. Santiago said, "We didn't have a rocking chair when Luis was a baby."

The clinician replied, "Maybe it's a feeling you can have together now. Do you think you could try it at home at times when Luis is crying and you feel frustrated by it?" Ms. Santiago nodded her head, without taking her eyes off Luis.

As this intervention demonstrates, helping very young children and their caregivers find ways to be alert and calm together can be foundational in recovery from traumatic stress. Regulation by a caregiver lays the groundwork for the developing infant's nascent capacity to self-soothe. In dyads where both caregiver and child have had their regulatory competencies derailed by the uncontrollable emotions that accompany a traumatic experience, the dyad is doubly challenged. First, the traumatized child faces a larger task in learning to regulate and modulate affects that does the child who is developing without the burden of being flooded by terrifying and overwhelming stimuli. Second, the caregiver, also overwhelmed, has more limited capacity to help the child meet the challenge of learning to self-regulate. Interventions that help the two attain moments of mutual calm and then help the caregiver reflect on the experience and find ways to repeat it are often an essential first step in Child-parent Psychotherapy.

Beginning to Make Meaning

In one early treatment session, Luis was sitting in his stroller screaming and crying. Ms. Santiago tried to calm him by rolling the stroller but when this did not work immediately, she asked to leave the room to make a phone call. She told the clinician that she would be right back, and asked her to stay with Luis. As Ms. Santiago got up and walked toward the door, Luis lunged forward in the stroller and his screaming intensified. The clinician asked Ms. Santiago to wait. She noted that as soon as it appeared that his mother would leave the room, Luis began to scream louder and appeared to be very frightened. She said, "He even seemed to try to throw himself out of the stroller to get to you. I think he needs you close to him to feel safe." She asked Ms. Santiago to stay in the room, or to take Luis with her to make her call. Ms. Santiago returned to her chair near the stroller and looked surprised when Luis stopped screaming as soon as she sat down. The clinician repeated that very young children need to keep their mothers close in order to feel safe, and said that when a child has been hurt or frightened, that need can be even more intense. She asked Ms. Santiago if it was hard to be around Luis so much because he was so demanding. Ms. Santiago replied that it was, but also noticed that it was easier to be near him when he wasn't screaming. The clinician nodded sympathetically and said that she understood what a burden a very young, dependent child with many needs and little ability to care for and entertain himself could be. She repeated that children who had been hurt and frightened had an even harder time seeing their mothers go away. She reminded Ms. Santiago that they had agreed that an important part of treatment would be helping her learn ways to teach Luis to be calmer so that he could be less aggressive. The clinician turned to Luis and said, "You're really listening to us. Your mommy and I are talking about how to help you feel better so you don't need to hit." Luis remained calm and Ms. Santiago reached out to him and rubbed his hand.

This session was a small turning point for Ms. Santiago. Before the intervention described above, she had little understanding of how important she was to Luis' sense of safety and well-being. She experienced him as a burden, and he was a difficult child for whom to care. But her own failure to see how she important she was to Luis kept Ms. Santiago from giving him the attention and reassurance that he needed to feel secure. In this moment, when it was dramatically clear that her leaving threw Luis into a panic and that her return restored him to a sense of calm, Ms. Santiago began to understand their relationship differently. She began to experience herself as potentially protective and to experience Luis as capable of responding positively to her care.

Progress In Treatment: Meeting the Caregiver's Needs

As Luis began to feel more secure in the playroom and more certain that his mother would stay with him, he was willing to get out of his stroller and begin to explore the toys. He seemed particularly drawn to the police car, exploring it and rolling it back and forth. The clinician commented that he was very interested in the police car and asked him if he was remembering the night his daddy was taken away by the police. Ms. Santiago replied that she was sure that he didn't remember that event, and took the car roughly from Luis who, predictably, began to scream. The clinician said that Luis and his mother had different needs at that moment. Luis wanted to play with the police car and cried when it was taken away. She said that she did not know for sure what he Luis was thinking about as he played with the car, and that possibly Ms. Santiago was right and he did not remember. She noted that the important thing happening right now was that Luis badly wanted to play with the car and something made his mother want to take it away from him. Ms. Santiago put the car down and Luis reached for it. The clinician said that his mommy would let him play with the car, but something made it hard for her. For the rest of the session, the three were quiet as Luis explored the car. As the time to leave came, the clinician asked if Ms. Santiago would be willing to meet with her alone to talk about what had happened.

In the collateral session, Ms. Santiago repeated her often-made statement that Luis might remember being hit and thrown by his father, but she was sure he did not remember anything else. She said firmly that he was in another room when the police came and did not know that his father had been taken by the police. The clinician said that she understood Ms. Santiago's position and asked if she could share something with her that researchers had learned about children and parents. Ms. Santiago agreed to listen, and the clinician told her that several studies suggested that children remember many more things than their parents think they do. She said that she could not know what Luis actually saw and what he remembered, but that she did know that it was very hard for parents to think that the children they love so much have been hurt and frightened. She offered developmental guidance, noting that Luis didn't have the words to tell the story of what he remembered and that all he could do was act out his strong feelings and use play to begin to tell a story about his experiences. She asked if she and Ms. Santiago might agree to simply watch Luis' play and discover what unfolded. Ms. Santiago agreed to this plan.

The clinician also used the collateral session to share some of her concerns about Luis' development. He had not yet spoken a word in the treatment sessions, and Ms. Santiago confirmed that he did not speak at home. The clinician also said that she worried about Luis' motor development because he spent so much time in the safety of his stroller. The clinician said that she believed that perhaps Luis was aggressive in part because he was so frustrated at not being able to explore, express himself, and make others understand him. She asked if Ms. Santiago might be willing to take Luis to another department in the hospital for a developmental assessment and Ms. Santiago agreed.

The developmental assessment revealed delays in language development and in gross and fine motor skills. Luis was eligible for speech and language services. The clinician helped Ms. Santiago make a connection with service providers for Luis' speech therapy, and also connected her with a home visiting service that helps parents of young children with delays learn specific skills to help their children's development.

Ms. Santiago's gratitude toward the clinician for offering this concrete help cemented the trust that was growing between them and assured Ms. Santiago's continuing engagement in the treatment. In addition, Ms. Santiago was better regulated during the collateral sessions, because she was not under stress from Luis' behavior. The clinician used these opportunities to help her learn affect regulation skills such as grounding, relaxation, and deep breathing. Ms. Santiago tried these techniques, with the clinician's support, during parent-child sessions at times when she found Luis' behavior difficult to manage. As she became more comfortable with them, she was able to use them at home, with the result that she became more confident of her ability to care for and calm Luis, and he became more confident that she would protect him from being overwhelmed by his feelings.

The Emergence of Trauma Themes

As Luis and his mother gradually became better regulated, his play, though still disorganized, expanded and became more symbolic. When Luis was rough with the toys or played aggressively, Ms. Santiago initially attempted to socialize him, telling him to "play nice." This tendency diminished gradually as the clinician worked with her in collateral sessions and in the parent-child sessions to process her own responses to his play. Ms. Santiago was able to acknowledge that she felt frightened by his aggression, and it took her some time to accept that the aggression in his play was not directed at her but was, instead, his attempt to communicate what he remembered about his life and to make meaning of his memories. Gradually, however, she became able to focus on the feelings that he was expressing in his play, and to notice that as he expressed his feelings symbolically through play, he was less enraged and aggressive in his behavior.

On one occasion, he took the police car and placed it inside the house, causing most of the furniture to fall out. The clinician commented that the police car had made a big mess in the house and turned everything upside down. She said, "You are showing us how you felt when the police came to your house." Ms. Santiago turned to him and comforted him. Luis and Ms. Santiago were unable to find words to communicate with one another, but she could see, with the clinician's support, how "upside down" Luis' life felt to him, and she could offer him physical comfort, if not verbal reassurance that things would be better.

Conclusion

When families are as deeply traumatized as were Ms. Santiago and her son, the work to help them recover is slow and may stretch over more than one episode of therapy. In cases where intergenerational trauma is present CPP clinicians are faced with both a parent and a child whose capacity to regulate affect is deeply impaired and whose basic assumptions about safety, their own value, and the reliability of others have been shattered (Janoff-Bulman, 1992). Both parent and child will need help to notice and tolerate their own emotional responses to one another and to events outside their relationship; both will need to be supported in letting down their defensive shields so that they can notice moments when the other individual is responding to them in warm and positive ways. Parents are generally expected to take the lead in helping young children learn to modulate their experience and expression of emotion. A parent who feels threatened by her child and overwhelmed by her own feelings will be less able to offer this needed developmental assistance. The tasks of Child-parent Psychotherapy in this case were to: (1) give Ms. Santiago and Luis some moments of mutual respite from the emotional overload that they both lived with from having been so repeatedly and frequently terrorized; (2) to help them find concrete and reliable ways to self-soothe and soothe one another; (3) to support them in finding new ways to experience themselves and one another so that Luis could feel that his mother could protect him and so that she could believe herself as competent to do so; and (4) to help them both begin to understand that trauma had a continuing effect on their feelings and behavior. Although there is much work left to do in this case, the first several months of Child-parent Psychotherapy allowed Luis and his mother to experience themselves and one another in different ways and to find some islands of calm in their overwhelming negative affect. These early positive experiences will lay a foundation for their growing capacity to trust and understand one another.

References

Bowlby, J. (1969/1982). *Attachment and loss: Vol. 1, Attachment*. New York: Basic Books.

Cicchetti, D., Rogosch, F. A., & Toth, S. L. (2006). Fostering secure attachment in infants in maltreating families through preventive interventions. *Development and Psychopathology, 18*, 623–650.

Cicchetti, D., Toth, S. L., & Rogosch, F. A. (1999). The efficacy of toddler-parent psychotherapy to increase attachment security in offspring of depressed mothers. *Attachment and Human Development, 1*, 34–36.

Fraiberg, S. (1980). *Clinical studies in infant mental health*. New York: Basic Books.

Freud, S. (1955). Beyond the pleasure principle. In J. Strachey (Ed. & Trans.), *The standard edition of the complete psychological works of Sigmund Freud* (Vol. 18). London: Hogarth Press. (Original work published 1920)

Ghosh Ippen, C., Harris, W. W., Van Horn, P., & Lieberman, A. F. (2011). Traumatic and stressful life events in early childhood: Can treatment help those at highest risk? *Child Abuse and Neglect, 35*, 504–513.

Janoff-Bulman, R. (1992). *Shattered assumptions: Toward a new psychology of trauma*. New York: Free Press.

Klatzkin, A., Lieberman, A. F., & Van Horn, P. (2013). Child-parent psychotherapy and the intergenerational transmission of historical trauma. In J. Ford & C. Courtois (Eds.), *Treating complex traumatic stress disorders in children and adolescents* (pp. 295–315). New York: Guilford Press.

Lieberman, A. F. (1992). Infant-parent psychotherapy with toddlers. *Development and Psychopathology, 4*, 559–574.

Lieberman, A. F. (2004). Child-parent psychotherapy: A relationship-based approach to the treatment of mental health disorders in infancy and early childhood. In A. J. Sameroff, S. C. McDonough, & K. L. Rosenblum (Eds.), *Treating parent-infant relationship problems* (pp. 97–122). New York: Guilford Press.

Lieberman, A. F., Ghosh Ippen, C., & Van Horn, P. (2006). Child-parent psychotherapy: 6-month follow-up of a randomized controlled trial. *Journal of the American Academy of Child and Adolescent Psychiatry, 45*, 913–918.

Lieberman, A. F., Padrón, E., Van Horn, P., & Harris, W. (2004). Angels in the nursery: The intergenerational transmission of benevolent parental influences. *Infant Mental Health Journal, 26*, 504–520.

Lieberman, A. F., Silverman, R., & Pawl, J. H. (2000). Infant-parent psychotherapy: Core concepts and current approaches. In C. H. Zeanah (Ed.), *Handbook of infant mental health* (2nd ed., pp. 472–484). New York: Guilford.

Lieberman, A. F., & Van Horn, P. (2005). *"Don't hit my mommy!": A manual for child-parent psychotherapy with young witnesses of family violence.* Washington, DC: ZERO TO THREE Press.

Lieberman, A. F., & Van Horn, P. (2008). *Psychotherapy with infants and young children: Repairing the effects of stress and trauma on early attachment.* New York: Guilford Press.

Lieberman, A. F., & Van Horn, P. (2009). Child-parent psychotherapy: A developmental approach to mental health treatment in infancy and early childhood. In C. H. Zeanah (Ed.), *Handbook of infant mental health* (3rd ed., pp. 439–449). New York: Guilford.

Lieberman, A. F., Van Horn, P., & Ghosh Ippen, C. (2005). Toward evidence-based treatment: Child-parent psychotherapy with preschoolers exposed to marital violence. *Journal of the American Academy of Child and Adolescent Psychiatry, 44*, 1241–1248.

Lieberman, A. F., Weston, D., & Pawl, J. H. (1991). Preventive intervention and outcome with anxiously attached dyads. *Child Development, 62*, 199–209.

Marans, S., & Adelman, A. (1997). Experiencing violence in a developmental context. In J. D. Osofsky (Ed.), *Children in a violent society* (pp. 202–222). New York: Guilford Press.

Marmar, C., Foy, D., Kagan, B., & Pynoos, R. (1993). In J. M. Oldham, M. B. Riba, & A. Talman (Eds.), *American psychiatry press review of psychiatry* (Vol. 12). Washington, DC: American Psychiatric Press.

Pynoos, R. S., Steinberg, A. M., & Piacentini, J. C. (1999). A developmental model of childhood traumatic stress and intersection with anxiety disorders. *Biological Psychiatry, 46*, 1542–1554.

Toth, S. L., Maughan, A., Manly, J. T., Spagnola, M., & Cicchetti, D. (2002). The relative efficacy of two interventions in altering maltreated preschool children's representation models: Implications for attachment theory. *Development and Psychopathology, 14*, 877–908.

Toth, S. L., Rogosch, F. A., Manly, J. T., & Cicchetti, D. (2006). The efficacy of Toddler-Parent Psychotherapy to reorganize attachment in the young offspring of mothers with major depressive disorder: A randomized prevention trial. *Journal of Consulting and Clinical Psychology, 74*(6), 1006–1016.

Part III
Interventions for Young Children

For pre-school and early school-aged children, the parent-child relationship has been shown to be a lynchpin in efforts to improve mental health. Research suggests that emotional dysregulation resulting from attempts to manage the anxiety of perceived threats is at the root of many mental health problems in young children, and that parenting seems to directly influence children's ability to manage this stress. When parenting is sensitive, it appears to buffer the effects of stress on children (Dozier, Lindheim, Lewis, Bick, & Bernard, 2009), promoting more healthy responses to stress. When parenting is ineffective and non-optimal, it magnifies the stressfulness of early traumatic experiences, possibly by increasing their perceived threat (Martorell & Bugental, 2006).

We present four interventions that focus on improving caregiving and the caregiver-child relationship as a way to improve emotional regulation and reduce children's behavior problems. In Chap. 6, Webster-Stratton describes the Incredible Years (IY); Triple P (PPP) is presented by Saunders and Pickering in Chap. 7; Urquiza and Timmer discuss Parent Child Interaction Therapy (PCIT) in Chap. 8; and Gilliam and Fisher describe Multidimensional Treatment Foster Care (MTFC) in Chap. 9. These interventions target slightly different populations of children at risk, and use different modes of delivery, showing the wide range of methods that can be used to achieve similar treatment goals.

References

Dozier, M., Lindhiem, O., Lewis, E., Bick, J., & Bernard, K. (2009). Effects of a foster parent training program on young children's attachment behaviors: Preliminary evidence from a randomized clinical trial. *Child & Adolescent Social Work Journal, 26*(4), 321–332.

Martorell, G. A., & Bugental, D. B. (2006). Maternal variations in stress reactivity: Implications for harsh parenting practices with very young children. *Journal of Family Psychology, 20–4,* 641–647.

Chapter 6
Incredible Years® Parent and Child Programs for Maltreating Families

Carolyn L. Webster-Stratton

History of Incredible Years (IY) Interventions and Conceptual Foundation

Thirty years ago, the Incredible Years (IY) Parent Program (Webster-Stratton, 1981, 1982) was first introduced as a new performance training group-based method for supporting parents, improving parenting practices, and strengthening parent-child attachment. The program was designed to promote responsive and nurturing parenting interactions and reduce harsh or coercive discipline methods. It was hypothesized that positive parent-child relationships and proactive child management skills would reduce children's behavior problems and strengthen their social and emotional competence. The IY Parent Program was designed to overcome limitations of existing parenting programs at that time that relied on verbal training (e.g., didactic lectures) and one-on-one therapy methods. The group format of delivering the IY program addressed parents' need for support as well as the cost and feasibility problems associated with other performance based methods such as individualized videotaped "bug-in- the ear" feedback. The IY Parent program, and all subsequent IY programs, were based on cognitive social learning (Patterson, Reid, & Dishion, 1992), modeling and self-efficacy (Bandura, 1982), attachment and relationship theories (Bowlby, 1988), cognitive brain developmental theories (Piaget & Inhelder, 1962) and problem solving methods (D'Zurilla & Nezu, 1982).

All IY parent programs have used training methods based on video-based and live modeling, active, experiential practice exercises, collaborative discussions and group support as key methods of promoting parent learning and maintaining emotion, cognitive and behavior change. Toward this end, a comprehensive DVD series of actual parent-child interaction video vignettes illustrating positive and less

C.L. Webster-Stratton, Ph.D., FAAN (✉)
Parenting Clinic, University of Washington, Seattle, WA, USA
e-mail: cws@u.washington.edu

S. Timmer and A. Urquiza (eds.), *Evidence-Based Approaches for the Treatment of Maltreated Children*, Child Maltreatment 3, DOI 10.1007/978-94-007-7404-9_6,
© Springer Science+Business Media Dordrecht 2014

effective parenting behaviors were developed as a tool for use by trained group leaders to facilitate parent group discussions, self-reflection, peer support and problem solving, practice exercises, and collaborative learning. Families involved in the program determine goals for themselves and their children informed by their cultural beliefs, self-manage their decisions regarding assigned home activities, participate in values exercises regarding their short and long term goals, and work with group leaders to recognize and overcome their personal barriers. The group format not only reduces costs associated with therapy but also strengthens parents' support networks and learning opportunities because of observing other parents using the parenting principles to manage behavior problems different from their own.

Since the 1980s, the IY Training Series has been expanded to include three complementary curricula for parents, teachers, and children, all of which utilize similar training methods and therapeutic processes. These programs were designed to reduce the multiple risk factors associated with the development of early-onset conduct problems and children's social and emotional difficulties and to strengthen family and school protective factors. The series has been the subject of extensive empirical evaluation and randomized control group studies for several decades with high-risk populations as well as with parents of children diagnosed with Oppositional Defiant Disorder (ODD), Conduct Disorder (CD) and ADHD (see review of research; (Webster-Stratton, 2012a, 2012c; Webster-Stratton & Mihalic, 2001; Webster-Stratton, Reid, & Beauchaine, 2011).

The purpose of this chapter is to describe the conceptual grounding and content of the evidence-based IY parent and child programs, including research evidence and to discuss the rationale for use of both these programs with families involved with child maltreatment. A brief summary of the methods for working with families involved with child welfare agencies and a case study is provided as well as references to other articles that provide more specific details for how to deliver the parent and child programs with fidelity to this population.

Summary of Incredible Years Parent Programs and Evidence-Base

The IY BASIC parenting series, consists of five curricula versions designed for different age groups: Baby Program (9–12 sessions; ages 6 weeks to 8 months), Toddler Program (12–13 sessions; ages 1–3 years), Preschool Program (18–20 sessions; ages 3–5 years), Early School Age Program (14 sessions +; ages 6–8 years) and the Pre-Adolescent Program (ages 9–12years) (16+ sessions). These programs are offered weekly to groups of 8–12 parents and emphasize developmentally age appropriate parenting skills, which help children accomplish their developmental milestones. Goals of the programs are tailored to each targeted child developmental stage. However, all programs include the following goals: (a) promoting parent competencies and strengthening parent-child relationships; (b) promoting a safe home environment with predictable routines; (c) reducing critical and physically violent discipline and increasing positive discipline strategies; (d) improving parental self-control, depression, anger management, communication skills, and conflict management skills; (e) increasing family support networks.

The IY Parenting Pyramid (shown below) serves as the roadmap for the content and parenting strategies discussed. The bottom of the pyramid focuses on parent tools designed to strengthen parent-child attachment and empathy through focused, child-directed play, academic, persistence, social and emotional coaching methods, sensitive responses, praise and encouragement. This bottom layer of the pyramid provides the foundational scaffolding and nurturing necessary to promote children's developmental growth and is applied liberally. A basic premise of the model is that a positive relationship foundation precedes discipline strategies, and parent attention to positive behaviors should occur far more frequently than attention negative behaviors. Only when this positive foundation is in place do later aspects higher on the pyramid work. Further up the pyramid the focus for toddlers is on predictable rules and routines, clear limit settings and proactive discipline such as ignoring, distracting, and redirecting. For the preschool and early school age programs, the top part of the pyramid also focuses on consequences such as Time Out and loss of privileges as well as teaching children beginning self-regulation and problem-solving skills. The school age programs include all the younger version content material plus additional information on monitoring after-school activities, and discussions of rules about TV, computer use and work chores, as well as drugs and alcohol. Additionally, these older age programs focus on ways to develop successful partnerships with teachers and coach children's homework assignments.

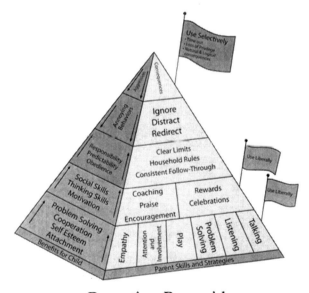

Parenting Pyramid

Additional parent training components include the ADVANCE parent program (9–12 sessions) which emphasizes parent interpersonal skills such as: effective communication skills, anger and depression management, ways to give and get support, problem solving with adults and with teachers, and ways to teach children problem-solving skills and have family meetings. Another optional adjunct training to the Preschool Program is the School Readiness Program (4–6 sessions) that is designed to help high-risk parents support their preschool children's reading readiness as well as their social and emotional regulation competence and language skills.

For a detailed review of research findings for the IY parent programs, see (Webster-Stratton, 2012a; Webster-Stratton & Reid, 2010). Briefly, research from eight randomized controlled trials (RCTs) by the developer and six RCTs by independent investigators with *treatment populations* and four RCTs by the developer and six RCTs by independent investigators with *high risk prevention populations* have found that the BASIC parenting program increases parents' use of positive attention (child directed play, coaching methods, praise, incentives) and positive discipline strategies, and reduces harsh, critical, and coercive discipline strategies. Across age groups, children's conduct problems or externalizing problems with their parents decreased while their positive affect, compliance, and cooperative behavior increased. In studies where parents were offered an extended parenting program utilizing the ADVANCE parent program with a focus on interpersonal communication, problem solving, and anger, depression, and stress management, concurrent improvements in marital relationships, parents' problem solving skills, and reductions in parental stress and depression were found as well as children's problem-solving skills (Webster-Stratton, 1994). The BASIC and ADVANCE programs have been found to be effective with diverse, multicultural populations including those representing Latino, Asian, African American, and Caucasian background in the United States (Reid, Webster-Stratton, & Beauchaine, 2001), and in other countries such as Denmark, Holland, Ireland, New Zealand, Norway, Russia, Sweden, and United Kingdom (Gardner, Burton, & Klimes, 2006; Hutchings, Gardner, et al., 2007; Larsson et al., 2009; McDaniel, Braiden, Onyekwelu, Murphy, & Regan, 2011; Posthumus, Raaijmakers, Maassen, Engeland, & Matthys, 2012; Scott, Spender, Doolan, Jacobs, & Aspland, 2001). It is hypothesized that the programs are easy to translate in other cultures because of the collaborative process and trained group leader's efforts to promote cultural diversity in discussions and vignettes chosen for participants (Webster-Stratton, 2009).

Application of Parent Interventions for Families Involved in Children Welfare

Each year over three million calls of concern about child maltreatment are made to child welfare service agencies in the U.S. (USDHHS, 2011). Almost 90 % of these children remain in their home, some with and many without, an active child welfare case opened. About one-in-four of these allegations of child maltreatment will be made about families who have had prior maltreatment reports filed. About one million allegations will eventually be substantiated and service cases opened. In about 75 % of those cases, these services will be provided to the families at home (Barth et al., 2005). Data suggest that 27–44 % of families with an open case will have parent training recommended or mandated (NSCAW Research Group, 2003) as a sole treatment to improve their children's safety and healthy development or as part of a multi-component service plan. Unfortunately, very few of the parenting programs recommended have empirical support or are evidence-based (Schoenwald & Hoagwood, 2001).

Although there are relatively few studies of parent training programs among families involved in child welfare, estimates indicate that 50–80 % of those parents involved with child welfare who begin parent training programs do not complete them (Chaffin et al., 2004; Lutzker, 1990; Lutzker & Bigelow, 2002). The drop out rate for child welfare clients may be so high because their life circumstances are generally stressful and take priority over parenting issues, and/or because even though the courts may have mandated attendance in a parenting group, cases are often closed before program completion resulting in parenting not feeling they need to complete them. In addition to issues with completion, parents who receive parent training as a result of their involvement with Child Welfare Services present other challenges to parent trainers. For example, parents may be resistant to attending a mandated group, especially if they don't feel they need parenting help. Or, they may have had their children removed and therefore are not able to practice new skills with their children at home. Parents may also have other mental health issues (depression or substance abuse) or stressful life circumstances (violent relationships, low income, lack of child care or transportation) that interfere with their ability to attend groups. They may see their problems in parenting to be a result of these external factors and not believe that parent training is necessary or valuable. However, the relevance of parent training for child welfare settings has been increasingly recognized (Barth et al., 2005). Recent field trials of EBPs for families of maltreated children ~ including Multisystemic Therapy, Safe Care, and Parent Child Interaction Therapy (PCIT) have had promising results (Corcoran, 2000). For example, a control group study found large reductions in physical abuse reports among parents who participated in PCIT, an individually coached program designed for parents of young children, in comparison with an existing community-based parent training program (Chaffin et al.).

Rationale for the Use of the IY Parent Programs for Families with Maltreated Children

Several aspects of the evidence-based IY BASIC parenting series make it particularly effective for families involved with child welfare due to maltreatment. First, the programs make extensive use of video modeling methods, showing vignettes of families from different cultural and socioeconomic backgrounds with a variety of parenting styles and child temperament and development. The diversity of the vignettes and settings allows most participating parents to identify with at least some of the parent and child models and therefore accept the vignettes as relevant. Moreover, the observational modeling and practice training approach is more effective learning for some of these families than the more cognitive, verbal training approaches. Second, the group-based program focuses on strategies for building support networks and decreasing the isolation and sense of alienation commonly found among these parents. In addition, the collaborative discussion approach helps parents to target their personal goals and strengths rather than their deficits, and group leaders place an emphasis on individualizing each group members' learning style, knowledge level and abilities. Third, the cognitive, behavioral, affective, and experiential methods of learning (cognitive restructuring, emotional regulation strategies, self-reflection and thought scripts, and behavioral rehearsal) are designed to bring about more sustained cognitive, emotion and behavior change leading to deeper relationship and interaction changes and more sustained results. Fourth, parenting programs are separated by children's developmental stage, which encourages more age-appropriate parenting strategies to be understood and utilized by parents. More detailed information on the group leader therapeutic methods and collaborative process can be found in a book for IY therapists/group leaders (Webster-Stratton, 2012b).

Core Content Components and Topic Objectives of the IY Basic Parent Program

This next section reviews the objectives and core components of the updated IY Parent Basic program (2006), particularly highlighting those that are relevant for the child welfare population.

Strengthen Parent-Child Relationships and Bonding

- Increase parents' empathy and responsiveness towards their children.
- Help parents to have age appropriate expectations and to be sensitive to individual differences in children's temperament, social, emotional and cognitive development.
- Promote parents' consistent monitoring and predictable supervision of children in order to keep them safe at all times.
- Increase parents' positive, coping thoughts and decrease their negative attributions about their children.
- Encourage parents to give more effective praise and encouragement for targeted prosocial behaviors.
- Help parents understand how to promote positive parent-child relationships and strengthen their attachment.

- Help parents learn to enjoy their children, play with their children, and follow their children's lead during play interactions.
- Help parents learn to become social, emotion, persistence, and academic "coaches" for their children.

Promote Routines, Effective Limit Setting, Non-punitive Discipline, and Problem Solving

- Help parents understand the importance of predictable schedules, routines and consistent responses, particularly in regard to separations and reunions with children.
- Help parents understand home safety, childproofing, and monitoring strategies are ongoing themes in sessions.
- Help parents learn anger management strategies and affect regulation so they can stay calm, controlled, and patient when disciplining their children.
- Help parents set up and communicate realistic goals for their children's social, emotional, and academic behavior.
- Help parents set up behavior plans and develop salient rewards for targeted prosocial behaviors.
- Help parents use non-punitive discipline and reduce harsh and physical discipline for misbehavior.
- Teach parents how to teach their children self-regulation skills by using brief Time Out to calm down.
- Teach parents to help their children manage anger and aggression by teaching them problem-solving and self-regulation strategies.
- Help parents to provide children with joyful and happy experiences and memories and reduce exposure to adult arguments, violent TV and computer games, and atmosphere of fear or depression.
- Teach parents how and when to use problem-solving strategies with their children.

Preliminary Research Evidence for Use of IY Parent Program for Maltreating Families with Young Children

As noted earlier the IY parent programs have been evaluated in RCTs as prevention programs in community samples, including socio-economically disadvantaged and multi-cultural groups of parents enrolled in Head Start (Webster-Stratton, 1998; Webster-Stratton & Reid, 2007; Webster-Stratton, Reid, & Hammond, 2001), as well as in UK with Sure Start families (Hutchings, Gardner, et al., 2007). In the Head Start studies, 20 % of parents reported prior involvement with child protective services for maltreatment (Webster-Stratton, 1998; Webster-Stratton et al., 2001).

Hurlburt (Hurlburt, Nguyen, Reid, Webster-Stratton, & Zhang, 2013) re-analyzed these data to determine if this subset of parents responded differently to the IY program than those whose parents had no prior child welfare system involvement. The results by independent observers in the home showed that, irrespective of whether or not parents were involved in the child welfare system, those who received the IY parenting group became significantly more positive, nurturing, and engaged with their children and less harsh and critical in their discipline compared with a control group of Head Start parents who received no parenting intervention. Overall, intervention outcomes did not differ in any significant way for parents with and without a history of involvement with child welfare and regardless of ethnic group. However, parents with such a history showed higher initial levels of negative and lower levels of positive parenting practices, consistent with other studies comparing matched samples of parents with and without a history of child maltreatment (Lutzker & Bigelow, 2002). The results of these analyses are promising in the sense that they provide further support for the use of the IY parent training model for helping to improve key parenting competencies in the child welfare population. However, because these parents participated in the program voluntarily and were not mandated by child welfare, it is unclear whether the results would be replicated with families who were court ordered or mandated by child protective services.

A pilot study (2007–2009) utilizing the toddler and preschool programs was conducted in Seattle, Washington where child welfare-referred, court mandated families or open cases in which parents mostly had their children at home (but were at risk of having them removed) were offered the updated BASIC parenting program. Fifteen parent groups with an average of 8–18 parents per group were delivered. Seventy percent of families (N = 136) who registered for the program completed the program. (In order to be classified as a program completer, families could miss no more than 4 of 16 sessions or they were asked to retake the program.) Day care and dinners were provided for parents and transportation when needed. There were 12 group leaders who co-facilitated delivery of the parent groups.

Parents were asked (but not required) to complete pre and post-treatment data on the Parenting Stress Index/Short Form (PSI-SF) (Abidin, 1990) which is a 36-item parent-report instrument of child behavior problems and parental adjustment. The PSI/SF includes four variables (a) a Total Stress score that provides an overall level of stress related to parenting and is derived from interactions with the child or as a result of children's behavioral characteristics; (b) Parental Stress subscale (PD) determines distress in the parent's personal adjustment directly related to parenting such as impaired sense of competence, conflict with child's other parent, lack of social support, restrictions in life and presence of depression; (c) Parent-child Dysfunctional Interaction subscale (P-CDI) focused on parents' view that the child does not meet their expectations and that parent-child interactions are not reinforcing to them. High scores indicate that the parent feels the child is a negative element in his/her life and suggests poor parent-child bonding and risk for neglect, rejection or abuse; and (d) The Difficult Child subscale (DC) focuses on behavioral

Fig. 6.1 Percentage of mothers and children in the clinical range pre and post treatment

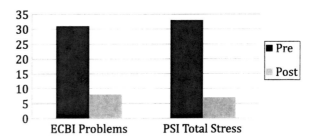

characteristics of the children that make them easy or difficult to manage. These are often a result of the temperament of the child and may include defiant, noncompliant, and demanding behaviors. Parents also completed the *Eyberg Child Behavior Inventory (ECBI*; Eyberg & Pincus, 1999) which is a 36-item informant report measure of conduct problems for children ages 2–16 years. Two scores are derived, the Total Behavior Problems score, which indicates the number of behaviors that a parent perceives as problematic and Total Intensity score, which indicates the degree to which those behaviors are a problem. Parents also completed a comprehensive consumer satisfaction questionnaire regarding the treatment they received.

Results showed that mothers who attended the IY parenting class reported significantly lower scores on the Total PSI Stress (t [57]$=6.53$, p$>.001$), Parent Distress (t[57]$=5.14$, p$>.001$), Dysfunctional Parent-child Relationship (t[57]$=4.50$, p$>.001$), and Difficult Child (t [57]$=5.03$, p$>.001$) from pre-test to post test. Results showed that fathers reported significantly lower Parent Distress (t[22]$=2.44$, p$>.02$) from pre-test to post-test. No other father changes were significant, although all scores were in the predicted direction. Results of the mother reports on the ECBI showed significant reductions in behaviors problems on both the Intensity Score (t [54]$=4.08$, p$>.001$) and Problem Score (t [51]$=3.22$, p$>.002$). Results of the father reports on the ECBI showed a significant reduction in behaviors problems on the Intensity Score (t [19]$=3.09$, p$>.006$).

In this study, the extent to which parents and children made clinically significant changes on both measures was analyzed by Chi-square analyses comparing the percentage of children and mothers in the clinical range on each measure at pre-test and post-test. Clinical significance analyses were not performed on the father data because of the small numbers of father reports available. Chi-square analyses showed that for the ECBI problem score, the percentage of children in the clinical range significantly decreased from pre-test to post-test. $\chi^2=3.98$ (1), p$<.05$. At pre-test 31 % of mothers reported that their children were in the clinical range compared to 8 % at post-test (Fig. 6.1).

Mothers showed clinically significant change on all subscales of the PSI. For ease of reporting, numbers are presented only for the Total Stress score; $\chi^2=8.82$ (1), p$<.003$. At pre-test 33 % of mothers reported stress levels in the clinical range compared to 7 % after treatment.

Parent satisfaction with the program was also high. Following treatment, parents' average satisfaction scores were 5.7 (1 ~ very low rating, 7 ~ very high rating) on reports of improvements in mother or father-child bonding, improvements in original problems, expectations for program success, confidence in handling current and future problems, and overall feelings. The highest scores (above 6.2) were for confidence in handling current and future child problems, and over all feelings were 6.35 for mothers and 6.04 for fathers. While there was no comparison group or control group in this program evaluation, the high attendance and satisfaction rates and the positive changes in parent and child behavior are very encouraging with respect to the use of the updated IY BASIC parent program for this population.

Finally, a recent study showed that the IY program resulted in attachment-based changes in sensitive parent responding compared with a control group indicating deeper level changes in the parent-child relationship. These results are highly relevant for working with maltreating parents (O'Connor, Matias, Futh, Tantam, & Scott, 2013).

Barriers to Providing Parent Training to Families Involved with Child Welfare

A number of barriers, noted above, may arise when working with families involved in the child welfare system. Below we will outline ways that the IY program can be used to overcome these barriers. In some cases, core components and therapy processes of the existing program are already well suited to working with this population. In other cases, program modifications or adjunct programs that are particularly relevant for the child welfare population are recommended.

One such barrier is that parents involved in the child welfare system may be difficult to engage because they are angry about being required to participate in parent education. The IY parent program, with its emphasis on collaboration rather than didactic prescriptions and its non-blaming and non-confronting focus on parent strengths instead of deficits is designed to counteract parent resistance. From the very first session, parents are involved in setting their own parenting goals as well as goals for their children's behavior. Therapists describe the group process as a partnership between the parents and the group leaders and emphasize that everyone in the group will be sharing ideas and learning from one another. This group process helps to diffuse parents' anger and sense of stigmatization because they receive validation from other group members who are struggling with similar difficulties in their day-to-day parenting experiences. Making new friends and sharing mutual problems and solutions is motivating and supportive for these parents, who often feel isolated and blamed (Coohey, 1996; Roditti, 2005). Moreover, the IY program's incorporation of motivational concepts such as individual goal setting, self-monitoring, reinforcing motivational self-talk, benefits and barriers exercises, peer buddy calls, and group leader coaching helps to promote demoralized parents' active engagement with the program. These program elements are theorized to help parents determine and accept responsibility for what they want to achieve, to empower parents and enhance attendance. A recent study with PCIT has indicated the usefulness of these concepts (Chaffin, Funderbunk, Bard, Valle, & Gurwitch, 2011).

A second barrier to group attendance is addressed by providing practical assistance for families by offering dinner, childcare, and transportation for the groups. These are offered in all of our community-based groups, not just to families involved in child welfare. Over and over, when families are asked to list reasons for not attending a group, childcare and transportation are among the top reasons listed. Families who do attend the groups always rate the social dinner time as a strong motivator for their ongoing participation.

A third difficulty in working with families involved with child welfare services is that parents are often experiencing multiple stressors that make it difficult for them to focus solely on parenting issues. For example, parents involved with Child Welfare Services have elevated rates of depression (Wilson, Dolan, Smith, Casanueva, & Ringeisen, 2012), have anger control difficulties (Ateah & Durrant, 2005), substance abuse problems, and conflictual relationships with partners that frequently escalate to domestic violence (Hazen, Connelly, Kelleher, Landsverk, & Barth, 2004). Many of these parents may also require other treatment for these co-morbid issues; however, it is difficult to compartmentalize treatment, and each of these issues is a significant barrier to effective parenting and to participation in a parenting group. For this reason it is recommended that the IY Parent ADVANCE Program be offered in addition to the BASIC Parent Program because it addresses interpersonal parent issues such as anger and depression management as they relate to parenting and also to parents' functioning in their adult environment. Themes of anger management, coping with stress, managing sad and discouraged feelings, problem solving and developing support networks are all incorporated into the IY ADVANCE parent program content. Parents are helped to learn elements of cognitive restructuring and self-regulation such as how to self praise, substitute coping thoughts for negative self-defeating thoughts, positive imagery, ways to develop positive supportive relationships through weekly buddy calls, strategies for using self-reinforcement when they achieve their goals and calm down strategies.

Helping Parents Whose Children Are in Foster Care

While nine out of ten children remain at home after investigation of abuse and/or neglect (Wulczn, Barth, Yuan, Jones Harden, & Landsverk, 2005), some will have had their children removed to foster care and parent training usually mandated as one of the conditions before family reunification can occur. Half of the small percentage of children who are removed from their biological home to foster care will be returned within 18 months of removal. The IY parent program is potentially useful for remediation of these parents' parenting difficulties but requires adaptations. For parents who may not have visitation rights or have only brief weekly supervised visitations, there are limited opportunities to practice the parenting skills they are learning with their children. According to the IY parent model, regular parenting practice with children at home between group sessions followed by group and leader feedback is a key component of behavior change. Therefore, for this population, group leaders need to show more video vignettes and set up many more coached practices during group sessions where parents alternate between the roles of parent and child in order to experience the perspective of their child as well as practice their parenting skills with other adults in the role of child. While this is typical practice for the IY program, spending more time on these practices helps enhance parents' empathy for their children as well as receive more coaching on their use of the parenting strategies. Additionally, the IY program's use of video modeling, group support, behavioral rehearsal, and in-group practice experiences provide opportunities for parents who are not living with their children to practice, watch, reflect on, discuss and learn appropriate parenting interactions and developmentally appropriate discipline. Expanding on these methods can help enhance the parents' modeling and experiential learning but also requires more time in treatment.

If these parents have visitation rights, they are asked to practice child-directed play and coaching skills during their visitations times. Parents are helped to plan activities to do with their child during visitation and to anticipate their child's response to seeing them after a separation. It is recommended that the visitation supervisors (and foster parents) be trained in the IY program so that their support will be consistent with what parents learn in the group, and they may even model some of the coaching skills themselves. While learning new parenting skills, parents also work on their own coping skills, their ability to manage anger and grief, on enhancing their support networks, and planning ahead for changes they will make when their children are returned home. Moreover, it is recommended that parents who do not have custody of their children when they take the program, repeat the IY group again after reunification so they can receive feedback and support while they are using the new parenting strategies at home with their children. Additionally, at this time group leaders help them strengthen their attachment with their child, a key foundational piece for their successful use of proactive discipline and responsive parenting. They work on the following: challenging negative and unrealistic thoughts and replacing them with positive coping thoughts and developmentally appropriate expectations; developing positive visualizations; determining self-care and pleasureable strategies; utilizing calm down strategies and their support network when needed. As they develop more confidence in themselves, their parenting approaches and understand their child's developmental milestones their relationships improve.

Ideally, foster parents will attend the parenting program with the biological parents. If this happens, foster parents can encourage parents' child-directed play and coaching interactions during their visitations, support parents' attachment and engagement with their children, and support children's emotional adjustment while in foster care. One randomized study has evaluated the use of the IY parent program offered jointly for foster parents and treatment mandated biological parents (whose children were removed due to child neglect or abuse) in comparison with a usual care condition. Findings indicated significant gains in positive parenting and collaborative co-parenting for both biological and foster parents in comparison with the usual care condition, and these results were maintained at 1-year follow-up. At follow-up, biological parents had sustained greater improvements and reported children with fewer behavior problems (Linares, Montalto, Li, & Vikash, 2006). IY attendance and completion rates for biological parents whose children were in foster care were similar to the Head Start IY study population, who had their children at home. Additionally, biological and foster parents who attended more than six sessions showed more improvement in positive parenting than those attending fewer sessions, indicating the importance of program dosage.

Adding the IY Home Coaching Model for Families Involved with Child Welfare

For child welfare referred parents who have their children at home, it is recommended that in addition to their group sessions, trained IY home visitor coaches work individually with them for a minimum of four home visits. Child welfare case managers, who are typically visiting these families anyway, may be trained to conduct coaching sessions in-home or their group leaders may schedule times for offering the sessions. These home visits are an opportunity to set up parent-child experiential practices and for parents to receive support and reinforcement for their efforts. A home visitor coaching manual with session protocols and parent workbooks are available. If parents cannot attend groups for some reason, the manual offers protocols for offering make up sessions at home or for delivering the entire program at home.

Summary of the IY Child Program and Evidence-Base (Dinosaur School)

The small group child treatment program (aka Dinosaur School) was originally developed in 1990 to directly focus on the social, emotional regulation, and problem-solving deficits of children diagnosed with ODD and externalizing problems (ages 4–8). This therapeutic group program (updated 2012) consists of a series of DVD programs (over 180 vignettes) that teach children problem-solving, emotional regulation, emotional literacy and social skills. The curriculum consists of 18–22 weekly, 2-h group sessions with 5–6 children per group. The two therapists for this program use comprehensive manuals that outline every session's content, objectives, video vignettes, role play practices, and descriptions of small group activities designed to practice key behaviors.

The Dinosaur program consists of seven main topic areas: Introduction and Rules; Empathy and Emotion; Problem Solving; Anger Control; Friendship Skills; Communication Skills; and School Skills. To enhance modeling and practice of child prosocial skills and feelings language, the DVD vignettes involve real-life conflict situations at home and at school (playground and classroom), such as teasing, being rejected, and destructive behavior. The goals of this program are to promote children's social and emotional competencies and reduce aggressive and noncompliant behaviors by doing the following: (a) strengthening social skills (turn taking, waiting, asking, sharing, helping, and complimenting); (b) promoting use of self-control and emotional self-regulation strategies (deep breathing, positive imagery, positive self-talk); (c) increasing emotional awareness by labeling feelings, recognizing the differing views of oneself and others, and enhancing perspective taking; (d) promoting children's ability to persist with difficult tasks; (e) improving academic success, reading, and school readiness; (f) reducing defiance, aggression, peer rejection, bullying, stealing, and lying and promoting compliance with adults and peers; (g) decreasing negative cognitive attributions and conflict management approaches; and (h) increasing self-esteem and self-confidence. More details on the therapeutic methods and process of delivering this program can be found in the following articles (Webster-Stratton & Reid, 2003, 2005, 2008).

Typically this 2-h child program is offered while the parents (biological and/or foster parents) attend the 2-h IY parent program. By offering these programs concurrently, the child group leaders are able to give feedback to parents at the end of the session about the skills children are learning and practicing and how they can expand this learning at home with the dinosaur home activities. In order to enhance generalization of the skills children are learning further, group leaders have regular telephone calls, emails, and communication with the children's teachers and collaborate with them on goals for behavior plans, share strategies that are working well and explain how the targeted prosocial behavior and self-regulation strategies can be encouraged and rewarded in the classroom. Child therapists can provide teachers with materials that may facilitate the learning at school such as the calm down thermometer, solution kit, dinosaur stickers, school rules cards and behavior plans. The Dinosaur School treatment program has been evaluated in three RCTs by the developer (Webster-Stratton & Hammond, 1997; Webster-Stratton et al., 2011; Webster-Stratton, Reid, & Hammond, 2004; Webster-Stratton, Reid, & Stoolmiller, 2008) and one RCT by an independent investigator (Drugli & Larsson, 2006). Several other studies with pre and post data have been reported by independent investigators (Hutchings, Bywater, Daley, & Lane, 2007; Hutchings, Lane, Owen, & Gwyn, 2004). Briefly, results have shown that children who participated in the Dinosaur School program showed more positive interactions with peers, improved emotion regulation literacy skills, more problem solving and friendship skills, and reductions in conduct problems and ADHD symptoms. Compared with the parent alone treatment program, combing the child program with the parent program resulted in significantly enhanced outcomes in regard to peer and school behavior as well as longer term child behavioral sustainability (Webster-Stratton & Hammond, 1997; Webster-Stratton et al., 2004).

Rationale for the Use of the IY Child Program for Maltreated Children

In addition to offering the IY parent group program, the small group therapeutic child treatment program is recommended for this population because research has indicated that children who have been neglected or abused and are in foster care have more behavior problems, self-regulation and emotional attachment difficulties, and other developmental, learning, and social difficulties than typical children (Crick & Dodge, 1994; Fantuzzo et al., 1991; Jaffee, Caspi, Moffitt, & Taylor, 2004; Knutson, DeGarmo, Koeppl, & Reid, 2005; Leslie, Hurlburt, Landsverk, Barth, & Slymen, 2004). In one study of children involved in the child welfare system in California, 42 % had a psychiatric disorder, mostly ADHD and ODD (Garland et al., 2001).

While this IY child program is being used clinically with this population, currently there are no RCTs evaluating its effectiveness with children who are in foster care or involved with child welfare. However, a study is underway in New York (Linares, Li, & Shrout, 2012) where foster children receive the child dinosaur small group treatment program while their biological parents and foster parents are participating together in the IY parent program.

Selecting IY Programs According to Population Risk Factors

Just as IY group leaders must help parents build strong foundations in their relationships with children in order to be successful, so must agencies or organizations be sure they provide adequate support and scaffolding according to the specific needs of the families. The BASIC parent programs are considered a mandatory or "core" component of the intervention with indicated or selective populations. The longer session protocols for the BASIC program delivery will be needed for high risk or treatment populations or new immigrant populations who find the content unfamiliar or who will need translators. Ideally, high-risk families will start by being offered the baby and toddler programs and continue with the age appropriate program for each developmental stage. This ongoing support is more likely to break the intergenerational transmission of child abuse and neglect than single shot program approaches. For families with mental health problems such as depression, marital conflict and anger problems it is recommended that they receive the ADVANCE curriculum after completing the BASIC program in order to address other family and interpersonal issues and to help support and maintain the changes they have made in their parenting interactions. For families who seem not to be grasping the concepts in group practices, or are reporting difficulty implementing the strategies at home, the home based IY model can be combined with the group training. This gives the parents a support group while also allowing them to have coached practice at home with their children and personalized, private feedback from IY coaches.

For families who have children with developmental problems or diagnoses such as ODD, CD, ADHD and Depression, it is recommended that the child also be offered the child treatment dinosaur program. Involving the child in a treatment group has several added advantages. First it permits therapists or group leaders to have a fuller understanding of a child's developmental needs when working with parents; it destigmatizes parents feeling the blame for their children's behaviors; and it allows parents to have practice exercises with the children in conjunction with group learning and support. Finally, research shows it improves out comes for children in terms of their behaviors with peers at school (Webster-Stratton & Hammond, 1997; Webster-Stratton et al., 2004).

Case Example: Robbie

Robbie is a 4-year-old boy who lives with his single mother, Melinda. Robbie's father left when he was 2 years old, and Melinda is unemployed and depressed. She tries to meet Robbie's needs and there are times when she lavishes attention on him; letting him stay up late watching TV with her and then allowing him to sleep with her at night. At other times she does not have the energy to engage with Robbie at all and frequently has left him unsupervised at home or on the playground. Still other times she asks him to do age inappropriate tasks such as make dinner, wash the dishes, or do the laundry and then gets very angry when he refuses or does it badly. He responds by throwing tantrums, which, in turn, fuel her anger or complete withdrawal. Melinda was reported to child protective services by a neighbor who was concerned about her explosive anger and neglectful behavior.

Robbie and his mother participated in treatment together with Melinda attending the weekly 2-h IY parent group at the same time that Robbie participated in the IY child treatment program, Dinosaur School. At the onset of treatment, Robbie had difficulty separating from his mother at the beginning of each dinosaur small group therapy session, and then he was clingy and almost inappropriately attached to the two child group therapists that he had just met. He was extremely volatile, easily irritated, and had dramatic mood swings. At times he was withdrawn and sad, at other times he seemed angry, defiant, oppositional, and noncompliant. In the small group he was interested in other children and seemed to want to make friends, but was easily jealous of any attention that other children were getting from the therapists. During unstructured play times he mostly played alone and rarely initiated verbal interactions with peers except to poke or push them, laugh at them and make unfriendly gestures.

Foundation of the Parenting Pyramid

For Melinda the IY parent group started with helping her understand the importance of providing Robbie with daily and predictable child directed play times where she consistently gave Robbie positive attention, consistent responses, and positive emotional and social coaching and praise. The goal of providing this predictable, undivided, focused attention was to help Robbie feel valued, respected, and more secure in his relationship with his mother. Robbie's mother was helped to understand his age appropriate developmental milestones ~ that of forming a secure attachment with her, developing beginning self-regulation skills as well as social friendship skills. She was encouraged to let him be a child rather than expect him to fill the male partner role, to comply with his ideas during play, as long as he was appropriate, and to engage in imaginary play so he could express is feelings. During practice sessions in the group, she was first asked to play the child role while another parent was in the parent role. This practice allowed her to see and experience the world from Robbie's viewpoint, to develop empathy and learn to appreciate Robbie's ideas and feelings such as his fears of abandonment. Melinda was also given many opportunities to practice in role as parent so that she could try out a new and more age appropriate way to interact and communicate. As Melinda continued these play times with Robbie using social and emotional coaching, she could see that Robbie enjoyed this form of attention from her and was imitating her words and behaviors. Her confidence in her skills as a parent began to increase, which, in turn, resulted in her feeling less depressed. In the parent group she also worked on challenging her negative, self-defeating thoughts and substituting positive coping thoughts. Other parents in the group also struggled with depressive and self-blaming attributions, and they provided a support network for each other. With her assigned parent buddy, another single mother from the group, she made a list of low-cost pleasurable activities she could engage in to refuel her energy. One of the ideas they came up with was to set a play date at the park where they met each week so their children could play together. They used this opportunity to practice some social coaching skills, which in turn gave Robbie a chance to practice his friendship skills. Melinda's support system began to increase, as did her hope.

Several home visits were set up so the parent group leader could coach Melinda's play interactions with Robbie at home. They focused on practicing social and emotional coaching which was a foreign language for this mother. As a result with the help of the therapist she developed scripts, written out and laminated on a ring, which she kept on her belt to refer to when she was playing or doing some activity with Robbie. With time this language became more comfortable and she started adding some of her own ideas to the script notes.

By the 6th session Melinda was feeling some success with her play sessions and began using stickers and hand stamps to reward Robbie's "positive opposite" behaviors; that is, when he was calm, used friendly words and complied with her requests. She learned to reduce the number of unnecessary commands and criticisms and instead to give positive and respectful commands as well as to set up a predictable bedtime routine. She called her buddy from the group each night after Robbie was in bed to share her success with this. While there were relapses with Robbie's behavior and times when she lost control, she learned these set backs were normal, indicating that Robbie was testing the limits to see how secure they were and how safe he was. Melinda felt she had a strategy to follow in terms of calming down, a support group to share with each week, and a buddy to call when needed. Her therapist called her each week to see how she was doing meeting her goal for the week and to provide support.

Child Dinosaur School

In the child dinosaur small group of six children, the therapists played with Robbie in ways that would model healthy relationships. Using puppets, therapists modeled setting boundaries on physical touch by teaching Robbie how to ask before touching someone else. He received hand stamps and praise for using friendly words and for gentle touch. Therapists worked on using emotion coaching with a focus on times he was calm, happy, and proud as well as pointing out how other children were enjoying playing with him. They paid little attention to Robbie's sulky or pouty behavior, but continued to model, prompt and encourage him to engage in friendly social interactions with other children. For example if Robbie was sulking, no direct attempts were made to cajole him out of his mood. Rather therapists might say to another child, "Billy, I'm really enjoying working on this art project with you. I bet that when Robbie is ready to join us he'll have some great ideas about what we should add to our drawing. He's a great artist and helpful friend."

Circle times during each child group session focused on watching DVD vignettes designed to model social skills such as sharing, waiting, taking turns, and giving complements. Puppets were an important part of Robbie's treatment plan. He seemed much more willing to share feelings and experiences with the puppets than directly with the therapists. Through puppet play, Robbie began to establish close and healthy relationships with the therapists. Therapists showed Robbie that they would continue to be positive and engage with him, even after he had rejected their attention or been oppositional. This attention was always given strategically so that Robbie received little attention when his behaviors were negative, but was quickly reinforced as soon as he was neutral or positive.

Initially Robbie sought attention from the other children in the group by being disruptive, silly, and loud. The other children were taught to ignore this inappropriate behavior and to give him privacy until he calmed down. Robbie was also put in charge of helping to monitor other children's friendly and positive behavior. This provided him with an opportunity to receive attention and positive approval from the other children. Children were taught to compliment things that they liked about the other children, and therapists repeatedly pointed out and reinforced every instance of friendly behavior they observed. After 4 sessions, Robbie began to report to his parents that he liked Dinosaur school. Two of the other boys in the group became friends with Robbie, and Robbie asked his mother if they could come over to play with him. From this point on, Robbie was consistently positive about coming to the group and Melinda reported that he seemed happy about a group-peer activity for the first time in his life.

In addition to the friendship skills taught in Dinosaur School, Robbie and the other children learned a series of problem solving steps (notice uncomfortable feelings, identify the problem, brainstorm solutions, try out and evaluate the best solution). The therapists tailored the problem solving scenarios to those that were relevant for children in the group, including Robbie. For Robbie, relevant problem-solving scenarios included communicating wants to others in appropriate ways, personal space, getting peer attention in positive ways, dealing with an adult's anger, and getting help from a safe adult. Another unit in the child group focused on self-regulation and calm down strategies for children to use (going into a turtle shell, taking deep breaths, using positive self talk). Robbie was happy to practice these strategies with the puppets during the group. The therapists also looked for times when they could see that he was beginning to become angry, and would coach him to use the calm-down thermometer and other strategies before he became too upset. Robbie was often receptive to this coaching, and as the group went on, he even began to initiate self-calming strategies without the therapists' prompts.

Top of Parenting Pyramid

The second half of the parenting program helped Melinda to use positive, proactive discipline. In this part of the program, one key strategy is strategic planned ignoring. Parents are taught to temporarily withdraw their attention at times when their children are engaging in behaviors such as whining, tantruming, rudeness, or back-talk. This was challenging for Melinda because, while she had reduced unnecessary commands and criticisms, it was very difficult for her to understand the rationale for the ignoring strategy. She worried that Robbie would not understand what was expected of him if she ignored his behavior and that ignoring was not a strong enough message, particularly for his rude verbal behaviors. However, given her success with the first part of the program, she was willing to give ignoring an experimental try. At first Robbie was persistent with his tantrums and would scream loudly that she didn't love him. Melinda worried that others hearing this would report her to child protective services. She was inclined to catastrophize the situation and worry that Robbie's behavior was irreversible, and he was on the path to becoming a delinquent like his father. She learned to change her negative thoughts by using her coping and reframing self-talk (e.g., "He will feel safer when he knows there are predictable limits." "He is only 4 and if I help him now, he won't become a delinquent). With support from the therapists and her buddy, Melinda was able to ignore several very violent temper tantrums, after which she could see that while Robbie still had tantrums, they were less intense and shorter. The therapists stressed the importance of giving positive attention back to Robbie as soon as the tantrum subsided. This, too, was difficult for Melinda because she was often still very angry and dysregulated herself and had trouble letting go of this anger once Robbie had calmed down. Again, her buddy was helpful in supporting her; the two mothers called and talked to each other whenever one of them was frustrated with her child's behavior. They were encouraged to remind each other that it was okay to vent to each other and to feel frustrated, but that they need to let go of the anger and move on in order to help their children see that positive behavior resulted in positive attention from their mothers.

Robbie's relationship with his mother had improved considerably, and he had learned more appropriate social behaviors and emotional language from his mother and in dinosaur school, but there were still times his behavior was aggressive or unsafe. Since it was clear that Robbie was desiring his mother's positive attention, the therapist then felt Melinda was ready to learn how to teach Robbie Time Out to calm down, reserved exclusively for aggressive behavior. This was practiced three to four times in parent group sessions with specific plans for what would happen if he refused to go or wouldn't sit in the chair. Additionally, since Robbie had learned and practiced this Time Out to calm down strategy in dinosaur school, Melinda learned to use the exact same script and language for sending him to Time Out at home. She reviewed calm down strategies with Robbie, including taking rocket breaths, thinking about his happy place, and using positive self-talk. Melinda was surprised how easily Robbie went to Time Out and noticed that he even reminded her of the words he could use (e.g., "I can calm down and try again"). The therapist called several times and let Melinda know she was available for any consultation needed. In week 17 of the program, Melinda learned how to teach Robbie problem solving steps, and they practiced using puppets how to solve hypothetical problem situations. Again since Robbie had learned problem solving and practiced many proactive solutions (e.g., sharing, helping, teamwork, ignoring, complimenting) in Dinosaur School he enjoyed helping teach his mother how this drama game worked to solve lots of problems.

Post Treatment Results

Robbie's behavior improved at home first as Melinda began to have a more predictable routine for meals and bedtimes, combined with frequent coaching and positive play interactions designed to build targeted emotion language and social skills. There continued to be explosive incidents throughout the treatment period, but they became less frequent, and Melinda became more confident in her ability to handle the problems. The Dinosaur child group quickly became a reinforcing activity for Robbie, and he made some of his first friends in the group. Melinda reported that he was proud of these friends and proud of his ability to help them. This was in sharp contrast to his negative feelings and resistance to attending these groups at the beginning of the program.

At the end of the group treatment, therapists recommended follow-up group booster sessions and therapist check-ins for Melinda to ensure that she had support to continue to use the skills that she had learned in the group and to help her cope with new issues that came up. Although Melinda had made huge changes during the group, her history of depression and isolation as well as Robbie's continued challenging behaviors made her vulnerable. While this was not mandated, when offered by her therapist Melinda was receptive to the idea of attending the ADVANCE parent program, stating that she was worried that without the support of the group, she would slip back into old habits with Robbie.

Assessment post treatment based on home observations and parent reports indicated that Robbie had significantly fewer behavior problems, and these improvements were maintained 1-year later. Melinda was actively reengaged in responsive parenting and strategic use of her attention for positive behaviors. She continued to meet monthly with a therapist and more informally with several other parents from the group, who became a close support network for her. One year after treatment, Robbie was observed to be compliant to approximately 60 % of his mother's commands, which was a huge increase. Melinda reported that she still experienced Robbie's behavior as overwhelming and challenging, at times, but that she was also able to step back from these feelings and to draw upon the strategies that she had learned in the group. *"Now, when I think about it, I know what I should do. That's a huge difference for me. Before I just yelled or gave up, and I felt that Robbie was winning. Now I feel like I know how to be in charge of him in a way that lets us both win in the end."*

Concluding Remarks

The Incredible Years (IY) parent and child programs are evidence-based programs, which seem relevant and offer promise for use with maltreating families with young children. These programs have demonstrated ability to improve parent-child relationships and to build parents' own sense of competence and self-control as well as strengthen their supportive family and community networks. While it is not uncommon for child welfare agencies to seek briefer interventions than IY, it is recommended that because these families are complex and are in the highest risk for re-abuse and maltreatment, they need a comprehensive treatment plan that addresses parenting training, family interpersonal and support needs, and children's problems with attachment, emotional regulation, social skills and cognitive development. With adequate support and training with the full array of IY treatment programs spanning children's developmental stages, it is hypothesized that, in the long term, these parents' improvements in parenting will lead to lower rates of re-abuse, fewer re-reports to child welfare services and more socially and emotionally competent children. Research documenting the effectiveness of the IY programs and other evidence based practices for this very high-risk population should be a national public health priority.

References

Abidin, R. (1990). *Parenting stress index* (2nd ed.). Odessa, FL: Psychological Assessment Resources, Inc.

Ateah, C. A., & Durrant, J. E. (2005). Maternal use of physical punishment in response to child misbehavior: Implications for child abuse prevention. *Child Abuse and Neglect, 29*(2), 169–185.

Bandura, A. (1982). Self-efficacy mechanisms in human agency. *American Psychologist, 84*, 191–215.

Barth, R. P., Landsverk, J., Chamberlain, P., Reid, J. B., Rolls, J. A., Hurlburt, M. S., et al. (2005). Parent-training programs in child welfare services: Planning for a more evidence-based approach to serving biological parents. *Research on Social Work Practice, 15*(5), 353–371.

Bowlby, J. (1988). *A secure base: Parent-child attachment and healthy development.* New York: Basic Books.

Chaffin, M., Funderbunk, B., Bard, D., Valle, L. A., & Gurwitch, R. (2011). A combined motivation and parent-child interaction therapy package reduces child welfare recidivism in a randomized dismantling field trial. *Journal of Consulting and Clinical Psychology, 79,* 84–95.

Chaffin, M., Silovsky, J. F., Funderburk, B., Valle, L. A., Brestan, E. V., Balachova, T., et al. (2004). Parent-child interaction therapy with physically abusive parents: Efficacy for reducing future abuse reports. *Journal of Consulting and Clinical Psychology, 72*(3), 500–510.

Coohey, C. (1996). Child maltreatment: Testing the social isolation hypothesis. *Child Abuse and Neglect, 20*(3), 241–254.

Corcoran, J. (2000). Family interventions with child physical abuse and neglect: A critical review. *Children and Youth Services Review, 22,* 563–591.

Crick, N. R., & Dodge, K. A. (1994). A review and reformulation of social information processing mechanisms in children's social adjustment. *Psychological Bulletin, 115,* 74–101.

D'Zurilla, T. J., & Nezu, A. (1982). Social problem-solving in adults. In P. C. Kendall (Ed.), *Advances in cognitive behavioral research and therapy* (Vol. 1). New York: Academic.

Drugli, M. B., & Larsson, B. (2006). Children aged 4–8 years treated with parent training and child therapy because of conduct problems: Generalisation effects to day-care and school settings. *European Child and Adolescent Psychiatry, 15,* 392–399.

Eyberg, S. M., & Pincus, D. (1999). *Eyberg child behavior inventory and Sutter-Eyberg behavior inventory-revised: Professional manual.* Odessa, FL: Psychological Assessment Resources.

Fantuzzo, J. W., DePaola, L. M., Lambert, L., Martino, T., Anderson, G., & Sutton, S. (1991). Effects of interpersonal violence on the psychological adjustment and competencies of young children. *Journal of Consulting and Clinical Psychology, 59,* 258–265.

Gardner, F., Burton, J., & Klimes, I. (2006). Randomized controlled trial of a parenting intervention in the voluntary sector for reducing conduct problems in children: Outcomes and mechanisms of change. *Journal of Child Psychology and Psychiatry, 47,* 1123–1132.

Garland, A. F., Hough, R. L., McCabe, K. M., Yeh, M., Wood, P. A., & Aarons, G. A. (2001). Prevalence of psychiatric disorders in youths across five sectors of care. *Journal of the American Academy of Child and Adolescent Psychiatry, 40,* 409–418.

Hazen, A., Connelly, C. D., Kelleher, K., Landsverk, J., & Barth, R. P. (2004). Intimate partner violence among female caregivers of children reported for child maltreatment. *Child Abuse and Neglect, 28,* 301–319.

Hurlburt, M. S., Nguyen, K., Reid, M. J., Webster-Stratton, C., & Zhang, J. (2013). Efficacy of Incredible Years group parent program with families in Head Start with a child maltreatment history. *Child Abuse and Neglect, 37*(8), 531–543.

Hutchings, J., Bywater, T., Daley, D., & Lane, E. (2007). A pilot study of the Webster-Stratton Incredible Years Therapeutic Dinosaur School Programme. *Clinical Psychology Forum, 170,* 21–24.

Hutchings, J., Gardner, F., Bywater, T., Daley, D., Whitaker, C., Jones, K., et al. (2007). Parenting intervention in Sure Start services for children at risk of developing conduct disorder: Pragmatic randomized controlled trial. *British Medical Journal, 334*(7595), 1–7.

Hutchings, J., Lane, E., Owen, R., & Gwyn, R. (2004). The introduction of the Webster-Stratton Classroom Dinosaur School Programme in Gwynedd, North Wales. *Education and Child Psychology, 21,* 4–15.

Jaffee, S. R., Caspi, A., Moffitt, T. E., & Taylor, A. (2004). Physical maltreatment victim to antisocial child: Evidence of environmentally mediated process. *Journal of Abnormal Psychology, 113,* 44–55.

Knutson, J. F., DeGarmo, D., Koeppl, G., & Reid, J. B. (2005). Care neglect, supervisory neglect and harsh parenting in the development of children's aggression: A replication and extension. *Child Maltreatment, 10,* 92–107.

Larsson, B., Fossum, B., Clifford, G., Drugli, M., Handegard, B., & Morch, W. (2009). Treatment of oppositional defiant and conduct problems in young Norwegian children: Results of a randomized trial. *European Child Adolescent Psychiatry, 18*(1), 42–52.

Leslie, L. K., Hurlburt, M. S., Landsverk, J., Barth, R., & Slymen, D. J. (2004). Outpatient mental health services for children in foster care: A national perspective. *Child Abuse and Neglect, 28*, 269–712.

Linares, L. O., Li, M., & Shrout, P. (2012). Child training for physical aggression?: Lessons from foster care. *Children and Youth Services Review, 34*(12), 2416–2422.

Linares, L. O., Montalto, D., Li, M., & Vikash, S. (2006). A promising parent intervention in foster care. *Journal of Consulting and Clinical Psychology, 74*(1), 32–41.

Lutzker, J. R. (1990). Behavioral treatment of child neglect. *Behavior Modification, 14*(3), 301–315.

Lutzker, J. R., & Bigelow, K. M. (2002). *Reducing child maltreatment: A guides for parent services*. New York: Guilford Press.

McDaniel, B., Braiden, H. J., Onyekwelu, J., Murphy, M., & Regan, H. (2011). Investigating the effectiveness of the Incredible Years Basic Parenting Programme for foster carers in Northern Ireland. *Child Care in Practice, 17*(1), 55–67.

O'Connor, T. G., Matias, C., Futh, A., Tantam, G., & Scott, S. (2013). Social learning theory parenting intervention promotes attachment-based caregiving in young children: Randomized clinical trial. *Journal of Clinical Child Psychology, 42*(3), 358–370.

Patterson, G., Reid, J., & Dishion, T. (1992). *Antisocial boys: A social interactional approach* (Vol. 4). Eugene, OR: Castalia Publishing.

Piaget, J., & Inhelder, B. (1962). *The psychology of the child*. New York: Basic Books.

Posthumus, J. A., Raaijmakers, M. A. J., Maassen, G. H., Engeland, H., & Matthys, W. (2012). Sustained effects of Incredible Years as a preventive intervention in preschool children with conduct problems. *Journal of Abnormal Child Psychology, 40*(4), 487–500.

Reid, M. J., Webster-Stratton, C., & Beauchaine, T. P. (2001). Parent training in head start: A comparison of program response among African American, Asian American, Caucasian, and Hispanic mothers. *Prevention Science, 2*(4), 209–227.

Roditti, M. G. (2005). Understanding communities of neglectful parents: Child caring networks and child neglect. *Child Welfare, 84*(2), 277–298.

Schoenwald, S. K., & Hoagwood, K. (2001). Effectiveness, transportability, and dissemination of interventions: What matters when? *Journal of Psychiatric Services, 52*(9), 1190–1197.

Scott, S., Spender, Q., Doolan, M., Jacobs, B., & Aspland, H. (2001). Multicentre controlled trial of parenting groups for child antisocial behaviour in clinical practice. *British Medical Journal, 323*(28), 1–5.

U.S. Department of Health and Human Services [USDHHS], Administration for Children and Families, Administration on Children, Youth and Families, & Children's Bureau. (2011). *Child maltreatment 2010*. Available from http://www.acf.hhs.gov/programs/cb/stats_research/index.htm#can

Webster-Stratton, C. (1981). Modification of mothers' behaviors and attitudes through videotape modeling group discussion program. *Behavior Therapy, 12*, 634–642.

Webster-Stratton, C. (1982). Teaching mothers through videotape modeling to change their children's behaviors. *Journal of Pediatric Psychology, 7*(3), 279–294.

Webster-Stratton, C. (1994). Advancing videotape parent training: A comparison study. *Journal of Consulting and Clinical Psychology, 62*(3), 583–593.

Webster-Stratton, C. (1998). Preventing conduct problems in Head Start children: Strengthening parenting competencies. *Journal of Consulting and Clinical Psychology, 66*(5), 715–730.

Webster-Stratton, C. (2009). Affirming diversity: Multi-cultural collaboration to deliver the Incredible Years Parent Programs. *The International Journal of Child Health and Human Development, 2*(1), 17–32.

Webster-Stratton, C. (2012a). *Blueprints for violence prevention, book eleven: The Incredible Years – Parent, teacher, and child training series*. Seattle, WA: Incredible Years.

Webster-Stratton, C. (2012b). *Collaborating with parents to reduce children's behavior problems: A book for therapists using the Incredible Years Programs Seattle*. Seattle. WA: Incredible Years Inc.

Webster-Stratton, C. (2012c). *The Incredible Years parents, teachers, and children's training series: Program content, methods, research and dissemination 1980–2011*. Seattle, WA: Incredible Years.

Webster-Stratton, C., & Hammond, M. (1997). Treating children with early-onset conduct problems: A comparison of child and parent training interventions. *Journal of Consulting and
Clinical Psychology, 65*(1), 93–109.

Webster-Stratton, C., & Mihalic, S. (2001). *Blueprints for violence prevention, book eleven: The
Incredible Years – Parent, teacher, and child training series*. Boulder, CO: Center for the Study
and Prevention of Violence.

Webster-Stratton, C., & Reid, M. J. (2003). Treating conduct problems and strengthening social
emotional competence in young children (ages 4–8 years): The Dina Dinosaur treatment
program. *Journal of Emotional and Behavioral Disorders, 11*(3), 130–143.

Webster-Stratton, C., & Reid, M. J. (2005). Treating conduct problems and strengthening
social and emotional competence in young children: The Dina Dinosaur treatment program.
In M. Epstein, K. Kutash, & A. J. Duchowski (Eds.), *Outcomes for children and youth with
emotional and behavioral disorders and their families: Programs and evaluation best
practices* (2nd ed., pp. 597–623). Austin, TX: Pro-Ed, Inc.

Webster-Stratton, C., & Reid, M. J. (2007). Incredible Years parents and teachers training series:
A head start partnership to promote social competence and prevent conduct problems. In P. Tolin,
J. Szapocznick, & S. Sambrano (Eds.), *Preventing youth substance abuse* (pp. 67–88).
Washington, DC: American Psychological Association.

Webster-Stratton, C., & Reid, M. J. (2008). Adapting the Incredible Years Child Dinosaur Social,
Emotional and Problem Solving intervention to address co-morbid diagnoses. *Journal of
Children's Services, 3*(3), 17–30.

Webster-Stratton, C., & Reid, M. J. (2010). The Incredible Years parents, teachers and children
training series: A multifaceted treatment approach for young children with conduct problems.
In A. E. Kazdin & J. R. Weisz (Eds.), *Evidence-based psychotherapies for children and adolescents* (2nd ed., pp. 194–210). New York: Guilford Publications.

Webster-Stratton, C., Reid, M. J., & Beauchaine, T. P. (2011). Combining parent and child training
for young children with ADHD. *Journal of Clinical Child and Adolescent Psychology, 40*(2),
1–13.

Webster-Stratton, C., Reid, M. J., & Hammond, M. (2001). Preventing conduct problems, promoting social competence: A parent and teacher training partnership in Head Start. *Journal of
Clinical Child Psychology, 30*(3), 283–302.

Webster-Stratton, C., Reid, M. J., & Hammond, M. (2004). Treating children with early-onset
conduct problems: Intervention outcomes for parent, child, and teacher training. *Journal of
Clinical Child and Adolescent Psychology, 33*(1), 105–124.

Webster-Stratton, C., Reid, M. J., & Stoolmiller, M. (2008). Preventing conduct problems and
improving school readiness: Evaluation of the Incredible Years Teacher and Child Training
Programs in high-risk schools. *Journal of Child Psychology and Psychiatry, 49*(5), 471–488.

Wilson, E., Dolan, M., Smith, K., Casanueva, C., & Ringeisen, H. (2012). *NSCAW child well-being
spotlight: Caregivers of children who remain in-home after a maltreatment investigation need
services* (OPRE Report #2012-48). Washington, DC: Office of Planning, Research and
Evaluation, Administration for Children and Families, U.S. Department of Health and Human
Services. Find this report and those on similar topics online at: http://www.acf.hhs.gov/
programs/opre/abuse_neglect/nscaw/

Wulczn, F., Barth, R., Yuan, Y., Jones Harden, B., & Landsverk, J. (2005). *Beyond common sense:
Child welfare, child well-being, and the evidence for policy reform*. New Brunswick, NJ:
Aldine Transaction.

Chapter 7
The Importance of Evidence-Based Parenting Intervention to the Prevention and Treatment of Child Maltreatment

Matthew R. Sanders and John A. Pickering

A Public Health Approach to the Prevention and Treatment of Child Maltreatment

Preventing the maltreatment of children should be given priority as a major public health challenge. The number of official reports of child maltreatment in most Western countries continues to rise each year (Australian Institute of Health and Welfare [AIHW], 2008; U.S. Department of Health and Human Services, 2008; World Health Organisation, 2009) and there is a general lack of consensus among researchers, policy makers and support workers about the best approach to take in combating the issue. Evidence clearly indicates that maltreated children are more likely to suffer antisocial outcomes including externalising behaviours (Kotch et al., 2008; Lansford, Berlin, Bates, & Pettit, 2007; Maas, Herrenkohl, & Sousa, 2008), and internalising problems (McHolm, MacMillan, & Jamieson, 2003; Widom, 1999; Widom, Dumont, & Czaja, 2007). Of particular concern, parents account for over 70 % of all persons believed to be responsible for perpetrating the majority of substantiated cases of child maltreatment (AIHW, 2005).

This chapter makes the case that improved parenting is the cornerstone of child maltreatment treatment and prevention and strengthening parenting and family relationships across the entire population is the approach most likely to reduce the unacceptably high rate of child maltreatment. We focus on the role of parenting programs in reducing the prevalence of child maltreatment and document the steps required to achieve population-level reductions in rates of child maltreatment. A parenting intervention, known as Pathways Triple P, is used to illustrate the

M.R. Sanders, Ph.D. (✉) • J.A. Pickering
Parenting and Family Support Centre, School of Psychology, The University of Queensland, Brisbane, St Lucia QLD 4072, Australia
e-mail: matts@psy.uq.edu.au; j.pickering@psy.uq.edu.au

S. Timmer and A. Urquiza (eds.), *Evidence-Based Approaches for the Treatment of Maltreated Children*, Child Maltreatment 3, DOI 10.1007/978-94-007-7404-9_7,
© Springer Science+Business Media Dordrecht 2014

complexities of working with parents at risk of harming their children through examination of a case study. Implications for policy makers, researchers, parents and their children are discussed.

Parents and Child Maltreatment

Maltreating parents tend to differ from non-maltreating parents in their inability to cope with anger provoking situations (Rodriguez & Green, 1997). Fortunately, significant inroads have been made in the last decade towards understanding how parents' cognitive factors influence their affect and behaviour towards their children (Azar & Weinzierl, 2005; Dix, Reinhold, & Zambarano, 1990; Kolko & Swenson, 2002; Sanders et al., 2004). Much of the research has centred on various forms of maladaptive schemas, unrealistic expectations, and negative attributional bias in interpreting child behaviour and negative parenting behaviour (Grusec & Mammone, 1995; Miller & Azar, 1996; Pidgeon & Sanders, 2009; Sanders et al., 2004).

A growing body of evidence has highlighted a clear link between parents who are at-risk of maltreating their children and the extent to which they possess faulty, causal attributional processes towards their explanations of their children's problem behaviours (Milner, 2003; Pidgeon & Sanders, 2009). It is reasoned that faulty attributions indirectly contribute to child maltreatment by increasing parental anger, overactivity and use of severe discipline strategies such as threats, yelling, hitting, grabbing and pushing (Dix, Ruble, & Zambarano, 1989; Nix et al., 1999). Parental anger is also a common factor underlying the act of parents physically abusing children (Kolko, 1996; Mammen, Kolko, & Pilkonis, 2002). It stands to reason, therefore, that if efforts can be made to address parental anger and negative attributional processes then improvements in rates of child maltreatment may occur. Parenting programs that address anger and attributional style, as well as other parenting skills more broadly, hold particular promise in reducing the rates of child maltreatment.

Why Parenting Programs Are Important

The quality of parenting that children receive has a major influence on their development, wellbeing, and life opportunities. Experimental clinical research has clearly demonstrated that structured parenting programs based on social learning models are among the most efficacious and cost-effective interventions available to promote the mental health and well-being of children, particularly children at risk of being maltreated (Collins, Maccoby, Steinberg, Hetherington, & Bornstein, 2000; National Research Council and Institute of Medicine, 2009). Evidence available with maltreating parents suggests that parent training leads to improvements in parenting competence and parent behaviour (James, 1994; Wekerle & Wolfe, 1998). These changes in parenting practice reduce the risk of further abusive behaviour towards children, reports to protective agencies, and visits to hospital. Beyond younger children, potentially modifiable family risk factors can also be targeted in order to reduce the rates of emotional and behavioral problems in adolescents (Dekovic, Janssens, & Van As, 2003). Although studies on parenting programs for parents of teenagers are far less extensive compared to studies with younger children (Kazdin, 2005), such programs have been demonstrated to improve parent-adolescent communication and reduce family conflict (Barkley, Edwards, Laneri, Fletcher, & Metevia, 2001; Dishion & Andrews, 1995), and reduce the risk of adolescents developing and maintaining substance abuse, delinquent behavior and other externalizing problems (Connell, Dishion, Yasui, & Kavanagh, 2007; Mason, Kosterman, Hawkins, Haggerty, & Spoth, 2003). Of note, parents of adolescents who participate in parenting programs have been found to report higher levels of confidence and use of more effective parenting strategies (Spoth, Redmond, & Shin, 1998).

Positive parenting programs based on social learning and cognitive-behavioral principles are the most effective in reducing problem behaviors in children and adolescents (Dretzke et al., 2009; Kazdin & Blase, 2011; Serketich & Dumas, 1996). These interventions typically provide active skills training to parents involving modeling and practice of skills, feedback, homework assignments in how to apply positive parenting (e.g., descriptive praise, incidental teaching, simple reward charts) and contingency management principles (e.g., logical consequences, non-exclusionary timeout). Different delivery formats have been successfully trialed including individual programs, small group programs, large group seminar programs, self-directed programs, telephone-assisted programs and more recently online parenting programs (see Dretzke et al., 2009; Nowak & Heinrichs, 2008; Sanders, 2012; Sanders, Baker, & Turner, 2012).

Numerous meta-analyses of parenting interventions attest to the benefits that parents and children derive (particularly children with conduct problems) when their parents learn positive parenting skills (Brestan & Eyberg, 1998; de Graaf, Speetjens, Smit, de Wolff, & Tavecchio, 2008a, 2008b; Nowak & Heinrichs, 2008). These benefits include children having fewer behavioral and emotional problems, more positive interactions with their parents and siblings, improved parental practices, improved mental health, and less parental conflict.

The Triple P System of Population-Level Parenting Intervention

The Triple P-Positive Parenting Program (see Sanders, 2012) is a system of parenting support and intervention that seeks to increase parents' confidence and skill in raising their children, thereby enhancing children's developmental outcomes. Triple P adopts a public health approach to parenting support which aims to make highly reliable, evidence-based parenting support available and accessible to all parents. This multilevel system of parenting support (see Fig. 7.1) is based on a public health model that provides five levels of intervention of increasing intensity geared towards

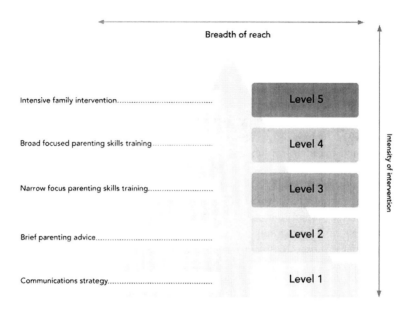

Breadth of reach

Intensive family intervention... Level 5

Broad focused parenting skills training........................... Level 4

Narrow focus parenting skills training............................ Level 3

Brief parenting advice.. Level 2

Communications strategy.. Level 1

Intensity of intervention

Fig. 7.1 The population multilevel, multiformat Triple P system of parenting support and intervention

normalising and destigmatizing parental participation in parenting education programs. The range of evidence-based tailored variants and flexible delivery options incorporate universal media messages for all parents (level 1), low intensity large group (level 2), topic-specific parent discussion groups and individual programs (level 3), intensive groups and individual programs (level 4), and more intense offerings for high risk or vulnerable parents (level 5). The program targets children at five different developmental stages: infants, toddlers, preschoolers, primary schoolers and teenagers. Within each developmental period the reach of the intervention can vary from being very broad (targeting an entire population) to quite narrow (targeting only high-risk children). Triple P targets modifiable family risk and protective factors causally implicated at the onset, and exacerbation or maintenance of adverse child development outcomes.

The rationale for Triple P's multilevel strategy is that there are differing levels of dysfunction and behavioral disturbance in children and adolescents, and parents have different needs and preferences regarding the type, intensity and mode of assistance they may require. The multilevel approach of Triple P follows the principle of selecting the 'minimally sufficient' intervention as a guiding principle to serving the needs of parents in order to maximise efficiency, contain costs, avoid over-servicing, and ensure that the program becomes widely available to parents in the community. The model avoids a one-size-fits-all approach by using evidence-based tailored variants and flexible delivery options (e.g., web, group, individual, over the phone, self-directed) targeting diverse groups of parents. The multidisciplinary nature of the program involves the utilisation of the existing professional workforce in the task of promoting competent parenting.

The Pathways Triple P-Positive Parenting Program

Pathways Triple P (PTP) is a specific variant within the larger Triple P system of intervention designed specifically for families with indicated risk factors for child abuse or neglect. When compared to other Triple P variants, the main variation of PTP is that it hones in on parental attributional and anger processes that place parents at risk of child maltreatment. Although the content of Pathways Triple P is relevant for all parents, this variant of the Triple P system has been developed as an intensive intervention program for parents who have difficulty regulating their emotions and as a result are considered at risk of physically or emotionally abusing their children. Consequently, it is viewed as an intervention for clients who are involved in the child protection system. Parents are generally referred to Pathways Triple P if the initial intake assessment and clinical interview reveal the following: (1) presence of coercive or harsh parenting or other elevated scores on standardized measures such as the Parenting Scale (Arnold, O'Leary, Wolff, & Acher, 1993) or the Parent's Attributions for Child's Behaviour Measure (Pidgeon & Sanders, 2004); (2) presence of dysfunctional attributions; (3) parent reports difficulty implementing positive parenting skills after exposure to either Group or Standard Triple P; (4) suspected or substantiated child abuse and neglect; (5) parent is literate and willing to participate.

Pathways Triple P targets the attributional processes parents have towards their child's and their own behaviour, as well as parental anger management deficits. Parents are taught a variety of skills aimed at challenging and countering their maladaptive attributions for parent-child interactions and to change any negative parenting practices they are currently using in line with these attributions. The attributional retraining strategies focus on teaching parents how to counter their misattributions regarding their child's negative behaviour, and their negative parenting behaviour towards their child. This involves teaching parents how to challenge their misattributions and generate more benign attributions regarding their child's negative behaviour and generate less anger-justifying attributions for their own negative behaviour. These sessions teach parents how to counter and alter not only their anger-intensifying attributional style for their child's behaviour, but also their anger justifying attributions for their negative parenting behaviour.

As described in Table 7.1, the Pathways Triple P intervention is typically delivered in conjunction with Group Triple P. The PTP specific components consist of four 2-h sessions where parents participate in discussion and exercises designed to orientate them towards the factors which are placing them at risk of maltreatment. Parents are asked to identify the reasons why they can react in negative ways towards children, the impact of negative or harsh discipline practices on children, and the causes of their own negative behaviour towards their child. The exercises are also designed to teach parents how to prevent anger escalation and negative parenting practices; a process which involves teaching parents to challenge and control their anger-intensifying attributions and mistaken explanations for their child's misbehaviour. Parents are also introduced to the emotion of anger, its physical effects, and parents

Table 7.1 The pathways Triple P system of Intervention

Pathways Triple P	Group Triple P sessions			
Intake session	Session 1	Session 2	Session 3	Session 4
Provide overview of program	Principles of positive parenting	**Parent-child relationship enhancement skills**	**Manage misbehaviour**	**Preventing problems in high-risk situations**
Explain what's involved	Identifying causes of child behaviour	Spending quality time	Establishing ground rules	Planning and advanced preparation
Obtain commitment	Monitoring children's behaviour	Talking with children	Using directed discussion	Discussing ground rules for specific situations
Conduct intake interview	Monitoring own behaviour	Physical affection	Using planned ignoring	Selecting engaging activities
Complete assessment booklet 1	Setting developmentally appropriate goals	**Encouraging desirable behaviour**	Giving clean calm instructions	Providing incentives
	Setting practice tasks	Giving descriptive praise	Using logical consequences	Providing consequences
	Self-evaluation of strengths and weaknesses	Giving non-verbal attention	Using quiet time	Holding follow-up discussions
	Setting personal goals for change	Providing engaging activities	Using time-out	
		Teaching new skills and behaviours		
		Setting a good example		
		Using ask, say, do		
		Using behaviour charts		

Pathways Triple P sessions				Group Triple P session
Module 1	Module 1	Module 2	Module 2	
Session 1	Session 2	Session 1	Session 2	Closure session
Parent traps	**How to get out of a parent trap**	**Understanding anger**	**Coping with anger**	Family survival tips
Identifying parent traps	Understanding the reasons parents get caught in parent traps	Recognising and understanding anger	Catching unhelpful thoughts	Phasing out the program
Understanding impact of own behaviour on children	Thought switching	Stopping anger from escalating	Developing personal anger coping statements	Strategies for maintaining change
Identifying dysfunctional attributions	Breaking out of a parent trap	Abdominal breathing and relaxation techniques	Challenging unhelpful thoughts	Problem solving for the future
		Planning pleasurable activities	Developing coping plans for high risk situations	Future goals
				Complete assessment booklet 2

are provided with a variety of techniques and strategies for becoming physically and mentally relaxed. Parents are also introduced to cognitive therapy concepts as they apply to anger management, which includes catching unhelpful thoughts, developing alternative coping statements in arousing situations, and challenging thoughts that lead to aggressive responses. Identifying high-risk anger situations and developing coping plans to manage anger in these situations are also covered.

Parents receive a copy of two workbooks, *Avoiding Parent Traps, and Coping with Anger*, which outline the principles taught in the two modules (focusing on the risk factors countering parents' misattributions for parent-child interactions and anger management). These parent workbooks have been published together with the existing practitioner's workbook (see Pidgeon & Sanders, 2005; Sanders & Pidgeon, 2005).

Evidence for Pathways Triple P

Several studies have demonstrated the effectiveness of Pathways Triple P in improving parenting practices and reducing the risk of child maltreatment. Sanders et al. (2004) randomly assigned 98 parents experiencing significant difficulties in managing their own anger in their interactions with their preschool-aged children to either Pathways Triple P which included attributional retraining, or a standard version of Triple P that provided training in parenting skills alone. At post-intervention, both conditions were associated with lower levels of observed and parent-reported disruptive child behaviour, lower levels of parent-reported dysfunctional parenting, greater parental self-efficacy, less parental distress, relationship conflict and similarly high levels of consumer satisfaction. Whereas the Pathways intervention showed a significantly greater short-term improvement on measures of negative parental attributions for children's misbehaviour, potential for child abuse and unrealistic parental expectation, at 6-month follow-up both conditions showed similarly positive outcomes on all measures of child abuse potential, parent practices, parental adjustment, and child behaviour and adjustment. Importantly, the Pathways intervention resulted in sustained and greater change in negative parental attributions.

In further support of the efficacy of the Pathways intervention, Wiggins, Sofronoff, and Sanders (2009) examined the effects of Pathways Triple P on parents who met the inclusion criteria of borderline to clinically significant relationship disturbance and child emotional and behavioural problems. Participants were randomly allocated into either an intervention or wait-list control group. The intervention was delivered in a group format for 9 weeks and consisted of parent skills training and cognitive behaviour therapy targeting negative attributions for child behaviour. Participants in the Pathways condition reported significantly greater improvement in parent-child relationship quality from pre- to post-intervention compared to participants in the control group with benefits maintained at 3-month follow-up. Participants in the intervention condition also reported a significant reduction in the use of dysfunctional parenting practices (laxness, verbosity and over-reactivity), blameworthy and intentional attributions for child behaviour and child externalising behaviour problems from pre- to post-intervention with reductions maintained at 3-month follow-up.

In a ground breaking study, Prinz, Sanders, Shapiro, Whitaker, and Lutzker (2009) examined the value of a public health approach to the prevention of child maltreatment in what was known as the US Triple P system population trial. Eighteen counties in South Carolina were randomly assigned to receive either the Triple P system or services-as-usual. Professional training for an existing workforce (over 600 service providers) in the Triple P counties was provided, and universal media and communication strategies pertaining to positive parenting were deployed via local newspapers, radio, school newsletters, mass mailings to family households, publicity at community events, and website information. These strategies implementing the system's universal facet are intended to destigmatize parenting and family support, make effective parenting strategies readily accessible to all parents, and facilitate help-seeking by parents who need higher intensity intervention.

Large improvements in the Triple P counties were found in three measured outcomes: substantiated child maltreatment, child out-of home placements, and child maltreatment injuries. The findings came from three separate sources: the Child Protective Services, the foster care system, and the hospital system respectively. This study is the first to randomize geographical areas and show the preventive impact of evidence-based parenting interventions on child maltreatment at a population level. This population trial demonstrated that offering parenting and family support via a broad system like Triple P, without singling out parents because of risk characteristics, could actually help prevent maltreatment and related problems.

The cumulative evidence clearly supports the efficacy and robustness of a tailored intervention for parents at risk of harming their children. However, the limited reach of most parenting programs ensures that these programs make little impact on prevalence rates of social and emotional problems of children and child maltreatment at a population level. The limited impact of available parenting interventions on children's problems at a population level underpins the need for implementation of Triple P as a public health system of parenting support and intervention (Sanders, 2012; Sanders & Murphy-Brennan, 2010).

The Implementation of Pathways Triple P Within the Child Welfare System

Pathways Triple P is applicable and relevant to the child welfare system services in several ways, including: (a) prevention of child maltreatment; (b) prevention of children's social, emotional, and behavioural problems; (c) family-based treatment of children's mental health problems for those who have endured abuse or neglect; (d) strengthening the parenting competence and confidence of foster parents; (e) treating parents who have maltreated their children or are at high risk of doing so; and

(f) assisting parents who seek voluntary services after having been referred for suspected maltreatment that did not rise to the level of substantiation or mandatory action. Although existing evidence supports the fit and acceptability of Pathways Triple P within the child welfare system (Petra & Kohl, 2010), an effective parenting support strategy needs to address two significant challenges within a robust implementation framework in order to succeed.

First, parenting interventions need to be delivered in a nonstigmatizing way. Currently, parenting interventions are perceived by many vulnerable/at risk parents as being for inadequate, ignorant, failed or wayward parents. To be effective, a whole-of-population approach to parenting support has to emphasise the universal relevance of parenting assistance so that the larger community of parents embraces and supports parents being involved in parenting programs. A nonstigmatized example is found in prenatal (birth) classes, which parents across a broad array of economic and cultural groups (and family configurations) find useful and do not perceive as stigmatizing.

Second, parenting support needs to be flexible with respect to delivery formats (e.g., group, individual, online) to meet the needs of parents in the child welfare system. Having every family receive an intensive intervention at a single location is not only cost ineffective but also unnecessary and undesirable from a family's perspective. Foster, Prinz, Sanders, and Shapiro (2008) estimated that the infrastructure costs associated with the implementation of the Triple P system in the US was $12 per participant, a cost that could be recovered in a single year by as little as a 10 % reduction in the rate of abuse and neglect. Flexibility would also make the intervention useful for mandated services, parenting support for foster and adoptive parents, and support for families within the child welfare system who are not involved with child protective services.

Case Study: James Family

Referral problem: The James family was referred to the first author to participate in Pathways Triple P by a social worker because of ongoing concerns regarding the parents' management of their son's uncooperative and aggressive behaviour. Ryan (aged 7 years) was the eldest child of Jane (36 years) and Edan (40 years). He also had a younger sister Amy (aged 5 years). On presentation, Jane described a recurring pattern of defiant, uncooperative, and aggressive behaviour that often (daily) escalated daily into physical aggression (pushing and punching) and verbal abuse (mainly threats of harm) towards his younger sister Amy. These conflicts usually occurred as a result of Amy trying to have a turn at using the family computer, game or to watch a specific TV program.

The social worker was particularly concerned about the father's coercive and ineffective methods of managing Ryan's behaviours and thought a parenting program may assist and prevent further involvement of the child protection system. Jane reported frequent (three to four times weekly) heated conflict between Ryan and his father in which the father used a variety of coercive tactics to get Ryan to cooperate. These behaviours included using verbal and gestural threats of physical punishment (closed fist), occasional episodes of severe physical publishment (grabbing around the throats, hitting Ryan with a leather strap), verbal abuse involving putdowns (*stupid, idiot*), and attempts to shame and humiliate Ryan in front of neighbours and his school friends (*You're such a girl. Not such a tough guy now are you?*). The father's conflict with Ryan often resulted in disagreements between the parents that escalated to shouting as Jane tried to become the peace maker and get Edan to calm down and to stop shouting at Ryan.

Relevant history and assessment: An intake interview with both parents and separately with the two children revealed that Edan had been a sergeant-major in the army and had become used to army style discipline since age 18. He expected his own kids to obey his commands immediately without question. He reported having a father who was a bully and unloving who used the belt to get his four brothers and himself to cooperate. Both parents agreed that their current methods of dealing with Ryan's behaviour were not working but were at a loss to know what else to do. Resistance was minimal and rapport was quickly established with the couple.

The clinical assessment comprised both parents completing a routine assessment package recommended for use in the delivery of Pathways Triple P (Sanders & Pidgeon, 2005) involving a selection of standardised measures and a structured within clinic family observation session involving both parents, as well as an interview with both Ryan and Amy. The observation tasks involved a free play activity (5 min), a joint parent and child task (5 min), a parent busy task (2 min), and a tidy away task (5 min). These tasks aimed to capture everyday family activities that could lead to conflict.

The assessment revealed a number of factors potentially contributing to the development or maintenance of Ryan's disruptive behaviour, including accidental rewards for misbehaviour (via attention), using vague, repetitive instructions, voice escalation by the father in particular during tidy up task, and a lack of positive engagement or attention for cooperative behaviour. The Eyberg Child Behavior Inventory (ECBI; Eyberg & Pincus, 1999) revealed that Ryan scored in the clinically elevated range on both the intensity and frequency subscales. Out of a possible 36 problem behaviours, 28 were seen as problems by Edan and 24 by Jane. On the Parenting Scale (PS; Arnold et al., 1993) Edan scored in the clinically elevated range for both overreactivity and verbosity and Jane for laxness and verbosity. These findings confirmed verbal reports and observational data showing that both parents had a dysfunctional parenting style. On the Parent Problem Checklist (PPC; Dadds & Powell, 1991) both Ryan and Jane's responses revealed frequent disagreement and arguing about parenting and discipline issues although on the Relationship Quality Index (RQI; Norton, 1983) there was a relatively high level of marital satisfaction.

On the measure of Parents Attributions for Misbehaviour (PACBM; Pidgeon & Sanders, 2004), Edan had a strong negative attributional style that supported quite punitive methods of discipline. Specifically he tended to blame Ryan for his misbehaviour and his attributions tended to be stable and negative. Jane's responses on the PACBM were in the nonclinical range. On the Parental Anger Inventory

(PAI, Hansen & Sedlar, 1998) Edan scored in the clinically elevated range on both the problem and intensity scale. Other notable findings were that both Edan and Jane were clinically elevated on the measures of depression and stress on the Depression Anxiety Stress Scales (DASS; Lovibond & Lovibond, 1995).

In summary, it was hypothesised that Ryan's conduct problem occurred in a context of significant family conflict and disharmony where the father's inadequate and highly coercive attempts to discipline Ryan were being maintained by an irrational belief system and family history that supported his use of corporal punishment and retribution, and intermittent success in stopping Ryan's aggressive behaviour. The father's attempts to deal with Ryan lead to frequent conflict with Jane. Jane's consequent compensatory behaviour resulted in inconsistent follow through. Edan had considerable anger management problems, and quite high stress likely resulting from a long history of living with family conflict. Of note, Edan reported considerable parent conflict in his family of origin. Both parents were somewhat depressed and overwhelmed by their struggles in dealing with problems parenting their children. But despite this conflict, both parents reported satisfaction with their marital relationship. This type of family with the combination of coercive parenting difficulties, attributional bias, and anger management problems, was deemed highly suitable for the Pathways Triple P intervention.

Description of the Intervention: Jane and Edan agreed to participate in Group Pathways Triple P with eight other parents. Jane and Edan were the only married couple (all other parents were a mixed gender group of lone parents). Six mothers and two fathers. As per Fig. 7.1, all parents were required to attend the four Group Triple P sessions where they were introduced to the 17 core positive parenting skills, and also to attend the four PTP sessions covering attribution retraining and anger management. The specific session content is described in Table 7.1. The group program made use of a mixture of brief didactic presentations of core content, group discussions, viewing DVD video demonstrations of specific positive parenting skills, role plays to practise specific skills taught and the setting of between session homework assignments.

Using a self-regulation framework each parent was asked to set their own goals and determine which of the skills introduced in the session were particularly relevant and meaningful to them. These goals were revised periodically throughout the intervention as new content was introduced. After the initial session, Edan's goals were to: (1) reduce the number of times per week he shouted at Ryan; (2) reduce the number of days that he lost his temper with anyone in the family; and (3) work with Jane to develop a parenting plan both could use in dealing with Ryan's disobedience and aggressive behaviour. From the initial session Edan realised the current situation was not working and he wanted to try a different way of dealing with the problem. Jane's goals were to: (1) stop criticising Edan for his poor parenting; (2) spend more positive time with Ryan; and (3) try to be more consistent in dealing with Ryan's aggression. After the intake interview Jane had realised that stepping in and rescuing Ryan from his father's anger was leading to very inconsistent ways of dealing with the problem and that they needed to work as a team.

Table 7.2 Evaluation of intervention outcomes[a]

Measures	Jane			Moved to normal range?	Edan			Moved to normal range?
	Time 1	Time 2	Time 3		Time 1	Time 2	Time 3	
ECBI intensity	**145**	112	114	Y	**152**	121	115	Y
ECBI problem	**26**	6	7	Y	**24**	12	8	Y
PS laxness	**3.2**	2.9	2.8	Y	**3.0**	2.8	2.4	Y
PS overreactivity	**3.8**	2.3	2.3	Y	**4.4**	3.0	2.8	Y
PS verbosity	3.0	2.5	2.4	N	**3.9**	3.3	3.2	N
PPC problem	**7.0**	5.0	4.0	Y	**8.0**	4.0	2.0	Y
PPC extent	**5.6**	3.4	3.0	Y	**6.1**	3.0	2.8	Y
PACBM	2.8	2.6	2.1	N	**4.2**	3.2	2.8	Y
DASS depression	**22**	14	9	Y	**18**	8	6	Y
DASS anxiety	6.0	6.0	5.0	N	7.0	7.0	5.0	N
DASS stress	**26**	15	15	Y	**24**	18	7	Y

[a]Bold indicates the score was in the clinical range at pre intervention

Table 7.2 shows the effects of the Pathways Triple P intervention on each scale. Inspection of Table 7.2 indicates that Jane's scores moved into the normal range on both subscales of the ECBI (Intensity and Problem); the Laxness and Overreactivity subscales of the Parenting Scale; both subscales of the Parent Problem Checklist (Problem and Extent); and each of the subscales of the DASS except for the Anxiety subscale. As for Edan, Table 7.2 indicates that he moved from the clinical to the nonclinical range in all outcome measures except for the Verbosity subscale of the PS, and the Anxiety subscale of the DASS. Overall, therefore, the intervention was very successful for both parents. The main findings were that both Edan and Jane developed a calmer, less explosive way of dealing with Ryan's misbehaviour. This in turn prevented conflict escalation with the mother and considerably reduced the level of conduct problems in Ryan. There were three critical moments during the intervention that were identified as major transition points. The first occurred prior to the first group session when the father realised that the approach he was using simply was not working. Prior to this he had not really confronted the issue of whether his parenting strategies actually worked in teaching Ryan to control his behaviour. The second transition point occurred in session one when the parents participated in an exercise that involved viewing video clips depicting possible reasons for a child behaviour problem (Exercise on *Causes of Misbehaviour*). There were three examples of parenting practices that Edan particularly related to (escalation traps, lack of attention for desired behaviour, and conflict between parents). The third transition point occurred in the first module of Pathways in the Module on *Avoiding Parent Traps*. It was a major insight to Edan when he recognised these traps were self-defeating and perpetuating the problem. Edan also found the last two sessions on anger management useful, but mainly to consolidate what he had already learned. By that stage, he had become much better at giving clear, calm instructions to Ryan and had learned to back up with more effective consequences (not threatening). He rarely became angry anymore. The first exercise in the

Avoiding Parent Traps module requires the parent to identify whether they are in any self-defeating parent traps. Edan recognised he was in two such traps: the *YOU'RE DOING IT ON PURPOSE* trap and the *YOU MADE ME DO IT* trap. This exercise involved sessions of attribution retraining. By the conclusion of the Pathways Triple P intervention, Edan's learning of positive parenting skills, and in particular the use of quiet time and time-out, enabled him to provide consistent consequences more calmly for behaviour he did not like, without the abusive escalation evident prior to the intervention. If the situation had not improved, or was making gradual improvements, one of three possibilities would have been considered: (1) Continue same treatment if progress is being made with extra sessions; (2) Explore reasons for non-response and address with other modules within the Enhanced Triple P suite of intervention (e.g., partner support, coping skills, more home feedback/coaching); or (3) Consider referral to specialist mental health service for child, parent, or both. In the current case, no such additional action was required and the intervention was associated with high levels of consumer satisfaction.

Conclusions and Implications

There is considerable scope for parenting interventions to improve children's developmental outcomes for any mental health, physical health, or social problem where potentially modifiable parenting and family variables have been causally implicated in the onset, maintenance, exacerbation or relapse of a problem. However, despite the weight of evidence indicating that parenting programs are among the most efficacious and cost-effective interventions available to promote the mental health and wellbeing of children and adolescents (Biglan, Flay, Embry, & Sandler, 2012), the majority of families who might benefit do not participate in parenting programs. The Triple P system adopted a public health approach to the delivery of universal parenting support with the goal of increasing parental self-efficacy, knowledge and competence in the use of skills that promote positive development in children and adolescents. This change in focus has enabled millions more children around the world to experience the benefits of positive parenting and family environments that promote healthy development and as a consequence fewer children have developed behavioral and emotional problems or episodes of maltreatment.

When parents are empowered with the tools for personal change they require to parent their children positively, the resulting benefits for children, parents and the community at large are immense. The Triple P system is the only parenting program shown to reduce the population level prevalence of child maltreatment. If fully implemented as a public health whole of community initiative it would reduce the level of child maltreatment. Effective dissemination needs to be based on a public health compatible system of interventions. Parents and service providers need intervention systems such as Triple P that transport readily from one setting to another, to better address the needs of children and families who touch the child welfare system.

References

Arnold, D. S., O'Leary, S. G., Wolff, L. S., & Acher, M. M. (1993). The parenting scale: A measure of dysfunctional parenting in discipline situations. *Psychological Assessment, 5*, 137–144.

Australian Institute of Health and Welfare [AIHW]. (2005). *Child Protection Australia 2003–2004* (Child welfare series no. 36). Canberra, Australia: Australian Institute of Health and Welfare.

Australian Institute of Health and Welfare [AIHW]. (2008). *Child Protection Australia 2006–2007* (Child welfare series no. 43). Canberra, Australia: Australian Institute of Health and Welfare.

Azar, S. T., & Weinzierl, B. S. (2005). Child maltreatment and childhood injury research: A cognitive behavioural approach. *Journal of Pediatric Psychology, 30*, 598–614.

Barkley, R. A., Edwards, G., Laneri, M., Fletcher, K., & Metevia, L. (2001). The efficacy of problem-solving communication training alone, behavior management training alone, and their combination for parent-adolescent conflict in teenagers with ADHD and ODD. *Journal of Consulting and Clinical Psychology, 69*(6), 926–941.

Biglan, A., Flay, B. R., Embry, D. D., & Sandler, I. N. (2012). The critical role of nurturing environments for promoting human well-being. *American Psychologist, 67*(4), 257–271.

Brestan, E. V., & Eyberg, S. (1998). Effective psychosocial treatments of conduct-disordered children and adolescents: 29 years, 82 studies, and 5,272 kids. *Journal of Clinical Child Psychology, 27*, 180–189.

Collins, W. A., Maccoby, E. E., Steinberg, L., Hetherington, E. M., & Bornstein, M. H. (2000). Contemporary research on parenting: The case for nature and nurture. *American Psychologist, 55*, 218–232.

Connell, A. M., Dishion, T. J., Yasui, M., & Kavanagh, K. (2007). An adaptive approach to family intervention: Linking engagement in family-centered intervention to reductions in adolescent problem behavior. *Journal of Consulting and Clinical Psychology, 75*(4), 568–579.

Dadds, M. R., & Powell, M. B. (1991). The relationship of interparental conflict and global marital adjustment to aggression, anxiety, and immaturity in aggressive and nonclinic children. *Journal of Abnormal Child Psychology, 19*, 553–567.

Dekovic, M., Janssens, J. M. A. M., & Van As, N. M. C. (2003). Family predictors of antisocial behavior in adolescence. *Family Process, 42*(2), 223–235.

Dishion, T. J., & Andrews, D. W. (1995). Preventing escalation in problem behaviors with high-risk young adolescents: Immediate and 1-year outcomes. *Journal of Consulting and Clinical Psychology, 63*(4), 538–548.

Dix, T., Reinhold, D. P., & Zambarano, R. J. (1990). Mothers' judgments in moments of anger. *Merrill-Palmer Quarterly, 36*, 465–486.

Dix, T., Ruble, D. N., & Zambarano, R. J. (1989). Mothers' implicit theories of discipline: Child effects, parent effects, and the attribution process. *Child Development, 60*, 1373–1390.

Dretzke, J., Davenport, C., Frew, E., Barlow, J., Stewart-Brown, S., et al. (2009). The clinical effectiveness of different parenting programmes for children with conduct problems: A systematic review of randomised controlled trials. *Child & Adolescent Psychiatric Mental Health, 3*, 1–10.

Eyberg, S. M., & Pincus, D. (1999). *Eyberg child behavior inventory and Sutter-Eyberg student behavior inventory – Revised: Professional manual*. Odessa, FL: Psychological Assessment Resources.

Foster, E. M., Prinz, R. J., Sanders, M. R., & Shapiro, C. J. (2008). The costs of a public health infrastructure for delivering parenting and family support. *Children and Youth Services Review, 30*(5), 493–501.

de Graaf, I., Speetjens, P., Smit, F., de Wolff, M., & Tavecchio, L. (2008a). Effectiveness of the Triple P Positive Parenting Program on parenting: A meta-analysis. *Family Relations, 57*, 553–566.

de Graaf, I., Speetjens, P., Smit, F., de Wolff, M., & Tavecchio, L. (2008b). Effectiveness of the Triple P Positive Parenting Program on behavioral problems in children: A meta-analysis. *Behavior Modification, 32*(5), 714–735.

Grusec, J. E., & Mammone, N. (1995). Features and sources of parents' attributions about themselves and their children. In I. N. Eisenberg (Ed.), *Social development: Review of personality and social psychology* (Vol. 15, pp. 49–73). Thousand Oaks, CA: Sage.

Hansen, D. J., & Sedlar, G. (1998). *Manual for the PAI: The parental anger inventory*. Lincoln, NE: University of Nebraska, Clinical Psychology Training Program.

James, J. E. (1994). Foundation education as a means of disseminating behavioural innovation to non-psychologists. *Behavior Change, 11*, 19–26.

Kazdin, A. E. (2005). *Parent management training: Treatment for oppositional, aggressive, and antisocial behavior in children and adolescents*. New York: Oxford University Press.

Kazdin, A. E., & Blase, S. L. (2011). Rebooting psychotherapy research and practice to reduce the burden of mental illness. *Perspectives in Psychological Science, 6*, 21–37.

Kolko, D. J. (1996). Clinical monitoring of treatment course in child physical abuse: Psychometric characteristics and treatment comparisons. *Child Abuse & Neglect, 20*, 23–43.

Kolko, D. J., & Swenson, C. C. (2002). *Assessing and treating physically abused children and their families: A cognitive-behavioural approach*. Thousand Oaks, CA: Sage Publications.

Kotch, J. B., Lewis, T., Hussey, J. M., English, D., Thompson, R., & Litrownik, A. J. (2008). Importance of early neglect for childhood aggression. *Pediatrics, 121*, 725–731.

Lansford, M. J., Berlin, D., Bates, J., & Pettit, G. S. (2007). Early physical abuse and later violent delinquency: A prospective longitudinal study. *Child Maltreatment, 12*, 233–245.

Lovibond, S. H., & Lovibond, P. F. (1995). *Manual for the depression anxiety stress scales* (2nd ed.). Sydney, Australia: Psychology Foundation Monograph.

Maas, C., Herrenkohl, T. I., & Sousa, C. (2008). Review of research on child maltreatment and violence in youth. *Trauma, Violence & Abuse, 9*, 56–67.

Mammen, O. K., Kolko, D. J., & Pilkonis, P. A. (2002). Negative affect and parental aggression in child physical abuse. *Child Abuse & Neglect, 26*(4), 407–424.

Mason, W. A., Kosterman, R., Hawkins, J. D., Haggerty, K. P., & Spoth, R. L. (2003). Reducing adolescents' growth in substance use and delinquency: Randomized trial effects of a parent-training prevention intervention. *Prevention Science, 4*(3), 203–212.

McHolm, A. E., MacMillan, H. L., & Jamieson, E. (2003). The relationship between childhood physical abuse and suicidality among depressed women: Results from a community sample. *American Journal of Psychiatry, 160*, 933–938.

Miller, L. R., & Azar, S. T. (1996). The pervasiveness of maladaptive attributions in mothers at-risk for child abuse. *Family Violence and Sexual Assault Bulletin, 12*, 31–37.

Milner, J. S. (2003). Social information processing in high-risk and physically abusive parents. *Child Abuse & Neglect, 27*, 7–20.

National Research Council and Institute of Medicine. (2009). Preventing mental, emotional, and behavioural disorders among young people: Progress and possibilities. Committee on the prevention of mental disorders and substance abuse among children, youth, and young adults: Research advances and promising interventions. In M. E. O'Connell, T. Boat, & K. E. Warner (Eds.), *Board on children, youth, and families, division of behavioural and social sciences and education*. Washington, DC: The National Academies Press.

Nix, R. L., Pinderhughes, E. E., Dodge, K. A., Bates, J. E., Pettit, G. S., & McFayden-Ketchum, S. A. (1999). The relation between mothers' hostile attribution tendencies and children's externalizing behaviour problems: The mediating role of mothers' harsh discipline strategies. *Child Development, 70*, 896–909.

Norton, R. (1983). Measuring marital quality: A critical look at the dependent variable. *Journal of Marriage and the Family, 45*, 141–151.

Nowak, C., & Heinrichs, N. (2008). A comprehensive meta-analysis of Triple P-Positive Parenting Program using hierarchical linear modeling: Effectiveness and moderating variables. *Clinical Child and Family Psychology Review, 11*, 114–144.

Petra, M., & Kohl, P. (2010). Pathways Triple P and the child welfare system: A promising fit. *Children and Youth Services Review, 32*, 611–618.

Pidgeon, A. M., & Sanders, M. R. (2004). *The parent's attributions for child behaviour measure*. Brisbane, Australia: The University of Queensland.

Pidgeon, A. M., & Sanders, M. R. (2005). *Pathways to positive parenting. Module 1: Avoiding parent traps*. Brisbane, Australia: Triple P International.

Pidgeon, A. M., & Sanders, M. R. (2009). Attributions, parental anger and risk of maltreatment. *International Journal of Child Health and Human Development, 2*(1), 57–69.

Prinz, R. J., Sanders, M. R., Shapiro, C. J., Whitaker, D. J., & Lutzker, J. R. (2009). Population-based prevention of child maltreatment: The US Triple P system population trial. *Prevention Science, 10*, 1–12.

Rodriguez, C. M., & Green, A. J. (1997). Parenting stress and anger expression as predictors of child abuse potential. *Child Abuse & Neglect, 21*, 366–377.

Sanders, M. R. (2012). Development, evaluation, and multinational dissemination of the Triple P-Positive Parenting Program. *Annual Review of Clinical Psychology, 8*, 345–379.

Sanders, M. R., Baker, S., & Turner, K. M. T. (2012). A randomized controlled trial evaluating the efficacy of Triple P Online with parents of children with early onset conduct problems. *Behaviour Research and Therapy, 50*, 675–684.

Sanders, M. R., & Murphy-Brennan, M. (2010). Creating conditions for success beyond the professional training environment. *Clinical Psychology: Science & Practice, 17*, 31–35.

Sanders, M. R., Pidgeon, A., Gravestock, F., Connors, M. D., Brown, S., & Young, R. M. (2004). Does parental attributional retraining and anger management enhance the effects of the Triple P- Positive Parenting Program with parents at risk of child maltreatment? *Behavior Therapy, 35*(3), 513–535.

Sanders, M. R., & Pidgeon, A. M. (2005). *Practitioner's manual for pathways Triple P.* Brisbane, Australia: Triple P International.

Serketich, W. J., & Dumas, J. E. (1996). The effectiveness of behavioral parent training to modify antisocial behavior in children: A meta-analysis. *Behavior Therapy, 27*, 171–186.

Spoth, R. L., Redmond, C., & Shin, C. (1998). Direct and indirect latent-variable parenting outcomes of two universal family-focused preventive interventions: Extending a public health-oriented research base. *Journal of Consulting and Clinical Psychology, 66*(2), 385–399.

U.S. Department of Health and Human Services. (2008). Administration on children youth and families. In *Child maltreatment 2006*. Washington, DC: US Government Printing Office.

Wekerle, C., & Wolfe, D. A. (1998). *Windows for preventing child and partner abuse: Early childhood and adolescence*. Washington, DC: American Psychological Association.

Widom, C. S. (1999). Posttraumatic stress disorder in abused and neglected children growing up. *American Journal of Psychiatry, 156*, 1223–1229.

Widom, C. S., Dumont, K. A., & Czaja, S. J. (2007). A prospective investigation of major depressive disorder and comorbidity in abused and neglected children grown up. *Archives of General Psychiatry, 64*, 49–56.

Wiggins, T. L., Sofronoff, K., & Sanders, M. R. (2009). Pathways Triple P-Positive Parenting Program: Effects on parent-child relationships and child behavior problems. *Family Process, 48*, 517–530.

World Health Organisation. (2009). *Preventing violence through the development of safe, stable and nurturing relationships between children and their parents and caregivers* (Series of briefings on violence prevention: The evidence). Geneva, Switzerland: Author.

Chapter 8
Parent-Child Interaction Therapy for Maltreated Children

Anthony Urquiza and Susan Timmer

There are many pathways that drive a family toward physical abuse – some of these pathways are easy to discern; while others are complex and reflect a series of interconnected behaviors, attitudes, and expectations. It has previously been argued that escalating coercive exchanges and harsh disciplinary strategies are primary contributors – and perhaps the most proximal – to physically abusive parent-child relationships (Cicchetti & Valentino, 2006; Urquiza & McNeil, 1996). It is suggested that negative coercive exchanges focus many, if not most, of the parent-child interactions that eventually lead to parental use of aggression to secure compliance (Milner, 2000). Chronic failure to comply with parental commands – even for common child expectations such as taking out the trash, doing homework, washing dishes – can lead to both reinforcement of negative attitudes about the child and increased anger with the child. Eventually, repeated instances of reinforced negative attitudes and continued non-compliance lead to parental aggression – as a means to secure child compliance and/or as an expression of parental frustration.

Neglectful parent-child dyads, like physically abusive, show a similar deficit in positive interactions, though their interactions typically are not characterized by the negative coercive cycle (Wilson, Rack, Shi, & Norris, 2008). In a meta-analysis of over 30 studies, Wilson and colleagues (2008) found that neglectful dyads could be discriminated from non-maltreated dyads by their lack of involvement, or detachment from each other, unlike physically abusive dyads.

To address the issue of child maltreatment, it is therefore essential to shift the fundamental characteristics of the negative coercive relationship and the detached relationship to contain a stable pattern of positive reciprocal cognitions and behaviors. This is an important intervention element, as both parent and child cognitions need

A. Urquiza, Ph.D. (✉) • S. Timmer, Ph.D.
CAARE Diagnostic and Treatment Center, Department of Pediatrics, University of California at Davis Children's Hospital, 3671 Business Dr., Sacramento, CA 95820, USA
e-mail: anthony.urquiza@ucdmc.ucdavis.edu; susan.timmer@ucdmc.ucdavis.edu

S. Timmer and A. Urquiza (eds.), *Evidence-Based Approaches for the Treatment of Maltreated Children*, Child Maltreatment 3, DOI 10.1007/978-94-007-7404-9_8,
© Springer Science+Business Media Dordrecht 2014

to be changed, as well as the sequences of behaviors that guide and are produced by these cognitions (i.e., the coercive cycle). So, the task of intervening with maltreated children should have several goals: improving parenting skills, decreasing child behavioral problems (i.e., increase in child compliance), and increasing the frequency of positive parent-child interactions. One evidence-based intervention that provides these elements is Parent-Child Interaction Therapy (PCIT), an intensive parenting intervention, classified by Chambless and Ollendick (2000) as an empirically supported treatment. When considering providing PCIT to maltreated children, one might legitimately ask, "How could a behaviorally-oriented, evidence-based, parenting program benefit a child who has been maltreated? What about the trauma?" On the following pages, we describe ways in which PCIT can benefit certain types of children and families who have experienced maltreatment – especially when children exhibit significant behavioral disruption. Following this, there is a discussion of the role in PCIT in addressing trauma symptoms in young children. The application of PCIT to young traumatized children is included because many maltreated children exhibit trauma symptoms; and because development of positive parent-child relationships may be one of the most effective and naturalistic trauma interventions for young children. Finally, we provide a description of a 'typical' case of an abused and severely traumatized young boy – incorporating many of the elements of the PCIT protocol (e.g., results of pre- and post-treatment assessments, development of treatment objectives, examples of efforts to enhance parent-child relationship quality, strategies to manage non-compliant behavior, and inclusion of coaching text from a PCIT treatment session). The goals of this chapter are to inform the reader of the value of PCIT in meeting the unique treatment needs of maltreating parent-child dyads, provide an overview of the evidence supporting PCIT with maltreating families, explain some of the mechanisms by which PCIT can benefit both abusive parents and maltreated children, and discuss the value of significant positive relationships in reducing child trauma symptoms in young children.

Theoretical Foundation

PCIT (Eyberg & Robinson, 1982) is one of several programs that emerged from Constance Hanf's lab at Oregon Health Sciences University in the late 1960s. Hanf's two-phase model was founded on the principles of operant conditioning, believing that through strategic social reinforcement it would be possible to change caregivers and children to modify maladaptive parent-child interactions (Reitman & McMahon, 2012). While focused on increasing discrete behaviors like parent's attention to the child and praise, Hanf, and subsequently Eyberg, also incorporated attachment theory's belief in the importance of maternal warmth and responsiveness (e.g., Ainsworth, 1979), Diana Baumrind's work (1966, 1967) which conceptualized healthy parenting as authoritative, with clear communication and firm limit setting, as well as the work of Virginia Axline (1947) and Bernard Guerney (1964), which promoted non-directive parental warmth and acceptance (Eyberg, 2004). Using Hanf's (1969) ideas of *in vivo* parenting and use the structure of a 'coaching' paradigm, Eyberg's innovation was to break down these skills into even more discrete parts – into specific verbalizations, which were behaviors she could easily teach parents. When combined together, the discrete behaviors could foster the construction of less tangible skills employed by child therapists, like nurturing, warmth, and responsiveness, and the skills needed for managing children's difficult behavior (like selective attention, positive reinforcement for compliance). Hanf's model was built on the belief that coaching parents in specific parenting skills was more effective way to change their behavior than psychoeducational, modeling, or role play.

What Is Parent-Child Interaction Therapy?

Parent-Child Interaction Therapy (PCIT) is a 14- to 20-week, manualized intervention founded on social learning and attachment theories. PCIT is designed for children between 2 and 7 years of age with disruptive, or externalizing, behavior problems (Eyberg & Robinson, 1983). The underlying model of change is similar to that of other parent-training programs. These programs promote the idea that through positive parenting and behavior modification skills, the parents themselves become the agent of change in reducing the child's behavior problems. However, unlike other parenting-focused interventions, PCIT incorporates both parent and child in the treatment sessions and uses live, individualized therapist coaching for an idiographic approach to changing the dysfunctional parent-child relationship.

PCIT is conducted in two phases. The first phase focuses on enhancing the parent-child relationship (Child-Directed Interaction; CDI), and the second on improving child compliance (Parent-Directed Interaction; PDI). Both phases of treatment begin with an hour of didactic training, followed by sessions in which the therapist coaches the parent during play with the child. From an observation room behind a two-way mirror, via a 'bug-in-the-ear' receiver that the parent wears, the therapist provides the parent with feedback on their use of the skills. Parents are taught and practice specific skills of communication and behavior management with the child. In addition to practicing these skills during clinic sessions, parents are asked to practice with the child at home for 5 min every day.

In CDI (typically 7–10 sessions), parents are coached to follow their children's lead in play by describing their activities, reflecting their appropriate verbalizations, and praising their positive behavior. The skills parents learn during this phase of treatment are represented in the acronym, PRIDE, which stands for Praise, Reflection, Imitation, Description, and Enjoyment. By the end of CDI, parents generally have shifted from rarely noticing their children's positive behavior to more consistently attending to or praising appropriate behavior. When caregivers master the skills taught in CDI by demonstrating that they can give ten behavior descriptions (e.g., "You are building a tall tower"), ten reflections (i.e., repeating back or paraphrasing the child's words), and ten labeled praises (e.g., "Thank you for playing so gently with these toys"), with fewer than three instances of asking a question, giving a command, and eliminate criticizing the child in a 5-min assessment, they move to the second phase of treatment. The following is an example of CDI coaching:

(Parent and child are playing with Legos; the therapist is watching from an adjacent observation room and talking to the parent through the 'bug-in-the-ear' system)

Therapist:	Describe what Robert is doing with his hands.
Robert:	(plays with blue Legos)
Parent:	You put all of the blue Legos on the table.
Therapist:	That was a great behavioral description!
Child:	Yes, I'm going to make a big blue tower.
Parent:	Oh… you're going to make a big blue tower
Coach:	You got it! That was a perfect reflection of what Robert said. He knows you are paying attention to what he is doing. When you give him praise and attention for his good behavior, he will do more of that behavior.
Child:	And I'm going to make a red barn too!
Therapist:	You make a red barn too, Mom.
Parent:	That's a great idea! I'm going to make a red barn just like you.
Therapist:	Great imitating! He really knows you're paying attention when you imitate his play.
Child:	Okay, you build yours right here, and the cow will go in it.
Therapist:	Robert is playing very gently with the toys today. And so creative!
Parent:	Robert, you are so creative with these Legos. You know just what to do!
Child:	Yeah!
Therapist:	Nice labeled praise, Mom.

In the example, you can see that therapists alternate between leading (and sometimes redirecting) the parent, following the parent, and giving brief psychoeducation: interpreting children's behavior, explaining the meaning and long term effects of using the skills. These coaching strategies gently lead the parent to try out, practice, and incorporate these skills into the fabric of their parenting.

In PDI (typically 7–10 sessions) therapists train parents to give only essential commands, to make them clear and direct, maximizing chances for compliance. Parents participating in PCIT traditionally learn a specific method of using time-out for dealing with noncompliance. Parents also may be taught "hands-off" strategies (e.g., removal of privileges) if indicated. These strategies are designed to provide caregivers tools for managing their children's behavior while helping them to avoid using physical power, focusing instead on using positive incentives and promoting children's emotional regulation. Mastery of behavior management skills during PDI is achieved when therapists observe that caregivers are able to use the behavior management strategies they were taught without being coached and when parents report that these strategies are effective in reducing problem behaviors. By the end of PDI, the process of giving commands and obtaining compliance are predictable and safe for parents and children. Increasing predictability and safety in families helps break the cycle of violence in abusive families (Dodge, Bates, & Pettit, 1990). The following script is an example of PDI coaching:

(Parent and child are playing with Legos; the therapist is watching from an adjacent observation room and talking to the parent through the 'bug-in-the-ear' system)

Therapist:	It is now time to clean up the toys. Tell Robert to put the Legos back in the box.
Parent:	Robert, it's time to clean up. Can you put the Legos back in the box? [Indirect Command]
Therapist:	Make it a direct command.
Parent:	Please put the Legos back in the box, Robert.
Therapist:	That was a perfect Direct Command. Now Robert knows exactly what he is supposed to do.
Child:	(Robert starts to put a couple of Legos in the box)
Therapist:	Now Robert is putting Legos away like you told him.
Parent:	Thank you for listening, Robert! [Labeled Praise]
Therapist:	Excellent labeled praise. That will help Robert want to listen more in the future.

As in CDI, the PCIT therapist alternates between leading, following and explaining to the parent. However, unlike CDI, the therapist is more corrective, never ignoring mistakes, and can be more directing, particularly in the midst of a child's time-out or time-out refusal. During these mini-crises, the therapist may give the parent the words to say, or prompt the parent with the beginning of a well-practiced phrase to keep the parent on track.

Therapists coach parents to recognize and provide appropriate responses for the child's behavior (e.g., recognizing and responding to praise for compliance; recognizing and ignoring minor inappropriate behavior – such as whining). As parents acquire these PCIT skills, therapists give fewer directives and instead use the coaching time to describe and praise the positive parenting they see, making connections between this behavior and the bigger picture of parenting and child development. An additional important element of PCIT coaching involves shifting *both* parent responses and cognitions about child behavior. While coaching, therapists often provide supplemental information about the child's behavior, to correct or minimize distortions in parent cognitions (especially negative or hostile cognitions). An example of this would be:

Child:	(Child is coloring with a marker and paper. In the process of coloring, the child accidentally moves the marker off of the paper and draws on the table.)
Therapist:	(Noticing that the child has colored on the table and the parent is irritated about the child drawing on the table) Oh… that happens all of the time. It is common for a child of his age to accidently draw on the table. The marker washes off the table easily – so no harm done. As soon as he starts to draw on the paper, give him a labeled praise for drawing on the paper.

Child: (Starts to draw on the paper again) I am drawing a truck.
Parent: That is an awesome truck [Labeled Praise]; and you are doing a great
              job drawing on the paper! [Labeled Praise]
Therapist: Awesome Labeled Praise, Dad! He wasn't misbehaving by drawing on
              the table – he is just not old enough to always draw on the paper. And
              now you've starting teaching him that it's good to draw on the paper.

Through the process of coaching, therapists can give parents immediate and accurate feedback about the child's behavior. We argue that when the therapist whispers into the parent's ear a different view of the child's behavior – a different interpretation of the child's intent – the therapist 'interrupts' the parent's previously held negative attribution (and negative affect) about the child's behavior. Over time, children's behaviors which were previously viewed through a lens of negative parental attributions and expectations shift to recognition and acknowledgement, then acceptance of the a more positive attribution of the child's behavior (prompted by therapist/coach's observation and positive attribution of the child's behavior).

Empirical Support for PCIT with Oppositional, Defiant Children

There have been numerous studies demonstrating the efficacy of PCIT for reducing child behavior problems (Eisenstadt, Eyberg, McNeil, Newcomb, & Funderburk, 1993; Eyberg, 1988; Eyberg & Robinson, 1982). Positive effects have been maintained for up to 6 years post-treatment (Hood & Eyberg, 2003). In addition, treatment effects have been shown to generalize to the home (Boggs, Eyberg, & Reynolds, 1990), school settings (McNeil, Eyberg, Eisenstadt, Newcomb, & Funderburk, 1991), and to untreated siblings (Eyberg & Robinson). In addition, there is research indicating that PCIT yields positive treatment outcomes with different types of cultural and language groups, including Spanish-speaking families (McCabe, Yeh, Garland, Lau, & Chavez, 2005), Chinese-speaking families (Leung, Tsang, Heung, & You, 1999), and African-American families (Fernandez, Butler, & Eyberg, 2011).

Empirical Support for PCIT with Abusive Families

While numerous studies demonstrated the value of PCIT with oppositional and defiant children, Urquiza and McNeil (1996) argued that some (if not many) of the symptoms of child victims of physical abuse or domestic violence were consistent with the disruptive behaviors of children in the PCIT studies. They proposed using PCIT with maltreated children and those exposed to domestic violence. There are many reasons to expect that PCIT would be a beneficial treatment for maltreating families. Effective treatments for these families should incorporate both the parent and the child because the behaviors of each contribute to the maladaptive responses of each, feeding a cycle of hostility and coercion. The treatment should also provide a means to directly decrease negative affect and coercive control, while encouraging (i.e., teaching, coaching) greater positive affect and discipline strategies. In the last decade, research findings have shown positive outcomes with maltreating parent-child dyads (Timmer, Urquiza, Zebell, & McGrath, 2005), children exposed to domestic violence (Timmer, Ware, Zebell, & Urquiza, 2008), and children with their foster parents (Borrego, Timmer, Urquiza, & Follette, 2004; Chaffin et al., 2004; Timmer, Borrego, & Urquiza, 2002; Timmer, Urquiza, & Zebell, 2006). In summary, while PCIT was initially developed as an intervention specifically for children with disruptive behavioral problems, there is currently ample research that identifies PCIT as an effective evidence-based parenting program for high-risk and abusive families.

Traumatized Children Have Behavioral Problems

It is not uncommon for maltreated children to have trauma symptoms in addition to problems with disruptive behavior. Trauma symptoms may derive from their experience of being physically abused and/or as a result from other traumatic events (e.g., exposure to domestic violence, community violence, sexual victimization). That is, children who experience traumatic events exhibit multiple symptoms consistent with Posttraumatic Stress Disorder (American Psychiatric Association, 2000), including nightmares, affective dysregulation, intrusive imagery, and intense distress related to internal or external cues associated with the traumatic event (Copeland, Keeler, Angold, & Costello, 2007). It is often more difficult to detect the effects of trauma in young children, because they do not recognize or cannot articulate the connection between the traumatic event and how they feel and behave (i.e., traumatic symptoms) – because of their developmental limitations (e.g., expressive language ability, social cognition, intellectual functioning). Although it can reasonably be argued that any type of traumatic event can lead to anger and defiance – the range of responses that lead to a specific child being labeled as defiant or oppositional can be complicated to determine. For example, we know that some traumatized children are also exposed to domestic violence or child physical abuse (Jouriles & Norwood, 1995). Further, there is a wealth of literature describing the experience of violence (i.e., being abused) and exposure to violence (i.e., exposure to domestic violence) as a significant predictor of aggressive, noncompliant, defiant behavior in children (e.g., Brown, 2005; Cohen, 2003; Milner, 2000). This pattern of disruptive child behavior appears to stem from a combination of parents' frequent modeling of aggressive and hostile behavior, and the child's own angry emotional responses and resulting oppositional behavior tied to being raised in such coercive and hostile environments.

One characteristic of many violent families that contributes to children's disruptive behavior problems is the absence of positive, warm, and nurturing parenting (Fantuzzo et al., 1991). When traumatized children live in families with chaotic lifestyles, in which consistent and positive parent-child relationships are infrequent or nearly nonexistent, their behavioral problems may be less related to their trauma than the overall chaotic and dysfunctional lifestyle in which they are being raised. The population of children who have disruptive behavioral problems resulting from inconsistent and poor parenting is the group for whom some type of intensive parenting intervention may be most effective (Kaminski, Valle, Filene, & Boyle, 2008); although it should be understood that this type of intervention may not *directly* address the cognitions and affect related to the child's trauma.

A Dyadic Parent-Child Intervention with Young Traumatized Children

Younger and older children respond differently to trauma, with younger children appearing to be more responsive to the stability (or lack of stability) of parental functioning and older children less likely to be adversely impacted by parent instability (Scheeringa & Zeanah, 2001). In particular, younger children (i.e., toddlers, preschool-age, elementary-age children) are highly responsive to parent cues of affective stability, instability, and distress related to adverse family events (e.g., interpersonal violence), often because their means of coping is still co-regulated by the parent (Chu & Lieberman, 2010; Fogel, Garvey, Hsu, & West-Stroming, 2006). In contrast, older children (i.e., school-age, adolescents) tend to rely more on their own coping skills and cognitions, may be more independent from distress experienced by a parent figure, and may develop other sources of support (e.g., peers, extended kin) (Werner, 1995). Because of these factors, approaches to treatment including both the parent and child are likely to be more effective with younger than older children (Runyon, Deblinger, Ryan, & Thakkar-Kolar, 2004).

PCIT and Traumatized Children

Recent research has shown that young traumatized children who complete PCIT show significant reductions in trauma symptoms (Mannarino, Lieberman, Urquiza, & Cohen, 2010). This finding – that participation in a behavioral, intensive parenting program is related to a reduction of trauma symptoms – may be initially puzzling to some. However, there are several reasons why young traumatized children would benefit from a parenting intervention – and especially PCIT.

Management of Disruptive Behavior

As stated earlier, some traumatized young children come from chaotic and dysfunctional families, experiencing poor and inconsistent parenting. They exhibit defiant, oppositional, and aggressive behavior. This family history and behavioral profile qualifies them as an appropriate clients for PCIT. There are also indications that externalizing behavior problems are symptoms of a traumatic response to a frightening event (Valentino, Berkowitz, & Stover, 2010). For some children, their traumatic response is exhibited through defiant and disruptive behaviors. It is therefore possible that by helping parents manage the child's disruptive behavior in a positive, consistent, and firm manner – a primary objective of PCIT – that the anxiety underlying that behavior may also subside, resulting in an overall decrease in trauma symptoms.

Improved Child Relationship Security and Stability with Their Primary Caregiver

Helping parents by enabling and supporting a more positive parent-child relationship is another primary objective of PCIT. One of the avenues to recovery from child trauma involves eliciting support from important caregivers. Supportive parenting is associated with positive child outcomes in many domains (Greenberg, 1999; Kim et al., 2003) – especially when a child is exposed to a traumatic event (Valentino et al., 2010). Therefore, it is essential to sustain a positive parent-child relationship and parental support in order to optimize the child's ability to deal with any adverse or traumatic experience. The combination of parental stress associated with child trauma and problematic child symptoms can erode a parent's ability to be supportive, warm, and understanding. One benefit of PCIT is that parents who used the PRIDE skills (i.e., parenting skills promoted within the first portion of PCIT) in their interactions with their children, particularly Praise and Reflection, are also more likely to be rated as sensitive, showing warmth and positive affiliation increase (Timmer & Zebell, 2006), which should strengthen the parent-child relationship. Throughout the course of PCIT, coaches focus on helping parents to recognize and attend to their children's positive behavior by describing and praising it. At the same time, parents are taught to ignore minor negative and inappropriate behaviors so that they can maintain a warm and supportive relationship with their children. As stated earlier, in the development of PCIT Eyberg incorporated play therapy goals and techniques proposed by the Axline's (1947) and Guerney's (1964) therapeutic approaches, because they promoted warmth and acceptance (Eyberg, 2004). An intervention that promoted warm, responsive, and authoritative parenting, and that combined nurturing, clear communication and firm limit-setting, may be an effective way to address a wide range of child mental health problems – including child trauma symptoms.

Parents as Therapists: Supporting Parent-Child Communication

Although there are many perspectives on what exactly constitutes psychotherapy, there is a rich literature describing the benefits of parents functioning in a supportive, therapeutic-like role with their children (see Guerney, 2000; Hutton, 2004). The central aspects of this type of filial therapy relationship include the following: (1) a positive relationship between a child and parent; (2) focus on development of appropriate and safe expression and communication; and (3) the use of play as a central theme (Urquiza, Zebell, & Blacker, 2009). In PCIT, parents are instructed about how to engage their children in positive and collaborative play (especially in the first component of PCIT). As a result, there is typically a more warm, supportive and affectionate relationship developed between the parent and child. Often, this includes positive verbal statements and physical affection exhibited by both the parent and the child. Similarly, the focus on safe and effective communication is a central tenet of PCIT. Parents are directed to communicate issues of safety, concern for the child's well-being, and positive regard for all appropriate and nonaggressive interactions. Because both parents and children generally perceive play activities as positive and enjoyable – sharing positive play experiences in PCIT sessions strengthens the communication between the dyad and helps rebuild a relationship history that is overall more positive and strengthening and less negative.

Management of the Traumatized Child's Affect

Traumatized young children have difficulty managing their feelings in emotionally difficult situations (Graham-Bermann & Levendoskly, 1998). These young children also have underdeveloped coping skills and a limited understanding of the traumatic experience they have endured (Eigsti & Cicchetti, 2004). These developmental limitations can hinder therapeutic efforts to directly address the child's trauma, traumatic symptoms, and help children to understand their responses (especially their feelings) to their trauma. In addition to developing a more positive and secure parent-child relationship, PCIT provides a mechanism to directly address many of the feelings that a child experiences – especially feelings associated with safety, fear, avoidance, and security. In the 'PCIT for Traumatized Children' protocol, a variation of PCIT for use with traumatized children (PCIT Training Center, 2012), therapists are instructed to help parents identify a child's thoughts, feelings, and behaviors, should the child act out the trauma in play or refer to the trauma during the treatment session. For example, if a child acted out an event, displaying anger, aggression, or fear – which are often shown by traumatized children – parents would be coached to respond appropriately to the child (A separate parent-only treatment session may be needed to assist the parent in common child responses to trauma and strategies to response to *their* traumatized child). In some cases with young children, the parent might be coached to play out a resolution to the traumatic event that involved keeping the child safe. With older children, the parent might be coached to recognize and identify the feelings the child was showing. Past research has shown that distressing events that are resolved appropriately are less distressing to children than unresolved events (McCoy, Cummings, & Davies, 2009). Additionally, cognitive-behavioral research has shown that when children have the experience of the feeling paired with the affect label presented by parents, they begin to understand the meaning of the distressing affect, which is one of the first steps to being able to discuss and manage these feelings (Widom & Russell, 2008). As children continue to understand these feelings, then parents can help them engage strategies to manage these feelings (e.g., safety planning, deep breathing, counting, progressive relaxation). An example of coaching to assist a child through this process might be like:

Child:	(A child who has been exposed to domestic violence is playing with a dollhouse, and simulates a father coming to the door and banging hard on the door – while yelling) Let me in! Let me in!
Therapist:	It looks like she is pretending through her play that she is afraid that her father is going to come back. Tell her that you understand that she is scared and remind her that there's a plan to keep you safe
Parent:	I think you get really scared when daddy comes over to our house and is angry. But we have a plan to stay safe. I call …
Parent & Child:	"9…1…1"
Parent:	Right! Then the police will come and we will be safe!
Therapist:	That was great. You are helping her to understand her feelings of being scared and that you can keep her safe– even if her father comes back. Maybe Mr. Potato Head can be a policeman, and you show her how the plan will work.
Parent:	Here comes Mr. Policeman! "Let's go Mister. No yelling and pounding doors is allowed here." [takes Dad doll away]. If daddy comes back and you get scared, you come and find me – I'll make sure you are safe.

In order to assist parents to be appropriately responsive to the child's concerns, the therapist may need to have a separate 'parent only' session or talk with the parent on the phone (between sessions) to educate them about the child's concerns and how they might be able to respond during the treatment sessions. As with traditional PCIT coaching processes, repetition of parental responses to child trauma increases the parents understanding and use of supportive resources to alleviate trauma behaviors (i.e., symptoms and cognitions).

Decreasing Child Behavioral Problems May Increase Parental Competence

For relationship-based interventions to be effective, the caregiver must be able to participate and implement the skills learned or ideas discussed during therapy sessions. When primary caregivers have other sources of stress and trying to cope with the effects of their own traumatic experiences, these problems can not only contribute to children's mental health problems, dampening parents' warmth and sensitivity and interfere with effective parenting (Lovejoy, Graczyk, O'Hare, & Neuman, 2000) but also can disrupt treatment effectiveness (Stevens, Ammerman, Putnam, & Van Ginkel, 2002). Symptoms of post-traumatic stress, such as depression, fatigue, dissociation and poor concentration can interfere with the acquisition of parenting skills (Reyno & McGrath, 2006). Furthermore, parental depression increases the likelihood of early treatment termination (Kazdin, 2000), completely removing the children from the possibility of being helped. However, research has shown that if traumatized parents can overcome their tendencies to drop out of treatment and participate in a relationship-based treatment, their own psychological symptoms can be relieved (Timmer et al., 2011).

In 'PCIT for Traumatized Children', parents are taught how to cope with the emotions that often accompany their children's disruptive behavior by using anxiety reduction skills such as deep-breathing and counting silently. They are coached to observe, notice, and react to their children's positive behavior. They are coached to show warmth, enthusiasm, and enjoyment in their interactions with their children. When traumatized parents repeatedly perform these positive and adaptive behaviors throughout the course of PCIT, it is thought that these adaptive responses may begin to generalize, or "spill over" into other parts of their lives, replacing maladaptive responses (Timmer et al., 2011).

PCIT Case Study

The family in treatment was a 30-year-old Latino father and his 7 year-old son, "Marco." The father reported that he had never married, but had been living with Marco's mother for approximately 9 years and had two children with her. The father sought treatment for his son because he believed that Marco had "a lot of anger issues with me and especially his mother," and felt that it was important to "get to the core" of his anger and resentment while he was young. The father reported that Marco was irritable, depressive, hyperactive, defiant, and aggressive towards him. He was also bossy and overbearing with his friends and other students at school.

Child History – Marco

At the time of the pre-treatment clinical intake interview, Marco lived with his father and 3-year-old sister in a homeless shelter, while Marco's mother was in an inpatient clinic for treatment of her alcohol and drug dependency. Their homelessness appeared to be a natural consequence of drug involvement and violence that ruled their lives up to that point. Marco's mother's history of alcohol and drug dependency dated back at least to Marco's birth. When Marco was 4, he was diagnosed with ADHD and Oppositional Defiant Disorder, and prescribed Adderall for treatment of the hyperactivity and attention deficit. For several years, the parents were mostly compliant with this treatment. Approximately a year earlier, the mother moved to Southern California. The father, Marco, and his baby sister followed. The mother was using methamphetamines and alcohol heavily during this time; the father reported using "some cocaine." The father told the therapist that during this time, Marco's behaviors were so disruptive they interfered with his schooling. He was often asked to leave school after 45 min. After 4 months, they moved back north. Shortly afterward, the father was arrested on possession of substances with intent to sell and was jailed for 60 days. While he was in jail, the father reported that the mother's substance use "got out of control," and they were evicted from their apartment. In addition to the drugs and housing insecurity, Marco was exposed to domestic violence between his parents. The last incidence of violence was approximately 5 months before coming into treatment: the mother and father began fighting while driving. The father pulled over to the side of the road, and the parents continued yelling, screaming, kicking and punching each other with the children looking on. The police were called to the incident and took the father into custody.

In the initial clinical interview, the father reported that Marco had been aggressive, destructive, defiant, and impulsive "for years." He believed that the child's behavioral problems resulted from his and the mother's drug and alcohol abuse and witnessing domestic violence. In addition to the disruptive behaviors, the father also reported that Marco wet the bed at night five out of seven nights. At this time, Marco was enrolled in the school associated with the homeless shelter. In the 3 weeks he had been attending school he had been suspended twice. The father reported some support from family and friends and being fairly happy living at the shelter, though he anticipated a move to transitional housing in the near future.

'PCIT for Traumatized Children' Assessment and Treatment Procedures

PCIT is an assessment driven treatment. Before beginning treatment and upon graduation, parents complete a battery of standardized assessments including the following measures: Child Behavior Checklist (CBCL, 1½–5 years; Achenbach & Rescorla, 2000) and the Eyberg Child Behavior Inventory (ECBI; Eyberg & Pincus, 1999), two standardized measures of the severity of children's behavior problems; the Trauma Symptom Checklist for Young Children (TSCYC; Briere et al., 2001), a measure of the severity of children's trauma symptoms; the Brief Symptom Inventory (BSI; Derogatis, 1993), a self-report measure of the parent's psychological symptoms; and the short form of the Parenting Stress Index (PSI; Abidin, 1995), a measure of the severity of three sources of stress in the parent role: parental distress, dysfunction in the parent-child relationship, and difficult child behavior.

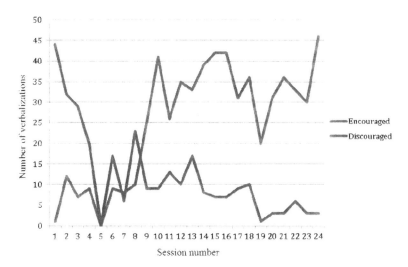

Fig. 8.1 Process of skill acquisition from pre- to post-treatment: numbers of encouraged and discouraged verbalizations in the weekly 5-min observational assessment

In addition, the therapist conducts a behavioral assessment pre- and post-treatment, observing the dyad as they play together in three semi-structured activities, using the Dyadic Parent-child Coding System-III (DPICS-III; Eyberg, Nelson, Duke, & Boggs, 2005), a micro-analytic coding system, designed by Eyberg and her colleagues (2005) to categorize parent verbalizations in parent-child interactions. The three play situations vary in the amount of control the parent is asked to use. In the first situation (Child Directed Interaction), parents are told to let the child pick an activity and to play along, following the child's lead in play. In the Parent Directed Interaction, parents are instructed to pick an activity and have the child play with the parent according to the parent's rules. In the third, and final situation, the parent is directed to have the child to 'clean up' without the parent's assistance.

In addition to the observational assessment of the parent and child in the DPICS sessions, the therapist uses the first 5 min of each weekly treatment session to observe the parent-child interactions in child-directed play. The therapist remains silent during this time, coding the parent verbalizations. Figure 8.1 summarizes the results of the therapist's weekly coding over the course of treatment.

Results

Course of Treatment in PCIT

Marco's intake assessment was conducted in September 2011. The father agreed with the therapist's suggestion that PCIT would fit their needs, and weekly sessions were scheduled. After the therapist conducted a didactic session, teaching the father about the skills he would need in the first phase of treatment and what to expect from treatment, once coaching sessions began. At the beginning of each session, the therapist talked briefly with the father, asking how Marco had behaved since they had last been seen, and how the father was doing.

Marco and his father made slow progress over the first 2 months of treatment. They consistently attended PCIT and did their "homework" (5 min of Special Time every day, practicing PCIT skills). Furthermore, the therapist reported that the father was responsive to coaching. However, Marco had a habit of trying to get the father's attention by asking "rapid fire" questions, swearing, or making critical comments during the 5-min behavioral observation at the beginning of the coaching session. The father would get upset, have a hard time recovering, and hence would not demonstrate much skill acquisition. At CDI 8, when the father mastered the skill of ignoring these disruptive behaviors, he made speedy progress in mastering encouraged verbalizations such as labeled praise, reflective statements, and behavioral descriptions. The dyad moved to the second phase of treatment three sessions after the father mastered the skill of ignoring.

The second phase of treatment (PDI) began in January and was completed in May. Altogether, the dyad received 10 PDI coaching sessions before the therapist was confident that the father could manage his son's behavior, and that his son's behavior problems were sufficiently diminished. During this time, the father learned to give clear, direct commands, and to react consistently, using time out when Marco was defiant. Marco was not always compliant with the time out, however. On two occasions, he was argumentative and defiant in response to his father's direct command, and refused to sit in the time-out chair. In these situations, the therapist used a "Swoop and Go" technique, in which the father picked up the toys and exited the room, and left Marco in the room alone until he sat in the chair. Once he sat in the chair, the father came back in the room, and the time out began. With a child Marco's age, the therapist considered using removal of privileges as a back-up, or incentive for taking the time out. However, with Marco's sassiness and love of an argument, the therapist decided that the Swoop and Go was the most expedient method for getting him to comply with the time out. Indeed, the session after his second (and final) Time Out-Swoop and Go, Marco's younger sister, who was participating in the session, required a time out. Marco happily demonstrated how to take the time out, showing off his time out expertise.

Mother's Involvement in PCIT

As noted above, Marco's mother was in an alcohol and drug rehabilitation program when Marco and his father began PCIT. She moved back home at about the 6th CDI coaching session (CDI 6). It is interesting to note that the father's skills showed a marked drop at CDI 7, just after the mother moved back with the family, but then recovered, showing the vulnerability of these skills to family stressors and the need for therapeutic support. Initially the mother showed no interest in participating in treatment, ridiculing the father's parenting behavior. Then, after living

Table 8.1 Scores on standardized assessments at pre-, mid-, and post-treatment

	Assessment point		
	Pre-treatment	Mid-treatment	Post-treatment
CHILD MEASURES			
ECBI (raw scores)			
Intensity scale (cutoff = 130)	158	144	125
Problem scale (cutoff = 15)	27	16	8
CBCL (T-scores)			
Internalizing	60		50
Externalizing	69		68
Total problems	70		52
TSCYC (T-scores)			
PTS total score	55		51
Depression	51		41
PSI (percentile scores)			
Parental distress	97	87.5	92.5
Parent-child dysfunctional relationship	90	70	55
Difficult child	97	97	85
PARENT MEASURES			
CAPI-abuse scale	338		251
BSI- depression	68		73

with the family for nearly 3 months, she expressed interest in having some PCIT training, realizing that Marco was much more responsive and compliant with his father than with her. The therapist quickly arranged for adjunct, in-home PCIT, so that the mother could also learn and practice the PCIT skills. After three in-home sessions, the number of the mother's encouraged verbalizations increased from 2 to 13; and discouraged verbalizations decreased from 27 to 0. However, shortly after her third session (at PDI 8 for Marco and his father), the mother was kicked out of the transitional housing program for substance use and re-entered a detoxification program.

Standardized Measures

Child Behavior Problems

The father's ratings of his son on the ECBI and the CBCL reflected behavior problems in the clinical range at pre-treatment (see Table 8.1). In particular, the father noted problems with Marco's oppositional and rule breaking behavior, his verbal expression (e.g., argumentative, yells, sassy), aggressiveness (e.g., provokes fights), and attention, yielding elevated scores on the externalizing and total behavior problems scales. The symptoms the father reported were consistent with the diagnoses of Oppositional-Defiant Disorder and ADHD.

By mid-treatment, the intensity of disruptive behavior problems reported on the ECBI had dropped a half of a standard deviation, but was still in the clinical range. By the end of treatment, the intensity of problems had dropped another half of a standard deviation to a level just below the clinical range. On the CBCL, the father reported decreases in the severity of Marco's internalizing and total behavior problems, but no significant change in the severity of his externalizing behaviors.

Child Trauma Symptoms

Marco's scores on the TSCYC pre-treatment per father's report showed clinical levels of arousal related to post-traumatic stress, and aggression. However, the most severe symptoms he reported on the arousal scale appeared to be related to his attention problems, which predated the most recent violent event he had witnessed. By post-treatment, however, all scales had dropped down into the normal range.

Parent Functioning

In addition to measures of his child's functioning, Marco's father completed the BSI, rating his own psychological symptoms, and the short form of the PSI, a measure of the severity stress in the parent role. Pre-treatment, his symptom profile on the BSI showed general symptomatic distress in the clinical range, endorsing among other things clinical levels of symptoms on the depression, anxiety, hostility, and phobic anxiety. Post-treatment, scores on these scales reflecting self-reported psychological symptoms decreased at least 1.5 standard deviations and were within normal limits. The father's response to questions on the PSI pre-treatment suggested that he was experiencing considerable stress in the parent role. He reported parental distress resulting from feelings of a lack of competence, of being restricted in other parts of his life because of being a parent, depression, and conflict with his spouse. He reported significant stress in his relationship with Marco, noting that he would "do things that bother him just to be mean." He also reported clinical levels of stress resulting from parenting a child with difficult behaviors. By post-treatment, the father's perception of stress resulting from Marco's difficult behaviors and dysfunction in the parent-child relationship decreased significantly. However, his parental distress remained elevated.

Summary of Gains

When Marco and his father came into treatment, Marco was sassy and mostly disrespectful to his father. He was aggressive towards him, grabbing toys from him, hitting him, appearing to try to dominate the play and provoke his father. Marco's father was not intimidated in the least by his aggressive behavior, but was upset by the sassy lack of respect, yelling, and swearing. The father was mostly irritated with Marco's behavior at pre-treatment; at his best, his tone with him was neutral and flat. Over the course of PCIT, Marco's father learned to attend to his positive behaviors and even more important, ignore his sassiness and rudeness. Marco, likely because he was 7 years old, was very sensitive to the genuine quality of his father's statements. As a rule, he was irritated by behavior descriptions and labeled praises unless the verbalizations showed attention to some aspect of his play that he valued. For example, when the father said, "you put the red gear next to the blue gear," Marco replied, "how about if we just play and don't talk?" The father (ignoring the sassy talk) followed by saying, "…and you put three orange gears together. I like that because it's so colorful!" Marco agreed with his father's observation, continuing to talk about the gears they were playing with. The father also was able to obtain Marco's compliance at least 75 % of the time, though in cases where Marco really did not want to comply (e.g., stopping playtime), the father still had to count and occasionally give him a time out. Overall, Marco's behaviors improved substantially. While he still was somewhat sassy and bossy post-treatment, the father was able to redirect his attention and engage him in relaxed, reciprocal play for long stretches of time. Marco's father showed that he understood Marco and could help him stay emotionally regulated. Marco's behavior and comments showed that he enjoyed being with his father, and above all, felt safe.

While we believe the potential gain of strengthening the parent-child relationship is great, the case presented within this chapter illustrates the complexity of people's lives and their ongoing vulnerability to risk. At several points in the course of treatment, this family could have terminated services. The father was depressed and not really making speedy positive changes; the mother re-entered the family's life and for a while was a destructive force in the fragile reconstruction of the father's relationship with his son. It is a tribute to the social worker, therapist, and – most of all – the father himself, that the family continued to participate in treatment. In the face of seemingly overwhelming obstacles, the father felt helped and supported, retaining his belief that the services would make a difference for his son's future.

Conclusion

A wealth of research over the last few decades testifies to the value of PCIT as a tool in improving parenting skills, decreasing child behavioral problems, and enhancing the quality of parent-child relationships. Replacing negative, hostile, and coercive parent-child interactions with a stable, predictable pattern of affection, praise, and other positive relationship-building behaviors appears to decrease behavior problems. The addition of effective behavior management skills insures that when troubles arise (as they always do), the parent will be able to handle them. However, even more than the curriculum content, PCIT uses coaching – an effective strategy for teaching and training parents. While coaching parents to adjust certain discrete behaviors in the moment, it is also possible reframe cognitions, point out competing attributions, and alter expectations. These are all important contributors to family's risk of abuse (Milner, 2000). However, simply viewing decreasing risk of abuse as a result of improvements in behavior change fails to appreciate the overall impact of PCIT on abusive parent-child relationships. Through repeated coaching related to parenting behaviors, therapists have an effective means to alter both parent and child cognitions (Dumas, 2005) – an element of treatment essential in abusive parent-child relationships. Further, the shift to more positive interactions and cognitions provide the foundation for changes the affective quality of the parent-child relationship (Timmer et al., 2011). It is suggested that the combination of Eyberg's formulation of PCIT as a means to improve parenting skill and decrease child behavior problems, combined with shifts in parental cognitions, lead to the decreases in risk of child maltreatment.

The case described in this chapter illustrates the ways in which PCIT can support and build a secure and nurturing parent-child relationship – which becomes the mechanism by which some abusive and high-risk families can shift to a position of relationship safety. Additionally, it is hoped that the case highlights that while PCIT can effect important behavioral change, there is much more to PCIT than simply changing behavior. As a powerful relationship teaching tool, *in vivo* coaching offers opportunities to extend interventions to the realm of automatic cognitions, attributions, and relationship expectancies.

References

Abidin, R. R. (1995). *Parenting stress index: Professional manual.* Odessa, FL: Psychological Assessment Resources.

Achenbach, T. M., & Rescorla, L. (2000). *Manual for the ASEBA preschool forms & profiles.* Burlington, VT: University of Vermont, Research Center for Children, Youth & Families.

Ainsworth, M. D. S. (1979). Infant-mother attachment. *American Psychologist, 34,* 932–937.

American Psychiatric Association. (2000). *Diagnostic and statistical manual of mental disorders* (IVth ed. – Text revision). Arlington, VA: American Psychiatric Association.

Axline, V. (1947). *Play therapy.* London: Ballantine Books.

Baumrind, D. (1966). Effects of authoritative parental control on child behavior. *Child Development, 37*(4), 887–907.

Baumrind, D. (1967). Child care practices anteceding three patterns of preschool behavior. *Genetic Psychology Monographs, 75*(1), 43–88.

Boggs, S., Eyberg, S., & Reynolds, L. A. (1990). Concurrent validity of the Eyberg Child Behavior Inventory. *Journal of Clinical Child Psychology, 91*(1), 75–78.

Borrego, J., Timmer, S., Urquiza, A., & Follette, W. (2004). Physically abusive mothers' responses following episodes of child noncompliance and compliance. *Journal of Consulting and Clinical Psychology, 72*(5), 897–903.

Briere, J., Johnson, K., Bissada, A., Damon, L., Crouch, J., Gil, E., et al. (2001). The Trauma Symptom Checklist for Young Children (TSCYC): Reliability and association with abuse exposure in a multi-site study. *Child Abuse & Neglect, 25,* 1001–1014.

Brown, E. J. (2005). Clinical characteristics and efficacious treatment of posttraumatic stress disorder in children and adolescents. *Pediatric Annals, 2,* 139–146.

Chaffin, M., Silovsky, J., Funderburk, B., Valle, L. A., Brestan, E., Balachova, T., et al. (2004). Parent–child interaction therapy with physically abusive parents: Efficacy for reducing future abuse reports. *Journal of Consulting and Clinical Psychology, 72*(3), 500–510.

Chambless, D. L., & Ollendick, T. H. (2000). Empirically supported psychological interventions: Controversies and evidence. *Annual Review of Psychology, 52*, 685–716.

Chu, A. T., & Lieberman, A. (2010). Clinical implications of traumatic stress from birth to age five. *Annual Review of Clinical Psychology, 6*, 469–494.

Cicchetti, D., & Valentino, K. (2006). *An ecological-transactional perspective on child maltreatment: Failure of the average expectable environment and its influence on child development* (pp. 129–201). Hoboken, NJ: Wiley.

Cohen, J. (2003). Treating acute posttraumatic stress reactions in children and adolescents. *Biological Psychiatry, 53*(9), 827–833.

Copeland, W. E., Keeler, G., Angold, A., & Costello, E. J. (2007). Traumatic events and posttraumatic stress in childhood. *Archives of General Psychiatry, 64*(5), 577–584.

Derogatis, L. R. (1993). *Brief symptom inventory (BSI): Administration, scoring, and procedures manual*. Minneapolis, MN: NCS Pearson, Inc.

Dodge, K., Bates, J. E., & Pettit, G. S. (1990). Mechanisms in the cycle of violence. *Science, 250*, 1678–1683.

Dumas, J. E. (2005). Mindfulness-based parent training: Strategies to lessen the grip of automaticity in families with disruptive children. *Journal of Clinical Child and Adolescent Psychology, 34*(4), 779–791.

Eigsti, I. M., & Cicchetti, D. (2004). The impact of child maltreatment of expressive syntax at 60 months. *Developmental Science, 7*, 88–102.

Eisenstadt, T., Eyberg, S., McNeil, C., Newcomb, K., & Funderburk, B. (1993). Parent–child interaction therapy with behavior problem children: Relative effectiveness of two stages and overall treatment outcome. *Journal of Clinical Child Psychology, 22*, 42–51.

Eyberg, S. (1988). PCIT: Integration of traditional and behaviour concerns. *Child and Family Behavior Therapy, 10*, 33–46.

Eyberg, S. M. (2004). The PCIT story–part one: The conceptual foundation of PCIT. *The Parent-Child Interaction Therapy Newsletter, 1*(1), 1–2.

Eyberg, S. M., Nelson, M., Duke, M., & Boggs, S. (2005). *Manual for the Dyadic parent-child interaction coding system* (3rd ed.). Unpublished manuscript.

Eyberg, S. M., & Pincus, D. (1999). *ECBI & SESBI-R: Eyberg child behavior inventory and Sutter-Eyberg student behavior inventory-revised, professional manual*. Odessa, FL: Psychological Assessment Resources.

Eyberg, S. M., & Robinson, E. A. (1982). Parent-child interaction therapy: Effects on family functioning. *Journal of Clinical Child Psychology, 11*, 130–137.

Eyberg, S. M., & Robinson, E. A. (1983). Conduct problem behavior: Standardization of a behavioral rating scale with adolescents. *Journal of Clinical Child Psychology, 12*, 347–354.

Fantuzzo, J. W., DePaola, L. M., Lambert, L., Martino, T., Anderson, T., & Sutton, B. (1991). Effects of interparental violence on the psychological adjustment and competencies of young children. *Journal of Consulting and Clinical Psychology, 59*(2), 258–265.

Fernandez, M. A., Butler, A. M., & Eyberg, S. M. (2011). Treatment outcome for low socioeconomic status African American families in parent-child interaction therapy: A pilot study. *Child and Family Behavior Therapy, 33*(1), 32–48.

Fogel, A., Garvey, A., Hsu, H., & West-Stroming, D. (2006). *Change processes in relationships: A relational-historical research approach*. Cambridge, UK: Cambridge University Press.

Graham-Bermann, S. A., & Levendoskly, A. A. (1998). The social functioning of preschool-age children whose mothers are emotionally and physically abused. *Journal of Emotional Abuse, 1*, 59–84.

Greenberg, M. T. (1999). Attachment and psychopathology in childhood. In J. Cassidy & P. R. Shaver (Eds.), *Handbook of attachment: Theory, research, and clinical applications*. New York: Guilford Press.

Guerney, B., Jr. (1964). Filial therapy: Description and rationale. *Journal of Consulting Psychology, 28*(4), 304–310.

Guerney, L. (2000). Filial therapy into the 21st century. *International Journal of Play Therapy,* *9*(2), 1–17.

Hanf, C. (1969, April). *A two stage program for modifying material controlling during mother-child interactions.* Paper presented at the meeting of the western Psychological Association, Vancouver, British Columbia, Canada.

Hood, K., & Eyberg, S. (2003). Outcomes of parent-child interaction therapy: Mothers' reports of maintenance three to six years after treatment. *Journal of Clinical Child and Adolescent Psychology, 32*, 412–429.

Hutton, D. (2004). Filial therapy: Shifting the balance. *Clinical Child Psychology and Psychiatry, 9*(2), 261–270.

Jouriles, E. N., & Norwood, W. D. (1995). Physical aggression toward boys and girls in families characterized by the battering of women. *Journal of Family Psychology, 9*, 69–78.

Kaminski, J. W., Valle, L. A., Filene, J. H., & Boyle, C. L. (2008). A meta-analytic review of components associated with parent training program effectiveness. *Journal of Abnormal Psychology, 36*, 567–589.

Kazdin, A. E. (2000). Perceived barriers to treatment participation and treatment acceptability among antisocial and their families. *Journal of Child & Family Studies, 9*, 157–174.

Kim, I. J., Ge, X., Brody, G. H., Conger, R., Gibbons, F. X., & Simons, R. I. (2003). Parenting behaviors and the occurrence and co-occurrence of depressive symptoms and conduct problems among African American children. *Depression, Marriage, & Families, 17*, 571–583.

Leung, C., Tsang, S., Heung, K., & You, I. (1999). Effectiveness of parent-child interaction therapy (PCIT) in Hong Kong. *Research on Social Work Practice, 19*(3), 304–313.

Lovejoy, M. C., Graczyk, P. A., O'Hare, E., & Neuman, G. (2000). Maternal depression and parenting behavior: A meta-analytic review. *Clinical Psychology Review, 20*, 561–592.

Mannarino, A., Lieberman, A., Urquiza, A., & Cohen, J. (2010, August). *Evidence-based treatments for traumatized children.* 118th annual convention of the American Psychological Association, San Diego, CA.

McCabe, K. M., Yeh, M., Garland, A. F., Lau, A. S., & Chavez, G. (2005). The GANA program: A tailoring approach to adapting parent-child interaction therapy for Mexican Americans. *Education and Treatment of Children, 28*, 111–129.

McCoy, K., Cummings, M., & Davies, P. (2009). Constructive and destructive marital conflict, emotional security and children's prosocial behavior. *Journal of Child Psychology and Psychiatry, 50*(3), 270–279.

McNeil, C. B., Eyberg, S. M., Eisenstadt, T. H., Newcomb, K., & Funderburk, B. (1991). Parent-child interaction therapy with behavior problem children: Generalization of treatment effects to the school setting. *Journal of Child Clinical Psychology, 20*, 140–151.

Milner, J. S. (2000). Social information processing and child physical abuse: Theory and research. In D. J. Hansen (Ed.), *Nebraska symposium on motivation, Vol. 46: Motivation and child maltreatment.* Lincoln, NE: University of Nebraska Press.

PCIT Training Center. (2012). *PCIT for traumatized children web course.* Retrieved from http://www.pcittraining.ucdavis.edu

Reitman, D., & McMahon, R. J. (2012). Constance "Connie" Hanf (1917–2002): The mentor and the model. *Cognitive and Behavioral Practice.* http://dx.doi.org/10.1016/j.cbpra.2012.02.005

Reyno, S., & McGrath, P. (2006). Predictors of parent training efficacy for child externalizing behavior problems – A meta-analytic review. *Journal of Child Psychology and Psychiatry, 47*, 99–111.

Runyon, M. K., Deblinger, E., Ryan, E. E., & Thakkar-Kolar, R. (2004). An overview of child physical abuse: Developing an integrated parent-child cognitive-behavioral treatment approach. *Trauma, Violence & Abuse, 5*(1), 65–85.

Scheeringa, M. S., & Zeanah, C. (2001). A relational perspective of PTSD in early childhood. *Journal of Traumatic Stress, 14*, 799–815.

Stevens, J., Ammerman, R., Putnam, F., & Van Ginkel, J. (2002). Depression and trauma history in first-time mothers receiving home visitation. *Journal of Community Psychology, 30*, 551–564.

Timmer, S. G., Borrego, J., & Urquiza, A. J. (2002). Antecedents of coercive interactions in physically abusive mother-child dyads. *Journal of Interpersonal Violence, 17*(8), 836–853.

Timmer, S. G., Ho, L. K. L., Urquiza, A. J., Zebell, N. M., Fernandez y Gracia, E., & Boys, D. (2011). The effectiveness of parent-child interaction therapy with depressive mothers: The changing relationship as the agent of individual change. *Child Psychiatry and Human Development, 42*, 406–423.

Timmer, S. G., Urquiza, A. J., & Zebell, N. (2006). Challenging foster caregiver-maltreated child relationships: The effectiveness of parent child interaction therapy. *Child & Youth Services Review, 28*, 1–19.

Timmer, S., Urquiza, A., Zebell, N., & McGrath, J. (2005). Parent-child interaction therapy: Application to physically abusive and high-risk dyads. *Child Abuse & Neglect, 29*, 825–842.

Timmer, S., Ware, L., Zebell, N., & Urquiza, A. (2008). The effectiveness of parent-child interaction therapy for victims of interparental violence. *Violence & Victims, 25*, 486–503.

Timmer, S. G., Ware, L. M., Urquiza, A. J., & Zebell, N. M. (2010). The effectiveness of parent-child interaction therapy for victims of interparental violence. *Violence and Victims, 25*, 4.

Timmer, S., & Zebell, N. (2006). *Mid-treatment assessment: Assessing parent skill acquisition and generalization.* Paper presented at the 2006 parent child interaction therapy conference, Gainsville, FL.

Urquiza, A. J., & McNeil, C. (1996). Parent-child interaction therapy: An intensive dyadic treatment for physically abusive families. *Child Maltreatment, 1*(2), 134–144.

Urquiza, A. J., Zebell, N. M., & Blacker, D. (2009). Innovation and integration: Parent-child interaction therapy as play therapy. In A. D. Drewes (Ed.), *Blending play therapy with cognitive behavioral therapy: Evidence-based and other effective treatments and techniques.* New York: Wiley.

Valentino, K., Berkowitz, S., & Stover, C. S. (2010). Parenting behaviors and posttraumatic symptoms in relation to children's symptomatology following a traumatic event. *Journal of Traumatic Stress, 23*(3), 403–407.

Werner, E. (1995). Resilience in Development. *Current Directions in Psychological Science, 4*(3), 81–85.

Widom, S., & Russell, J. (2008). Children acquire emotions gradually. *Cognitive Development, 23*, 291–312.

Wilson, S., Rack, J., Shi, X., & Norris, A. (2008). Comparing physically abusive, neglectful, and non-maltreating parents during interactions with their children: A meta-analysis of observational studies. *Child Abuse & Neglect, 32*, 897–911.

Chapter 9
Multidimensional Treatment Foster Care for Preschoolers: A Program for Maltreated Children in the Child Welfare System

Kathryn S. Gilliam and Philip A. Fisher

Maltreated children are at risk for many challenges across the lifespan, including behavioral and health problems (Burns et al., 2004), developmental delays (Landsverk, Garland, & Leslie, 2002), and psychopathology (Briggs-Gowan, Horwitz, Schwab-Stone, Leventhal, & Leaf, 2000). Although not every maltreated child will end up on a negative developmental trajectory, many will. Early intervention is essential in mitigating the negative effects of maltreatment and other forms of "toxic stress" in childhood (Shonkoff, 2010). Experiences of maltreatment in infancy and early childhood can be particularly damaging and are unfortunately a frequent occurrence for young children in the child welfare system. During the first few years of life, children develop maternal attachment, begin to learn how to regulate emotions, and experience dramatic physical and cognitive development. This is a time of great growth. However, it is also accompanied by vulnerability. Foster children who have experienced maltreatment early in life are at higher risk for deficits in executive functioning and developmental delays (Pears & Fisher, 2005; Pears, Fisher, Bruce, Kim, & Yoerger, 2010). Therefore, evidence-based early interventions targeting this young group are likely to have a substantial impact on the developmental trajectories of these children, shifting them in a more positive direction.

Mitigating these risks is the goal of the Multidimensional Treatment Foster Care for Preschoolers program (MTFC-P; Fisher, Ellis, & Chamberlain, 1999). MTFC-P targets three focal areas in this population of young maltreated children: behavior problems, emotion regulation, and developmental delays (Landsverk et al., 2002; Maughan & Cicchetti, 2002; Pears & Fishers, 2005). Deficits in these areas are related to various negative outcomes both during childhood and beyond, including increased risk for placement disruptions (Newton, Litrownik, & Landsverk, 2000),

K.S. Gilliam (✉)
Department of Psychology, University of Oregon, Eugene, OR, USA

P.A. Fisher, Ph.D.
Department of Psychology, University of Oregon, Eugene, OR, USA

Oregon Social Learning Center, Eugene, OR, USA
e-mail: kgilliam@uoregon.edu; philf@uoregon.edu

S. Timmer and A. Urquiza (eds.), *Evidence-Based Approaches for the Treatment of Maltreated Children*, Child Maltreatment 3, DOI 10.1007/978-94-007-7404-9_9,
© Springer Science+Business Media Dordrecht 2014

further development of internalizing and externalizing behaviors and school-failure (Zima et al., 2000). One of the major mechanisms of change in MTFC-P lies in training the foster parents and long-term placement caregivers in parenting skills that, once acquired and frequently used with the child, can have profound effects on child behavior and development. The focus on parent training as a means for effecting change in the child arises from the research findings and subsequent conceptual model developed by Patterson and colleagues at the Oregon Social Learning Center. A short history of the development of the MTFC-P intervention is provided below, followed by a description of the conceptual model underpinning MTFC-P, a detailed description of the intervention, and a review of MTFC-P's evidence base. The chapter concludes with a case study of an MTFC-P participant.

History of MTFC Interventions

Adapted for use with young foster children, MTFC-P is an extension of Multidimensional Treatment Foster Care (MTFC), an evidence-based intervention designed to treat children in the juvenile justice system. The MTFC family of interventions evolved from research on the development of antisocial behavior at the Oregon Social Learning Center beginning in the 1960s (Patterson, 1982; Patterson, Debaryshe, & Ramsey, 1989; Patterson & Fagot, 1967). The cornerstone of this research involved a social learning–based model of familial interactions and parenting practices. Extensive longitudinal research on families revealed key elements of parenting to be highly predictive of child and adolescent problem behavior, particularly antisocial behavior (Loeber & Dishion, 1983; Patterson, Dishion, & Bank, 1984). These parenting practices led to coercive patterns of interaction between parents and children that escalated over time, reinforcing aversive and negative behaviors in all family members.

Although parenting variables were a major focus of the work of Patterson and colleagues, a variety of other variables thought to be involved in the development, maintenance, and escalation of child antisocial behavior were also assessed. Many of these variables demonstrated a relationship with child problem behavior and its associated negative outcomes. For example, parents from a low-income background with high levels of daily stress (DeGarmo, Forgatch, & Martinez, 1999), those with depression (Gartstein & Fagot, 2003) or those who have a child with a difficult temperament (Leve, Kim, & Pears, 2005) often experience more child problem behavior. However, researchers have consistently shown that these variables exert a distal influence over the development of antisocial behavior: that is, they affect child behavior and outcomes primarily through their tendency to disrupt parenting (Bank, Forgatch, Patterson, & Fetrow, 1993; Conger et al., 1992; Conger, Patterson, & Ge, 1995; Larzelere & Patterson, 1990). In other words, a parent being depressed or having a temperamentally difficult child is primarily associated with child problem behavior to the extent that it leads parents to employ parenting strategies most predictive of negative outcomes. Thus, parenting continues to be identified as one of the most proximal determinants of child behavior (Patterson, Forgatch, & DeGarmo, 2010; Patterson, Reid, & Dishion, 1992) and is a main target for intervention within the models developed at the Oregon Social Learning Center.

Based on the knowledge that parenting practices strongly predict child outcomes, Patterson and colleagues developed strategies that formed the basis of interventions to assist parents in transforming how they interact with their child. The initial intervention product of this research was Parent Management Training (PMT; Forgatch & Patterson, 2010), which involved training parents to practice consistent discipline, set clear limits, and give adequate positive reinforcement for prosocial behaviors. Overall, PMT, as the first of the social learning–based parenting interventions, has been employed with thousands of families, and numerous randomized controlled trials have established PMT as an evidence-based family intervention (Dishion, Patterson, & Kavanagh, 1992; Ogden & Hagen, 2008; Patterson, Chamberlain, & Reid, 1982; Walter & Gilmore, 1973; Wiltz & Patterson, 1974).

Following successful development of PMT, researchers became interested in applying this social-learning-based model to more high-risk samples, specifically to families with adolescents at risk for juvenile delinquency and incarceration (Chamberlain & Reid, 1998). In line with this aim, in the early 1980s, Oregon state policy makers issued a call for community-based alternatives to residential care for adolescents involved with the juvenile justice system who had severe emotional and behavioral problems (Leve, Fisher, & Chamberlain, 2009). Multidimensional Treatment Foster Care (MTFC) was developed in response to this need.

MTFC is based on the assumption that in a family with severe problems such as juvenile delinquency, child aggression, or an inability of the parents to provide adequate support to the child, parenting training was an inadequate intervention (Bank, Marlowe, Reid, Patterson, & Weinrott, 1991; Chamberlain & Reid, 1998; Patterson, 2002). In contrast, within MTFC, children were placed with foster families receiving specialized training and ongoing support in behavioral parenting approaches (Chamberlain, 2003). While each child was in foster care, the family of origin received training in the same parenting techniques. This facilitated successful reintegration of the child with the family of origin (Fisher, Kim, & Pears, 2009).

MTFC (Chamberlain, 2003) has been found to positively impact outcomes across several randomized clinical trial studies (Chamberlain, Leve, & DeGarmo, 2007; Chamberlain & Reid, 1998; Eddy & Chamberlain, 2000; Eddy, Whaley, & Chamberlain, 2004). As mentioned previously, MTFC is intended for children in foster care and juvenile justice programs who would otherwise require placement in more restrictive settings such as residential care. MTFC allows children and youths to receive services in the naturalistic context of a family setting and remain in the communities in which they live.

The core components of MTFC involve the training of both foster care parents and the individuals likely responsible for permanent care to provide consistent parenting and limit-setting (Chamberlain, 2003). During the intervention, children and adolescents experience these positive parenting practices in the foster placement while also receiving additional services from both an individual therapist and a behavioral specialist. At the conclusion of the intervention, children and adolescents transition to a permanent placement in which the same parenting techniques seen in the foster care home are employed, providing a consistent structure conducive to maintenance of intervention gains. Although MTFC was originally developed in Oregon, the program has been successfully implemented at over 50 sites in the United States, more than 15 sites in England, and more than 20 sites in Norway, Denmark, Sweden, the Netherlands, and New Zealand.

MTFC-P, developed as an extension of MTFC for preschool aged children, is particularly relevant for this volume considering its focus on children with histories of maltreatment. Beginning in the late 1990s, Fisher et al. (1999) adapted the MTFC program to meet the needs of this younger population (ages 3–5 years). A variety of factors, including early disruption of attachment relationships, prenatal drug and alcohol exposure, abuse, and neglect, make this a particularly high-risk population (Fisher, Burraston, & Pears, 2005; Fisher et al., 1999; Klee, Kronstadt, & Zlotnick, 1997). Consideration of these risk factors informed the adaptations employed in the development of MTFC-P. Key differences between the MTFC and MTFC-P programs reflect an emphasis on developmental considerations in the preschool population targeted by MTFC-P. Whereas the original MTFC contains an individual child therapy component, MTFC-P includes a therapeutic playgroup to help children prepare for success at school entry (Pears, Fisher, & Bronz, 2007). This therapeutic playgroup focuses on developmentally salient skills related to socio-emotional competence and emotion regulation that become increasingly important during school.

Conceptual Foundation of MTFC-P

The philosophy behind the MTFC-P program, like that of the original MTFC program, is that long-term outcomes for maltreated foster children might be most improved when treatment occurs in the context of family and community. Rather than removing the child from these naturalistic settings and placing him/her in residential care, MTFC-P services are delivered in the context of specially trained and highly supervised foster parents and through school consultation. As such, the child learns what is expected from him/her in a typical family situation, and, while the child is in foster care, the individuals who will be providing the long-term care for the child (i.e., the biological family, relatives, or others with whom the child will live after completing treatment) are instructed in the parenting strategies to which the child is being exposed in the foster home. By maintaining consistency in the discipline strategies and in the support for positive behavior across these contexts, the program greatly increases the potential for the child to function in family and school settings over the long term (Fisher et al., 2005, 2009).

Research findings related to the deleterious effects of early adversity on development informed the design of MTFC-P. The emphasis on emotion regulation was guided by research findings suggesting that experiences of early adversity such as neglect and placement disruption negatively affect both the development of physiological systems for stress regulation, particularly the hypothalamic-pituitary-adrenal (HPA) axis (Fisher, Gunnar, Dozier, Bruce, & Pears, 2006) and also executive functioning, including inhibitory control (Pears & Fisher, 2005; Pears et al., 2010). Responsive parenting is a critical component of the development of successful regulation skills in the face of stress. From infancy through middle childhood, children are dependent on external regulation from caregivers to buffer their developing stress regulatory systems from insult (Fisher & Gunnar, 2010). In situations where the child does not receive developmentally supportive, responsive caregiving, the HPA axis appears to have the potential to become dysregulated as demonstrated by both patterns of hypocortisolism and hypercortisolism (Fisher & Gunnar, 2010). Additionally, poor inhibitory control, a component of executive function, is common amongst maltreated foster care children and contributes to the maintenance of problem behaviors through a reduced ability to process feedback and inhibit responses appropriately (Bruce, McDermott, Fisher, & Fox, 2009; Pears et al., 2010).

Interventions that keep the child within a family context are uniquely suited to bring about sustainable change in behavior and also neurobiological systems like the HPA axis due to the significant influence of family environment on behavior in parents and children, as demonstrated by Patterson and colleagues' early research (Patterson & Fagot, 1967; Patterson et al., 1992). For the maltreated child, the environment of his or her family of origin has been characterized by a lack of security that undermines typical development, particularly that of the stress response system and related neural systems such as the prefrontal cortex which is implicated in executive function and inhibitory control. Considering the links both between parenting practices and child behavior, and also those between early adversity and neurobiological functioning, interventions targeting consistent parenting in both the foster home and the permanent placement hold promise for mitigating the effects of early adversity on both behavior and neurobiology. In MTFC-P, the child's birth family (or adoptive family if parental rights have been terminated) is involved in treatment to increase the likelihood that an environment of consistent discipline, limit-setting, and positive reinforcement is maintained when the child leaves the foster home and enters the long-term placement, thus increasing the child's chances of attaining a more positive developmental trajectory.

Finally, MTFC-P is focused on issues specific to young children who have experienced abuse and neglect, such as developmental delays and emotion regulation (Landsverk et al., 2002; Maughan & Cicchetti, 2002). The intervention is intended to provide the children and parents with the tools for these high-risk children to begin to make adequate developmental progress. An integral part of this approach is making a smooth transition to kindergarten. MTFC-P uses a therapeutic playgroup to target this potentially difficult developmental time by providing a safe and structured environment in which children can develop the socioemotional and academic skills necessary for school success. In playgroup, the children learn and practice regulating their emotions and engaging in positive social interactions with peers. Additionally, children are taught early literacy skills that they may not have received in their foster homes but that have been demonstrated to be critically important for success in school (Senechal & LeFevre, 2002). Increasing the likelihood of a smooth transition to kindergarten by promoting emotion regulation skills and prosocial behaviors that are critical for future school success (Blair, 2002) is especially important for this population given their increased risk for behavioral problems in school and also school failure (Zima et al., 2000). If the children enter kindergarten prepared for the transition, they stand to benefit greatly from the structured learning environment and opportunities for social interactions provided in school.

Program Components

MTFC-P is a multicomponent program that includes services to children, foster parents, and long-term placement caregivers (e.g., birth families and adoptive families). After a child is placed in an MTFC foster home, services begin not only for the child but also for the foster parent as well as for the permanent placement caregiver. Services for the foster parent include parent training, daily phone calls assessing the child's problem behavior and the foster parent's level of stress, weekly support groups, and 24-h crisis support. Services for the child include a behavior support specialist who assists the child in naturalistic settings in which the child may have behavioral difficulties, such as on the playground or in the grocery store, and also the therapeutic playgroup. Permanent placement caregivers receive parent training similar to that provided to the foster parents. A key underlying principle of MTFC-P is that services should be delivered in a proactive manner. That is, rather than waiting until child problems reach a point where his or her placement might be compromised, program staff members work collaboratively with the foster parents to prevent small problems from escalating. Another key principle of MTFC-P is the stratification of roles among the intervention staff members to increase efficient administration of the intervention. Though MTFC-P is an intensive intervention requiring a number of staff members, the clearly defined and stratified role of each member maximizes the case load of each individual due to the efficiency achieved by parceling out responsibility for one relationship and/or component (i.e., foster parent trainer, Parent Daily Report (PDR) caller, etc.) to one individual, with little overlap in responsibilities across staff members. In this section, we describe both the various program components and also the corresponding staff roles.

Recruitment of Foster Parents

MTFC-P foster parents are recruited in a variety of ways, including advertisements in local newspapers, postings in public places such as community centers and schools, and word-of-mouth. One of the most effective strategies employed for recruiting MTFC-P foster parents is through the participating parents. Current MTFC-P foster parents know what kinds of skills the program requires, are familiar with the support provided, and are often strong advocates for the program.

The recruitment of foster parents begins with a screening telephone call by the foster parent recruiter and is followed by a home visit. During a home visit, the details of the program are presented to prospective foster parents. The home visit also allows the recruiter to determine if the home environment would be appropriate for caring for a high-needs child.

MTFC-P foster parents are a diverse group. Over the several decades in which this program has been operating, they have included married couples, single parents, individuals with and without parenting experience, and individuals with varying economic statuses, sexual orientations, and cultural backgrounds. The main quality that distinguishes MTFC-P foster parents is their interest in being part of a treatment team and having a considerable amount of contact with the program staff. Individuals who are not interested in such a high level of contact, who are unwilling to participate in the program activities (described below), or whose schedules preclude them from participating in these kinds of activities do not make good MTFC-P foster parents. Otherwise, there are no specific criteria for individuals to be selected to participate.

Foster Parent Training

The foster parent training consists of 20 h of instruction over the span of 1 weekend and a following weekday evening. During the training, they are introduced to the specific behavioral management models employed with children in the age group that they are planning to have in their home. Details of the program staffing structure and the services available to parents and children are also provided. Considerable emphasis during the training is placed on providing children with positive support for prosocial behavior, including the use of concrete reinforcement strategies. Some prospective foster parents are extremely resistant to the idea of rewarding children for positive behavior. In many instances, it is possible to work through this concern by helping the foster parents understand that such measures are necessary for reversing the negative patterns of interaction to which the child has grown accustomed. However, individuals unwilling to provide a high level of positive reinforcement are discouraged from continuing to participate in training. Essentially, the goal of training is to identify individuals who share the philosophy of the program, even if it is not one that they have a great deal of experience employing.

Ongoing Services to Foster Parents

After the child is placed in the MTFC-P foster home, direct services begin in earnest. Based on information available in the child's case file, an initial individualized daily treatment program is developed by program staff members in consultation with the foster parents. From the first day of placement, foster parents have daily contact with the program in the form of a 5- to 10-min daily telephone call to collect information about problem behaviors that have occurred in the past 24 h. The caller uses a standardized checklist called the Parent Daily Report (PDR; Chamberlain & Reid, 1987). The foster parents are asked if each behavior on the PDR checklist occurred and, if so, whether it was stressful. The information collected via this telephone call is critical for ongoing case planning. It allows program staff members and foster parents to identify the most stressful commonly occurring behaviors, providing clear targets for the child behavior management program. In addition, because numbers of problem behaviors can be summed for each day (total problem behavior score), the PDR provides a method for assessing treatment progress over time. Finally, if foster parents report a great deal of stress or distress on a particular day, a program staff member can follow-up with more intensive contact to support the family.

In addition to daily telephone contact, all foster parents participate in a weekly support group meeting. At this meeting, program staff members review each child's progress using PDR data. The foster parents have a chance to present situations that were particularly challenging or positive for them. Other foster parents provide peer support and assistance in problem solving difficult child behavior. The meeting lasts for approximately 2 h, and childcare is provided along with snacks or a light meal.

The program staff provides support for emergency or crisis situations at all times. Although accommodations have been made to comply with a country's labor laws in some locations in which MTFC-P has been implemented, the idea that someone from the program is always available to help with difficult situations is a critical component of the program's success. Moreover, because MTFC-P uses a proactive approach to crisis management, the foster parents may feel less overwhelmed and alone when dealing with difficult circumstances, which might contribute to the low placement disruption rates that have been observed among MTFC-P foster homes (Fisher et al., 2009).

Services to Children

The MTFC-P foster children receive a comprehensive program of services. All children are placed on a behavior management program that is developmentally appropriate and targets both problem behaviors to be reduced and also prosocial behaviors to be increased. The behavior management program includes immediate tangible reinforcement for positive behavior, such as stickers or the use of star charts. The program expectations are that foster parents will maintain this reinforcement program with the children for the duration of their program participation.

Individual behavior programs are adjusted over time to meet the needs of the child. Foster parents provide input to the program staff via the aforementioned individual and group meetings to identify specific problems that require attention and to provide information about particularly effective methods for reinforcing positive behavior. The high degree of contact between the program staff and the foster parents allows each child's needs to be addressed on an ongoing basis. In addition to the behavior management program, a therapeutic playgroup is provided to help the children learn the skills they will need to be successful in school from both social and academic perspectives.

Services to Birth and Adoptive Families

During the time that the child is in MTFC-P, the program collaborates with the child welfare caseworker to identify the most likely long-term placement resource for the child. In many instances, this is the birth family from which the child came prior to entering foster care. In other instances, depending on the circumstances of the child, long-term care may be provided by close relatives or a nonrelative adoptive family. Program staff members work with birth and adoptive families to help teach them the parenting and behavior management skills that are being employed in the foster home. For example, they are taught how to implement a concrete system for reinforcing children's prosocial behavior and to use effective strategies to set limits around negative behavior without being overly harsh and coercive. Program staff members support these families during the child's transition into the permanent home. It is noteworthy that, in some instances, children stay with the MTFC-P foster family indefinitely rather than moving to another family. When this situation does occur, it is typically the best option due to the secure relationship likely already established over the course of the intervention. Services to the long-term placement caregivers continue until the child is stable in the home, as assessed by PDR data and the judgment of the treatment team, at which point services are discontinued.

Program Staffing Structure

One of the unique aspects of the MTFC-P program is the use of a team approach to providing services. Each treatment team contains a group of staff members with clearly defined roles. These roles are stratified and contain very little overlap. This set-up allows team members to focus primarily on the family needs related to their expertise. The treatment teams usually work with 12–15 children concurrently and their roles are as follows:

The program supervisor is responsible for coordinating the activities of all other team members and for serving as liaison between the program and any other services that the child and family is receiving. This individual is also the primary authority figure for the child and the foster family regarding limit setting or enforcing program rules. The program supervisor runs foster parent support group meetings and is available on an on-call basis at all times to manage crises.

The foster parent consultant provides additional support to the foster family and is often a former foster parent. The foster parent consultant delivers services via a home visit and frequent (at least weekly) telephone contact and participates as a co-leader in the weekly foster parent support group meetings. When the PDR caller indicates that foster parents have experienced a high level of stress on a given day, the foster parent consultant calls the foster parent to offer support. The foster parent consultant serves as an on-call backup if the program supervisor is not available.

The child receives support via individual sessions with the behavior support specialist, often a university student or other young person who is able to establish rapport with the children in the program. As noted above, behavior support specialists often deliver services in the context of community settings (e.g., home, school, playground, grocery stores, etc.) to help the child learn prosocial skills in their naturalistic environment. The behavior support specialist is the primary individual service provider for children in the MTFC-P program, while in the original MTFC program both a behavior support specialist and individual child therapist work with the child one-on-one.

A family therapist works with the long-term placement caregivers to prepare them to receive the child following foster care. The specific strategies employed are described above and are derived directly from parent training approaches that were developed at the Oregon Social Learning Center. The family therapist is usually a masters or doctoral level professional.

The PDR caller maintains daily contact with the foster families. This individual is often a clerical-level staff member. It is essential that they establish good rapport with the foster families and take information accurately over the telephone. Moreover, this individual needs to be able to understand when foster parents are having a difficult time so that other program staff members can follow up as appropriate.

A consulting psychiatrist is employed to manage the child's medication. Although not all children in the program receive psychiatric medications, many of these children do, so it is helpful to have a single provider coordinating care in this area. The consulting psychiatrist works with the child and with the program staff to flesh out a complete picture of the child's needs.

Playgroup staff includes a playgroup lead teacher and an assistant teacher. These individuals run the weekly therapeutic playgroup, helping the children to develop socioemotional skills during peer interactions and to learn early literacy skills. They usually have early childhood education experience or are in university programs to train teachers.

MTFC-P Evidence Base

The results presented in multiple peer-reviewed articles document how MTFC-P participants show positive change in important outcome measures, particularly young, maltreated children. For example, in a comparison between MTFC-P and regular foster care, participation in the intervention predicted greater improvements in the behavioral adjustment of the participating children (Fisher, Gunnar, Chamberlain, & Reid, 2000). In fact, whereas the MTFC-P children showed reductions in behavioral problems from pre- to post-intervention, the regular foster children showed increases in behavioral problems over the same time period, indicating that MTFC-P might buffer against the further development of problem behavior (Fisher et al., 2000). Furthermore, these positive changes in the MTFC-P children were coupled with the MTFC-P parents' increased use of the positive parenting practices targeted by the program, including consistent discipline, monitoring, and positive reinforcement. Thus, participation in MTFC-P is associated with improvements in child problem behaviors, likely achieved by the provision of support necessary to increase positive parenting practices within the long-term caregiver's home to improve the child's chances of future positive outcomes.

Although not directly targeted by intervention, participation in MTFC-P has also predicted increases in secure attachment behaviors (Fisher & Kim, 2007). Many maltreated young children, like those referred to MTFC-P, display disorganized or insecure attachment styles (e.g., Carlson, Cicchetti, Barnett, & Braunwald, 1989). Both the experience of maltreatment and also removal from the family of origin contribute to difficulties in forming secure attachments with current and future caregivers. The multiple placement disruptions common in high-risk foster care populations further jeopardize the child's ability to exhibit behaviors to foster the development of a secure attachment. Though clearly a relevant factor for maltreated young children in foster care, attachment can be challenging to assess in this population since the Strange Situation Paradigm (Ainsworth, Blehar, Waters, & Wall, 1978) most often used requires participation from an individual the child clearly views as a primary caretaker, which a foster child with a history of multiple placements may not have. To address this limitation in their investigation of the effect of MTFC-P on attachment behaviors, (Fisher and Kim, 2007) used the Parent Attachment Diary (PAD; Stovall-McClough & Dozier, 2000). The PAD asks the foster parent to report on the child's behavior over the past 2 weeks in response to situations that are frightening or distressing to the child, and these attachment-related behaviors are then coded in to secure, resistant, and avoidant categories of behavior. These assessments occurred every 3 months for 12 months post-intervention (Fisher & Kim, 2007). Results revealed that participation in MTFC-P is associated with an increase in the number of secure attachment behaviors (specifically, in the likelihood that the child will seek out the proximity of their caregivers when hurt, frightened, or separated from them). Conversely, foster care children not in the intervention showed a decrease in secure attachment behavior over time (Fisher & Kim, 2007). It is noteworthy that MTFC-P affects this important outcome variable, though the intervention is not attachment-focused. Thus, the key target variables of MTFC-P – the child's socioemotional development and the primary caregivers' consistent parenting – appear to be important components for the development of secure attachment behaviors over time.

The MTFC-P children also exhibit increased placement stability (Fisher et al., 2009). This outcome variable is particularly important from a prevention standpoint considering the literature documenting increases in risks for permanent placement failure related to a higher number of previous placements (Fisher et al., 2005; Wells & Guo, 1999). Fisher et al. (2009) found that the MTFC-P children, despite having experienced a significantly greater number of placements than foster children not receiving the intervention, had a significantly greater number of successful permanent placements over the 2-year period following participation in MTFC-P. Given the strong predictive power of placement stability for negative outcomes, the fact that MTFC-P can improve the likelihood of successful placement in young children is strong evidence for its potential for changing developmental trajectories in these children.

It is important to note that there is also evidence of MTFC-P's effectiveness at impacting neurobiological systems that have been negatively affected by early life stress (e.g., Bruce, Fisher, Pears, & Levine, 2009; Fisher et al., 2000; Fisher, van Ryzin, & Gunnar, 2011). One such system is that underlying stress regulation, often indexed by the stress hormone cortisol. In typically developing children, cortisol release peaks in the morning and decreases over the course of the day. In early childhood, regulation of this system is achieved primarily from the environment. Responsive caregiving characterized by consistent and appropriate responses to a child's distress provides external regulation of stress early in life and promotes the eventual development of the child's self-regulatory abilities. However, young foster children often do not have sufficient or consistent external regulation. As a result of this young foster children often show an abnormal diurnal cortisol rhythm, suggesting neurobiological effects associated with their histories of maltreatment specifically related to stress regulation (Bruce et al., 2009).

Fisher and colleagues (2007) have shown MTFC-P to have a preventative effect on this process. Specifically, while foster children not participating in the intervention showed a significant increase in HPA axis dysregulation over time, children in MTFC-P did not show this dysregulation but rather exhibited patterns of cortisol release more closely resembling those of community control children (Fisher et al., 2000, 2006; Fisher, Stoolmiller, Gunnar, & Burraston, 2007). Fisher and colleagues also found that MTFC-P children showed less cortisol dysregulation during transitions from one home to another, suggesting that the intervention may make this particularly vulnerable time less stressful for the child (Fisher et al., 2011).

Furthermore, MTFC-P appears to buffer the effects of caregiver stress on the HPA-axis regulation of the child (Fisher & Stoolmiller, 2008). When a caregiver experiences high levels of stress, the caregiver's ability to employ consistent parenting strategies is often diminished (Halme, Tarkka, Nummi, & Astedt-Kurki, 2006). This situation is particularly salient in the foster care context in which foster parents often must manage high levels of problem behaviors exhibited by high-risk foster children. In a randomized controlled trial of MTFC-P compared to regular foster care, the MTFC-P parents showed reduced levels of self-reported stress in response to child problem behavior, and this effect was maintained at a 1-year follow-up (Fisher & Stoolmiller, 2008). Additionally, the self-reported stress levels of the regular foster care parents increased over this time period, suggesting that MTFC-P may serve a protective function in the context of caregiver stress. Importantly, the increased levels of caregiver stress observed in foster parents not receiving the intervention were associated with lower morning cortisol levels in the child (Fisher & Stoolmiller, 2008), indicating the potential for caregiver stress to impact a child's stress regulatory system. MTFC-P might affect children's HPA axis regulation by supporting the caregivers and, thus, decreasing caregiver stress levels. On the whole, the evidence suggests that participation in MTFC-P predicts positive change in a child's stress regulatory system, partially through improvements in parents' stress levels.

In sum, evaluations of MTFC-P have incorporated a variety of outcome measures (behavioral and neurobiological) to demonstrate the intervention's capacity to facilitate positive changes and mitigate the negative effects associated with remaining in foster care. These results support the importance and the promise of early intervention with young maltreated children. MTFC-P, by supporting effective parenting and consistency for the child, can be considered an evidence-based family intervention that alleviates the risks associated with foster children who have histories of maltreatment.

MTFC-P Case Study

The following case study illustrates how MTFC-P can be used as an effective treatment for preschool-aged foster children. "*Gabriel*" was a 4-year-old male with a history of significant physical abuse and neglect when he was referred to the program. Gabriel had been raised by a single mother who had two other younger children, each of whom had a different father. Gabriel's mother had a history of drug and alcohol abuse as well as involvement in relationships that included domestic violence. She had never graduated from high school, experienced unemployment and housing instability, and was dependent on public assistance for financial support. When Gabriel entered foster care, Gabriel's mother was well known to the child welfare system caseworkers because of her maltreatment of the children and involvement in domestic violence.

Prior to being referred to the MTFC-P program, Gabriel had been in several foster homes. However, his aggressive and defiant behavior made him difficult to manage, and the foster parents in these homes had requested Gabriel's removal due to this behavior. Although only a preschooler, Gabriel was quite large for his age and very strong. As such, when he became aggressive, he could destroy a considerable amount of property and pose a risk of physical harm to his caregivers. Gabriel's caseworker believed that if she were unable to stabilize him in a treatment foster care home, the only alternative would be residential treatment. This profile is not uncommon for children referred to the MTFC-P program. The standardized mental health assessment conducted at the time revealed that Gabriel met criteria for conduct disorder (unusual for such a young child) as well as for attention deficit and hyperactivity disorder. It was not clear whether some of this aggression was a manifestation of post-traumatic stress disorder, which is difficult to diagnose at this age, so PTSD was listed as a rule-out diagnosis. The diagnostic information obtained from this assessment was employed to develop Gabriel's initial treatment plan.

Gabriel was placed in a foster home with new foster parents. These foster parents had raised their biological children, but these children were now grown and no longer living in the home. Although MTFC-P placements are sometimes made in foster families in which there are younger children, such a placement for Gabriel was deemed risky because of the potential harm that could be caused by his aggressive behavior.

Gabriel's initial transition to the MTFC-P foster home did not go smoothly. Although foster children often show relatively limited negative behavior when first placed in a new home (this is sometimes referred to by clinical staff who work with the children as a "honeymoon period"), Gabriel began to exhibit problem behaviors almost immediately. He was noncompliant with his foster parents' requests and was often quite defiant in his tone. When pressed to complete a task such as clearing his plate or cleaning his room, he escalated quickly from defiance to violence. This violence included destruction of property (plates and other ceramic objects, wooden furniture, walls and doors) and physical aggression towards the foster parents.

During this initial adjustment period to the foster home, Gabriel's foster parents required considerable support from program staff members. Gabriel's foster parents were instructed in the appropriate use of consistent and nonaggressive discipline strategies, including timeout and privilege removal. They were also given a positive reinforcement program to implement. Because of Gabriel's high rate of negative behavior, the program staff felt it was necessary for the parents to reinforce Gabriel's positive behavior frequently and immediately.

Although the foster parents were observed to implement these behavioral strategies quite effectively during home visits and reported employing them frequently, Gabriel's behavior problems continued to escalate. The on-call staff availability and the staff role stratification proved instrumental in getting past these initial difficulties. The program supervisor served in an authority role and made frequent visits to the house to enforce limits. This made it possible for the foster parents to assume a more supportive and less power-assertive role. The foster parent consultant provided emotional support to the foster parents during this time, which was clearly needed. The foster parents also received considerable support via the daily PDR calls. In addition, the foster parents attended weekly support group meetings; through these meetings, they were able to hear from other, more experienced foster parents about the challenges involved in children transitioning to a new home. Although this did not take away from the difficulties of caring for Gabriel, it normalized these difficulties.

After approximately 6 weeks of this pattern of aggressive and noncompliant behavior, Gabriel began to respond more positively to his foster parents. He gradually became more compliant and was slower to escalate into aggression when frustrated or upset. However, whenever the foster parents became less structured in response to these improvements, Gabriel had significant setbacks, becoming destructive towards property and aggressive towards the foster parents. As such, it was necessary for the foster parents to continue to implement the MTFC-P behavior program with a high degree of fidelity. Gabriel was a regular participant in the program playgroup, and this increased his use of prosocial behavior with peers.

After several months of treatment in this foster home, Gabriel's behavior was stable enough and his aggression had decreased to the degree that his caseworker made the decision to place his two younger siblings (both brothers) with him. This change produced yet another episode of extremely challenging behavior on Gabriel's part. By this time, however, the foster parents continued to consistently use the behavior program with Gabriel and his siblings, believing that this would ultimately produce the most positive changes. Gabriel's behavior again stabilized.

After Gabriel had been in care for approximately 8 months, proceedings to terminate his biological mother's parental rights were initiated as a result of her lack of compliance with the conditions set forth by her caseworker and her ongoing drug use. The court determined that terminating parental rights for Gabriel and his siblings was the appropriate decision, and Gabriel was made eligible for adoption.

The foster parents who had been caring for Gabriel and his siblings considered becoming adoptive parents but decided that they were too old to take on this role. However, their friends from church who were much younger and knew the children were interested in adopting them. This proved to be an excellent situation that allowed Gabriel and his siblings to remain in contact with the foster parents and to stay in their community of origin. Although Gabriel and his brothers continued to require a high level of support and structure, MTFC-P was terminated once the children were stable in the adoptive home.

Concluding Remarks

This chapter provides an overview of the MTFC-P program, describes its origins at the Oregon Social Learning Center, provides details about the program's components, elaborates on the evidence base for MTFC-P, and provides a case study demonstrating how MTFC-P helped one child with a significant history of maltreatment move in a more positive direction. Programs like MTFC-P have the potential to transform the lives of many troubled children. Nevertheless, financial and programmatic barriers continue to exist regarding early intervention programs for young foster children. More work is needed for programs like MTFC-P to become standard practice in community settings. This work will require collaborative efforts on the part of policymakers, child welfare leaders and caseworkers, researchers, and community members. Only through such collaborative efforts is progress likely.

References

Ainsworth, M. D. S., Blehar, M. C., Waters, E., & Wall, S. (1978). *Patterns of attachment: A psychological study of the strange situation*. Hillsdale, NJ: Lawrence Erlbaum.

Bank, L., Forgatch, M. S., Patterson, G. R., & Fetrow, R. A. (1993). Parenting practices of single mothers: Mediators of negative contextual factors. *Journal of Marriage and Family, 55*, 371–384.

Bank, L., Marlowe, J. H., Reid, J. B., Patterson, G. R., & Weinrott, M. R. (1991). A comparative evaluation of parent training for families of chronic delinquents. *Journal of Abnormal Child Psychology, 19*, 15–33.

Blair, C. (2002). School readiness: Integrating cognition and emotion in a neurobiological conceptualization of children's functioning at school entry. *American Psychologist, 57*(2), 111–127.

Briggs-Gowan, M. J., Horwitz, S. M., Schwab-Stone, M. E., Leventhal, J. M., & Leaf, P. J. (2000). Mental health in pediatric settings: Distribution of disorders and factors related to service use. *Journal of American Academy of Child and Adolescent Psychiatry, 39*, 841–849.

Bruce, J., Fisher, P. A., Pears, K. C., & Levine, S. (2009). Morning cortisol levels in preschool-aged foster children: Differential effects of maltreatment type. *Developmental Psychobiology, 51*, 14–23.

Bruce, J., McDermott, J. M., Fisher, P. A., & Fox, N. A. (2009). Using behavioral and electrophysiological measures to assess the effects of a preventive intervention: A preliminary study with preschool-aged foster children. *Prevention Science, 10*, 129–140.

Burns, B. J., Phillips, S. D., Wagner, H. R., Barth, R. P., Kolko, D. J., Campbell, Y., et al. (2004). Mental health need and access to mental health services by youth involved with child welfare: A national survey. *Journal of the American Academy of Children and Adolescent Psychiatry, 43*, 960–970.

Carlson, V., Cicchetti, D., Barnett, D., & Braunwald, K. (1989). Disorganized/disoriented attachment relationships in maltreated infants. *Developmental Psychology, 25*, 525–531.

Chamberlain, P. (2003). The Oregon Multidimensional Treatment Foster Care model: Features, outcomes, and progress in dissemination. *Cognitive and Behavioral Practice, 10*, 303–312.

Chamberlain, P., Leve, L. D., & DeGarmo, D. S. (2007). Multidimensional Treatment Foster Care for girls in the juvenile justice system: 2-year follow-up of a randomized clinical trial. *Journal of Consulting and Clinical Psychology, 75*, 187–193.

Chamberlain, P., & Reid, J. B. (1987). Parent observation and report of child symptoms. *Behavioral Assessment, 9*, 97–109.

Chamberlain, P., & Reid, J. B. (1998). Comparison of two community alternatives to incarceration for chronic juvenile offenders. *Journal of Consulting and Clinical Psychology, 6*, 624–633.

Conger, R. D., Conger, K. J., Elder, G. H., Jr., Lorenz, F. O., Simons, R. L., & Whitbeck, L. B. (1992). A family process model of economic hardship and adjustment of early adolescent boys. *Child Development, 63*, 526–541.

Conger, R. D., Patterson, G. R., & Ge, X. (1995). It takes two to replicate: A mediational model for the impact of parents' stress on adolescent adjustment. *Child Development, 66*, 80–97.

DeGarmo, D. S., Forgatch, M. S., & Martinez, C. R., Jr. (1999). Parenting of divorced mothers as a link between social status and boys' academic outcomes: Unpacking the effects of SES. *Child Development, 70*, 1231–1245.

Dishion, T. J., Patterson, G. R., & Kavanagh, K. (1992). An experimental test of the coercion model: Linking theory, measurement, and intervention. In J. McCord & R. Tremblay (Eds.), *The interaction of theory and practice: Experimental studies of intervention* (pp. 253–282). New York: Guilford.

Eddy, J. M., & Chamberlain, P. (2000). Family management and deviant peer association as mediators of the impact of treatment condition on youth antisocial behavior. *Journal of Consulting and Clinical Psychology, 68*, 857–863.

Eddy, J. M., Whaley, R. B., & Chamberlain, P. (2004). The prevention of violent behavior by chronic and serious male juvenile offenders: A 2-year follow-up of a randomized clinical trial. *Journal of Emotional and Behavioral Disorders, 12*, 2–8.

Fisher, P. A., Burraston, B., & Pears, K. C. (2005). The Early Intervention Foster Care Program: Permanent placement outcomes from a randomized trial. *Child Maltreatment, 10*, 61–71.

Fisher, P. A., Ellis, B. H., & Chamberlain, P. (1999). Early intervention foster care: A model for preventing risk in young children who have been maltreated. *Children's Services: Social Policy, Research, and Practice, 2*(3), 159–182.

Fisher, P. A., & Gunnar, M. R. (2010). Early life stress as a risk factor for disease in adulthood. In R. A. Lanius, E. Vermetten, & C. Pain (Eds.), *The impact of early life trauma on health and disease* (pp. 133–141). Cambridge, UK: Cambridge University Press.

Fisher, P. A., Gunnar, M. R., Chamberlain, P., & Reid, J. B. (2000). Preventive intervention for maltreated preschool children: Impact on children's behavior, neuroendocrine activity, and foster parent functioning. *Journal of the American Academy of Child and Adolescent Psychiatry, 39*, 1356–1364.

Fisher, P. A., Gunnar, M., Dozier, M., Bruce, J., & Pears, K. C. (2006). Effects of a therapeutic intervention for foster children on behavior problems, caregiver attachment, and stress regulatory neural systems. *Annals of the New York Academy of Sciences, 1094*, 215–225.

Fisher, P. A., & Kim, H. K. (2007). Intervention effects on foster preschoolers' attachment-related behaviors from a randomized trial. *Prevention Science, 8*, 161–170.

Fisher, P. A., Kim, H. K., & Pears, K. C. (2009). Effects of Multidimensional Treatment Foster Care for Preschoolers (MTFC-P) on reducing permanent placement failures among children with placement instability. *Child and Youth Services Review, 31*, 541–546.

Fisher, P. A., & Stoolmiller, M. (2008). Intervention effects on foster parent stress: Associations with child cortisol levels. *Development and Psychopathology, 20*, 1003–1021.

Fisher, P. A., Stoolmiller, M., Gunnar, M. R., & Burraston, B. (2007). Effects of a therapeutic intervention for foster preschoolers on diurnal cortisol activity. *Psychoneuroendocrinology, 32*, 892–905.

Fisher, P. A., Van Ryzin, M. J., & Gunnar, M. R. (2011). Mitigating HPA axis dysregulation associated with placement changes in foster care. *Psychoneuroendocrinology, 36*, 531–539.

Forgatch, M. S., & Patterson, G. R. (2010). The Oregon Model of Parent Management Training (PMTO): An intervention for antisocial behavior in children and adolescents. In J. R. Weisz & A. E. Kazdin (Eds.), *Evidence based psychotherapies for children and adolescents* (2nd ed., pp. 159–178). New York: Guilford.

Gartstein, M. A., & Fagot, B. I. (2003). Parental depression, parenting and family adjustment, and child effortful control: Explaining externalizing behaviors for preschool children. *Applied Developmental Psychology, 24*, 143–177.

Halme, N., Tarkka, M.-T., Nummi, T., & Astedt-Kurki, P. (2006). The effect of parenting stress on fathers' availability and engagement. *Child Care in Practice, 12*(1), 13–26.

Klee, L., Kronstadt, D., & Zlotnick, C. (1997). Foster care's youngest: A preliminary report. *American Journal of Orthopsychiatry, 67*, 290–299.

Landsverk, J., Garland, A. F., & Leslie, L. K. (2002). Mental health services for children reported to child protective services. In J. E. B. Meyers, L. Berliner, J. N. Briere, C. T. Hendrix, T. A. Reid, & C. A. Jenny (Eds.), *APSAC handbook on child maltreatment* (2nd ed., pp. 487–507). Thousand Oaks, CA: Sage.

Larzelere, R. E., & Patterson, G. R. (1990). Parental management: Mediators of the effect of socioeconomic status on early delinquency. *Criminology, 28*, 301–323.

Leve, L. D., Fisher, P. A., & Chamberlain, P. (2009). Multidimensional Treatment Foster Care as a preventive intervention to promote resiliency among youth in the child welfare system. *Journal of Personality, 77*, 1869–1902.

Leve, L. D., Kim, H. K., & Pears, K. C. (2005). Childhood temperament and family environment as predictors of internalizing and externalizing trajectories from ages 5 to 17. *Journal of Abnormal Child Psychology, 33*, 505–520.

Loeber, R., & Dishion, T. J. (1983). Early predictors of male delinquency: A review. *Psychological Bulletin, 94*, 68–99.

Maughan, A., & Cicchetti, D. (2002). Impact of child maltreatment and interadult violence on children's emotion regulation abilities and socioemotional adjustment. *Child Development, 73*(5), 1525–1542.

Newton, R. R., Litrownik, A. J., & Landsverk, J. A. (2000). Children and youth in foster care: Disentangling the relationship between problem behaviors and number of placements. *Child Abuse & Neglect, 24*(10), 1363–1374.

Ogden, T., & Hagen, K. A. (2008). Treatment effectiveness of parent management training in Norway: A randomized controlled trial of children with conduct problems. *Journal of Consulting and Clinical Psychology, 76*, 607–621.

Patterson, G. R. (1982). *A social learning approach: 3. Coercive family process.* Eugene, OR: Castalia.

Patterson, G. R. (2002). The early developmental of coercive family process. In J. B. Reid, G. R. Patterson, & J. Snyder (Eds.), *Antisocial behavior in children and adolescents: Developmental theories and models for intervention* (pp. 25–44). Washington, DC: American Psychological Association.

Patterson, G. R., Chamberlain, P., & Reid, J. B. (1982). A comparative evaluation of parent training procedures. *Behavior Therapy, 13*, 638–650.

Patterson, G. R., Debaryshe, B., & Ramsey, E. (1989). A developmental perspective on antisocial behavior. *American Psychologist, 44*, 329–335.

Patterson, G. R., Dishion, T. J., & Bank, L. (1984). Family interaction: A process model of deviancy training. *Aggressive Behavior, 10*, 253–267.

Patterson, G. R., & Fagot, B. I. (1967). Selective responsiveness to social reinforcers and deviant behavior in children. *The Psychological Record, 17*, 369–378.

Patterson, G. R., Forgatch, M. S., & DeGarmo, D. S. (2010). Cascading effects following intervention. *Development and Psychopathology, 22*, 949–970.

Patterson, G. R., Reid, J. B., & Dishion, T. J. (1992). *A social learning approach. IV. Antisocial boys*. Eugene, OR: Castalia.

Pears, K. C., & Fisher, P. A. (2005). Developmental, cognitive, and neuropsychological functioning in preschool-aged foster children: Associations with prior maltreatment and placement history. *Journal of Developmental and Behavioral Pediatrics, 26*, 112–122.

Pears, K. C., Fisher, P. A., & Bronz, K. D. (2007). An intervention to promote social emotional school readiness in foster children: Preliminary outcomes from a pilot study. *School Psychology Review, 36*, 665–673.

Pears, K. C., Fisher, P. A., Bruce, J., Kim, H. K., & Yoerger, K. (2010). Early elementary school adjustment of maltreated children in foster care: The roles of inhibitory control and caregiver involvement. *Child Development, 81*, 1550–1564.

Senechal, M., & LeFevre, J.-A. (2002). Parental involvement in the development of children's reading skill: A five-year longitudinal study. *Child Development, 73*(2), 445–460.

Shonkoff, J. P. (2010). Protecting brains, not simply stimulating minds. *Science, 333*, 982–983.

Stovall-McClough, K. C., & Dozier, M. (2000). The development of attachment in new relationships: Single subject analyses for 10 foster infants. *Development and Psychopathology, 12*, 133–156.

Walter, H., & Gilmore, S. K. (1973). Placebo versus social learning effects in parent training procedures designed to alter the behaviors of aggressive boys. *Behavior Therapy, 4*, 361–371.

Wells, K., & Guo, S. (1999). Reunification and reentry of foster children. *Children and Youth Services Review, 21*, 273–294.

Wiltz, N. A., Jr., & Patterson, G. R. (1974). An evaluation of parent training procedures designed to alter inappropriate aggressive behavior of boys. *Behavior Therapy, 5*, 215–221.

Zima, B. T., Bussing, R., Freeman, S., Yang, X., Belin, T. R., & Forness, S. R. (2000). Behavior problems, academic skill delays and school failure among school-aged children in foster care: Their relationship to placement characteristics. *Journal of Child and Family Studies, 9*(1), 87–103.

Part IV
Interventions for School Aged Children

Research findings suggest that emotions are often dysregulated or poorly regulated in maltreated youth (Cicchetti & Toth, 2000). Emotional dysregulation interferes with good decision-making, and increases the likelihood of making risky decisions that support "good feelings" (Blakemore & Choudhury, 2006). Understanding when and how executive functions develop, and the role emotions play in decision-making during childhood and adolescence suggests that successful interventions for these children will involve cognitive-behavioral strategies for managing emotions, and improve impulse control. We present two different types cognitive-behavioral therapies, showing the flexibility of these treatment systems. Mannarino, Cohen, and Deblinger describe the effectiveness and function of Trauma-Focused Cognitive Behavioral Therapy (TF-CBT) in Chap. 10, and Kolko and his colleagues describe Alternatives for Families- A Cognitive Behavioral Therapy (AF-CBT) in Chap. 11.

References

Blakemore, S.-J., & Choudhury, S. (2006). Development of the adolescent brain: Implications for executive function and social cognition. *Journal of Child Psychology and Psychiatry, 47*(3), 296–312.

Cicchetti, D., & Toth, S. (2000). Developmental processes in maltreated children. In D. Hansen (Ed.), *Nebraska symposium on motivation* (Motivation and child maltreatment, Vol. 46, pp. 85–160). Lincoln, NE: University of Nebraska Press.

Chapter 10
Trauma-Focused Cognitive-Behavioral Therapy

Anthony P. Mannarino, Judith A. Cohen, and Esther Deblinger

Introduction

Over the past two decades, there has been a proliferation of research on children and families exposed to traumatic life events. Major national disasters like the September 11 terrorist attacks and Hurricane Katrina have focused national attention on the impact of such monumental events, how to identify children most affected, and what kinds of immediate and longer-term interventions could be of benefit. Despite the obvious tragedy of these large scale events and the media attention which they garner, many more children and families experience sexual abuse, physical abuse, domestic violence, community violence, bullying, and other types of interpersonal violence on a daily basis in our country.

Trauma-Focused Cognitive-Behavioral Therapy (TF-CBT) was originally developed for children who had been sexually abused and their non-offending caretakers (Cohen, Mannarino, & Deblinger, 2006). Research has demonstrated that TF-CBT is superior to comparison treatments in reducing a variety of symptoms and problems in child victims and their non-offending caretakers (Cohen, Deblinger, Mannarino, & Steer, 2004). Additional studies have now demonstrated that TF-CBT is effective for children who have experienced domestic violence, traumatic loss, and multiple traumas (Cohen, Mannarino, & Deblinger, 2010). (The research supporting TF-CBT will be reviewed later in this chapter.) In fact, in a recent

A.P. Mannarino, Ph.D. (✉) • J.A. Cohen, MD
Department of Psychiatry, Center for Traumatic Stress in Children and Adolescents,
Drexel University College of Medicine, Allegheny General Hospital, Four Allegheny Center,
Room 860, Pittsburgh, PA 15212, USA
e-mail: amannari@wpahs.org; Jcohen1@wpahs.org

E. Deblinger, Ph.D.
CARES Institute, University of Medicine & Dentistry of New Jersey, Stratford, NJ, USA
e-mail: deblines@umdnj.edu

S. Timmer and A. Urquiza (eds.), *Evidence-Based Approaches for the Treatment of Maltreated Children*, Child Maltreatment 3, DOI 10.1007/978-94-007-7404-9_10,
© Springer Science+Business Media Dordrecht 2014

meta-analysis of evidence-based psychosocial treatments for children and adolescents exposed to traumatic events, TF-CBT was the only intervention that achieved the "well-established" criteria for efficacy (Silverman et al., 2008).

Development and Theoretical Underpinnings of TF-CBT

TF-CBT is an evidence-based treatment for children and families who have experienced traumatic events. The model draws from a variety of theoretical approaches, including family systems, neurobiology, developmental theory, attachment theory, and client-centered humanistic treatment principles. For example, family systems and attachment theory influence both our belief in the importance of and how non-offending (non-perpetrator) parents are included in TF-CBT treatment. Specifically, our understanding of the critical role of parents for providing meaning and context, modeling effective coping and support, and providing a safe environment for emotional expression for children after traumatic experiences, influenced our decision to include parents during parallel individual TF-CBT sessions. Accordingly, both parents and children can freely express the impact of the child's traumatic experiences in individual sessions and subsequently during conjoint parent-child TF-CBT sessions in order to enhance positive child-parent attachments, communication and support. Since perpetrating parents typically deny their role in causing the child's trauma and undermine the above supportive parenting functions, as well as serving as ongoing trauma reminders, these parents are not included in TF-CBT treatment.

Neurobiological and developmental models of trauma have influenced our understanding of how psychotherapy can impact the traumatic changes in children's brain structure and functioning (Cohen, Perel, DeBellis, Friedman, & Putnam, 2002), and that trauma reminders serve as triggers for trauma symptoms to recur throughout the course of treatment. These trauma reminders need to be carefully monitored and addressed through the use of appropriate coping skills and exposure strategies throughout the course of treatment. Client-centered principles of active listening and accurate reflection influence our belief in the critical importance of establishing trust and safety in the therapeutic relationship after child trauma. However, the essential theoretical underpinnings of TF-CBT are cognitive-behavioral principles; specifically, the ability to reflect on, make connections among and change maladaptive trauma-related thoughts, feelings and behaviors. In particular, TF-CBT is focused on helping children to overcome the avoidance that commonly occurs after exposure to traumatic events and which is the hallmark of posttraumatic stress disorder (PTSD). Indeed TF-CBT is based on the theoretical concept of gradual exposure as children are encouraged over time to gradually and increasingly overcome their avoidance of the traumatic event(s). It is a short-term treatment approach that typically takes 8–16 sessions to complete (Cohen et al., 2006). However, as the model has been applied with adolescents with complex trauma and/or youth placed in residential settings, the length of treatment may be up to 25 sessions (Cohen, Mannarino, & Navarro, 2012; Kliethermes & Wamser, 2012).

TF-CBT is a components- and phase-based, hierarchical treatment model in which the early treatment components set the foundation for the subsequent components. The three phases of TF-CBT include (1) an initial stabilization/skill-building phase; (2) a trauma narrative and processing phase; and (3) a treatment consolidation and closure phase. In typical practice, each phase takes approximately the same number of sessions. For example, if the entire TF-CBT treatment takes 15 sessions, the stabilization/skills-building phase, trauma narrative and treatment consolidation phases would each take about 5 sessions.

The stabilization/skills building phase includes the TF-CBT components psychoeducation, parenting skills relaxation, affective regulation, and cognitive coping. These skills serve the purpose of helping the child to manage affective, behavioral or interpersonal dysregulation including that occurring in response to trauma reminders. If the child is experiencing avoidance of trauma reminders in the environment that are impeding daily functioning (e.g., refusing to attend school or sleep in his own bed), an in vivo exposure program is often started in this phase since this exposure program typically takes several weeks to complete. The second phase of TF-CBT includes the trauma narrative and cognitive processing. The purpose of this phase is to help the child gain additional mastery over personal trauma memories as he describes his own trauma experiences. The final TF-CBT phase includes completion of the in vivo exposure component, conjoint parent-child sessions, and enhancing safety. The purpose of this phase is to consolidate previous treatment gains, including bringing the child and parent together in order to integrate their treatment experiences and enhance positive attachment and communication. Together these components spell the acronym PRACTICE which signifies the importance of the TF-CBT skills being practiced both in and outside of treatment sessions in order to achieve mastery. These components are delivered in parallel treatment sessions for the child and parent. (If a child has been placed in foster care as may be the case for children who have experienced maltreatment, the foster parent would ordinarily participate in TF-CBT.)

Although the PRACTICE components are the essential ingredients of TF-CBT, the developers firmly believe in the importance of the therapeutic relationship with both the child and caretaker. As with other evidence-based treatments, TF-CBT could not be implemented successfully without a strong, safe, and empathic therapeutic alliance. Sexual abuse and other forms of child maltreatment often engender intense feelings of shame and embarrassment which are only worsened by the typical secrecy of these events. The support and strength of the therapeutic relationship are critical if children are going to have the courage to progress through the TF-CBT components and overcome their avoidance and fear.

Empirical Support for TF-CBT

Research conducted over two decades ago examining the therapeutic needs of children and their families in the aftermath of child sexual abuse provided the impetus for the development of an evidence-based treatment model for traumatized children and their families (Cohen & Mannarino, 1988; Deblinger, McLeer, Atkins, Ralph, & Foa, 1989; Mannarino & Cohen, 1986; Mannarino, Cohen, & Gregor, 1989; McLeer, Deblinger, Atkins, Foa, & Ralph, 1988). The authors initially developed strikingly similar treatment models and conducted independent randomized trials at their respective institutions examining the evidence-based treatment referred to today as Trauma-focused Cognitive Behavioral Therapy (TF-CBT) for children and adolescents (Cohen et al., 2006).

Cohen and Mannarino (1996) first examined the efficacy of an early version of TF-CBT in a randomized trial in which preschool children with a history of having been sexually abused, along with their non-offending parents, were randomly assigned to TF-CBT or a nondirective supportive therapy. The results documented the superior efficacy of TF-CBT over the nondirective therapy with regard to internalizing symptoms and overall behavior problems. Furthermore, the findings of a 1-year follow-up to this investigation documented the maintenance of symptom improvement over the follow-up period with clinical findings also demonstrating greater benefits of TF-CBT with respect to reducing age inappropriate sexual behaviors in this population. TF-CBT was next compared to a nondirective approach with children ages 7–14 who had been sexually abused (Cohen & Mannarino, 1998). The findings of this investigation demonstrated that children assigned to TF-CBT as opposed to the nondirective supportive treatment exhibited significantly greater improvements on measures of social competence and depression with clinical findings also suggesting the superiority of TF-CBT over nondirective therapy in the treatment of sexually inappropriate behaviors.

After conducting preliminary pre-post investigations of early versions of TF-CBT in individual and group therapy formats (Deblinger, McLeer, & Henry, 1990; Stauffer & Deblinger, 1996), Deblinger and colleagues conducted several independent randomized trials as well. In the first of these investigations, Deblinger hypothesized a critical role of including parents in TF-CBT treatment based on the theoretical role of parents in treatment described above. Families facing the crisis of child sexual abuse were randomly assigned to one of three experimental TF-CBT conditions – child only, mother only, mother and child – or to a community control condition (Deblinger, Lippmann, & Steer, 1996). The findings documented that families assigned to conditions that included active participation of the mother (i.e., mother only or mother and child conditions) demonstrated significantly greater reductions in children's externalizing behavior problems and significantly greater increases in effective parenting skills. On the other hand, significantly greater improvements with respect to PTSD symptoms were found among the children assigned to the experimental conditions in which the children were actively engaged (i.e. child only or mother and child conditions) as opposed to the community control or mother only condition. This investigation not only documented the critical importance of both child and caregiver participation but also demonstrated the maintenance of symptom improvement over a 2-year follow-up period (Deblinger, Steer, & Lippmann, 1999).

Deblinger and colleagues also examined the differential efficacies of supportive therapy and TF-CBT delivered via group treatment formats. For this investigation, young children (ages 2–8) and their non-offending mothers were randomly assigned to alternative group therapy conditions (Deblinger, Stauffer, & Steer, 2001). The results demonstrated that mothers assigned to the TF-CBT groups exhibited significantly greater reductions in intrusive, abused-related thoughts and negative parental emotional reactions as compared to mothers assigned to the supportive therapy groups. In addition, children assigned to the TF-CBT groups demonstrated greater improvements with regard to body safety knowledge and skills as compared to children assigned to the supportive therapy groups.

The authors' first collaborative investigation was a multisite randomized trial in which children (ages 8–14 years) who had been sexually abused and their non-offending caregivers were randomly assigned to TF-CBT or a child-centered therapy approach. The results of this investigation replicated earlier findings documenting the superior efficacy of TF-CBT (Cohen, Deblinger, Mannarino, & Steer, 2004). More specifically, children assigned to TF-CBT as compared to those assigned to child-centered supportive treatment demonstrated significantly greater improvement with respect to PTSD, depression, behavior problems, shame and abuse-related attributions. Similarly, parents assigned to TF-CBT demonstrated greater improvement in their own levels of depression, abuse-specific distress, support for their child, and effective parenting skills. These findings too were maintained over a 1-year follow-up period (Deblinger, Mannarino, Cohen, & Steer, 2006).

The most recent collaborative investigation examined the effects of TF-CBT delivered in 8 vs. 16 sessions with or without the trauma narrative (TN) component. In this multisite investigation, children ages 4–11 were randomly assigned along with their caregivers to one of four conditions: 8 sessions with no TN, 8 sessions with TN, 16 sessions with no TN, and 16 sessions with TN. While children and caregivers across all four conditions exhibited significant pre- to post-treatment improvement across all 14 outcome measures, the eight session condition that included the TN component seemed to be significantly more effective and efficient in ameliorating parents' abuse-specific distress as well as children's abuse-related fear and general anxiety. On the other hand, parents assigned to the 16 session, no narrative condition were found to exhibit a significantly greater increase in effective parenting practices and their children demonstrated fewer externalizing behavioral problems than those assigned to the other conditions. These findings highlighted the importance of tailoring the focus and length of TF-CBT to the child's pre-treatment symptom profile (Deblinger, Mannarino, Cohen, Runyon, & Steer, 2011).

It should also be noted that additional TF-CBT treatment outcome studies, including randomized trials and quasi-experimental studies, have been conducted by the authors as well as other investigators with children exposed to other types of traumas and with diverse populations around the world. For example, in a recent randomized trial, TF-CBT was compared to usual community care (i.e., nondirective supportive therapy) with children exposed to intimate partner violence (Cohen, Mannarino, & Iyengar, 2011). The results indicated that TF-CBT delivered in a community setting and in only eight sessions led to significant improvement with respect to PTSD and anxiety suffered by children exposed to domestic violence. Another recently completed randomized trial examined the benefits of TF-CBT with- and without pre-treatment engagement strategies for children placed in foster care (Dorsey, Cox, Conover, & Berliner, 2011). The preliminary results suggest that foster families randomly assigned to the engagement condition were less likely to drop out of treatment prematurely, though no significant treatment differences were found regardless of assigned condition among families who completed TF-CBT. In general, dropout rates from TF-CBT are about 10–20 %, which is low for a community clinic setting. Maltreated children are no more likely to drop out of TF-CBT than other traumatized children in our experience. In addition, randomized trials further documenting the efficacy of TF-CBT in individual and group formats have been conducted in Australia (King et al., 2000), Canada (Konanur & Muller, 2012) and the Democratic Republic of Congo (O'Callaghan & McMullen, 2012) with each of these studies documenting the superior efficacy of TF-CBT over comparison conditions.

Several other important quasi-experimental studies have been conducted examining TF-CBT with children who have suffered traumatic grief, children in foster care as well as children suffering traumatic stress secondary to the September 11 terrorist attacks and Hurricane Katrina. The findings suggest the value of TF-CBT for children experiencing traumatic grief symptoms after the loss of loved ones (Cohen, Mannarino, & Knudsen, 2004). In addition, the results of a quasi-experimental study with children in foster care not only documented the benefits of TF-CBT in alleviating traumatic stress symptoms but further suggested the superior efficacy of TF-CBT as compared to standard systems of care in improving placement stability and reducing runaway attempts (Lyons, Weiner, & Scheider, 2006). TF-CBT also appears to be of considerable benefit to children and their families affected by man-made and natural disasters as documented by the results of treatment outcome studies conducted in the aftermath of the September 11 terrorist attacks (CATS Consortium, 2010; Hoagwood & The CATS Consortium, 2007) and Hurricane Katrina (Jaycox et al., 2010). In these studies TF-CBT was used successfully for primarily low income, Hispanic and African American populations with positive outcomes. TF-CBT applications for diverse cultural groups have been developed and implemented and are described elsewhere (Cohen, Mannarino, & Deblinger, 2012).

In sum, to date there have been over 25 scientific investigations conducted examining the efficacy of TF-CBT, including 13 randomized controlled trials. While there is still much to be learned about the optimal implementation of TF-CBT with different populations in diverse settings, the aforementioned research provides strong support for the therapeutic benefits of TF-CBT with diverse populations of children and their families in the aftermath of abuse and other forms of trauma. Given the above findings, important areas for future TF-CBT research may include (1) the continued identification of factors that enhance TF-CBT outcomes for specific populations; (2) the impact of TF-CBT on biological and social development over longer follow- up periods as well as (3) the evaluation of alternative methods for the dissemination of TF-CBT training to therapists working with traumatized children and their families.

Target Populations, Settings and Symptoms

Although TF-CBT can be used after exposure to a variety of traumatic events, including domestic violence and traumatic loss, the focus in this chapter is on child maltreatment. In this regard, the major emphasis of TF-CBT has been on child sexual abuse through the participation of both the child victim and non-offending caretaker in treatment. TF-CBT can be used to treat victims of physical abuse; particularly to address PTSD symptoms and behavioral problems. However, this model is not intended for offending caretakers who have been physically coercive or abusive. In the latter instance, we would recommend a different evidence-based treatment such as "Alternatives for Families: A Cognitive-Behavioral Treatment- AF-CBT" (Kolko & Swenson, 2002) or Combined Parent-child Cognitive Behavioral Therapy-CPC-CBT (Runyon & Deblinger, 2013).

TF-CBT can be used with children and adolescents from ages 3 to 17. One of the earliest TF-CBT treatment outcome studies was with preschool children (Cohen & Mannarino, 1996). Later studies have demonstrated the efficacy of the model with adolescents (Cohen, Deblinger, Mannarino, & Steer, 2004). Through the numerous TF-CBT trainings that the developers have conducted, they have also heard anecdotally that the model is being implemented with 18–19 year-olds, although there is no empirical data at this time to support its efficacy with this older group. One frequently asked question is whether TF-CBT can be used with children who have developmental delays (e.g., autism; mild mental retardation). Through collaborations and consultation with many child mental health programs across the country, the developers have learned that the model is indeed being used with these populations, particularly for those children who have reasonable verbal skills. When treating these groups, there is a greater emphasis on repetition and practice in order to achieve basic mastery in the skills-based components and use of non-verbal techniques (e.g., art; drawings; play materials) for the trauma narrative and processing (Cavett & Drewes, 2012; Grosso, 2012).

Since TF-CBT strongly encourages strong parental involvement, another question is whether this treatment model can work effectively with parents who have personal mental health difficulties. Some evidence suggests that TF-CBT is effective in improving mild to moderate parental depressive and PTSD symptoms. For example, in one randomized controlled treatment study, parents who participated in their children's TF-CBT treatment experienced significantly greater improvement in their personal depressive symptoms as assessed by the Beck Depression Inventory-II (BDI-II; Beck, Steer, Ball, & Ranieri, 1996) than parents who participated in their children's child-centered therapy (Cohen, Deblinger, Mannarino, & Steer, 2004). In an initial TF-CBT effectiveness study for traumatically bereaved children, participating parents who were initially symptomatic with regard to PTSD and depression as measured by the PTSD Scale-Self Report (Foa, Cashman, Jaycox, & Perry, 1997) and BDI-II, respectively, experienced highly significant improvements in these symptoms (Cohen, Mannarino, & Knudsen, 2005). In a second TF-CBT effectiveness study for this population, participating parents who were initially symptomatic with regard to PTSD experienced significant improvement (Cohen, Mannarino, & Staron, 2006). These positive outcomes may be due to parents receiving a substantial proportion of individual time with TF-CBT therapists and finding the TF-CBT skills applicable to their personal mild to moderate depressive or PTSD symptoms. However, when parents have more severe mental health problems or when these problems are not directly related to the child's trauma experiences, therapists most often find it important to encourage parents to receive additional individual mental health services. A positive therapeutic relationship with the TF-CBT therapist will greatly facilitate this referral process.

The treatment outcome studies for TF-CBT have taken place in clinic office settings. However, over the past decade, TF-CBT is now being implemented in a variety of settings, including home-based services, schools, residential centers, and inpatient programs. A common barrier for home-based TF-CBT is locating a private place where the treatment can be implemented confidentially and without interruption. In the schools, one advantage is that children are easily accessible, although it is important to help children transition from a treatment session with calming activities so that they can concentrate on subsequent academic tasks. Ideally when TF-CBT is provided in school settings, the parents also participate in treatment. However, it is sometimes challenging to engage parents in school-based treatment as they might find it difficult to attend sessions or would prefer that the school deal with the child's problems (Rivera, 2012). If feasible strategies for including the parent in school-based treatment are unsuccessful, the therapist may opt to provide TF-CBT to the student without ongoing parental involvement. In this situation, the therapist typically still tries to engage the parent in treatment through periodic phone contact.

In residential treatment facilities, parents may not be available either because they live at great distance from the institution or have significant conflict with their children and do not want to participate in treatment. When this occurs, a direct care staff member may participate in TF-CBT with the child's consent and provided that they understand the importance of keeping the child's treatment confidential. Also, it has been the experience of the developers that when direct care staff members have been trained in the impact of trauma and have knowledge of the TF-CBT skills that children are learning that the model can be implemented more successfully (Cohen, Mannarino, & Navarro, 2012). One major drawback of acute inpatient hospital programs (as opposed to residential treatment facilities) is that the length of stay is typically very brief, often 1 week or less. In these facilities, as with other short-term acute programs lasting a month or less, the best approach would be to introduce the client to the impact of trauma and perhaps to stabilization skills, then transfer the client to a TF-CBT provider in the community for full TF-CBT treatment. However, some long term inpatient programs continue to have lengths of stay as long as 4–6 months which would allow enough time for TF-CBT to be completed.

For maltreated children, particularly those victimized by sexual abuse, PTSD symptoms are a major focus of TF-CBT. Deblinger's earliest treatment outcome studies addressed PTSD symptoms as the primary treatment target (Deblinger et al., 1989, 1990). It should be noted that in their treatment outcome studies the TF-CBT developers have never required that children meet full criteria for PTSD in order to be included. Instead the criteria have been at least one symptom in each of the three symptom clusters (i.e., re-experiencing; avoidance; hyperarousal). This decision reflects that the *Diagnostic and Statistical Manual* criteria for PTSD (DSM–IV-TR, 2000) were developed based on field trials with adults and the self-report nature of PTSD symptoms. Thus, many children, especially very young children, could have significant PTSD symptoms without meeting full criteria. In these circumstances, we would still strongly recommend that TF-CBT be implemented.

As reviewed in a preceding section, TF-CBT research has demonstrated that this approach is effective in treating a variety of other symptoms and problems. These include internalizing and externalizing behavioral difficulties, sexual behavior problems, general anxiety, abuse-related fears, depressive symptoms, and shame in child victims. Additionally, caretakers who participate in TF-CBT experience significant reductions in their own depression and abuse-related distress while becoming more supportive of their children who have been abused and increasing their parenting skills (Cohen, Deblinger, Mannarino, & Steer, 2004; Deblinger et al., 2011). Thus, TF-CBT can be implemented with children and adolescents who have developed a wide range of psychological problems after their abuse experiences with the added value of parents/caretakers making significant gains as well.

In their treatment outcome studies with sexually abused children, the TF-CBT developers have noted that most of their subjects had experienced multiple traumas. In fact, the average number of traumas has been between 3 and 4 (Cohen, Deblinger, Mannarino, & Steer, 2004; Deblinger et al., 2011). Although it was not determined in these studies how many of the children would be considered to have complex trauma (i.e., early repeated interpersonal trauma involving an attachment figure), many of these subjects exhibited the characteristics commonly associated with complex trauma, including significant affective dysregulation, difficulties with trust in interpersonal relationships, cognitive distortions about their traumatic experiences, and somatic symptoms. Thus, it is the developers' perspective that TF-CBT can be used successfully with children and adolescents with complex trauma (Cohen, Mannarino, Kliethermes, & Murray, 2012). Since complex trauma by its nature involves the traumatic disruption of an attachment relationship, developing a new trusting relationship often serves as a trauma trigger. Thus, when treating this population, therapists may need to particularly emphasize trust and safety during the initial TF-CBT stabilization phase. Establishing a trusting relationship with youth who have complex trauma typically takes longer than with other youth, because these youth repeatedly are re-triggered by the relationship itself, test the attachment, and also have more behavioral and emotional regulation problems than other youth so they need more time to learn and practice the initial skills. Thus, the usual proportionality of TF-CBT (with equal proportions devoted to each phase of TF-CBT treatment) is altered with this population such that the stabilization phase takes up to half of the entire TF-CBT treatment., Also, TF-CBT may require as many as 25 treatment sessions for youth with complex trauma such that 12 sessions might be devoted to the stabilization phase and 13 sessions to the trauma narrative and treatment consolidation phases (Cohen, Mannarino, & Navarro, 2012;

Kliethermes & Wamser, 2012). We would add that the great majority of adolescents with a trauma history who have been placed in residential centers likely have complex trauma and would require these TF-CBT treatment modifications.

Contraindications for TF-CBT

The implementation of TF-CBT requires that there be an identifiable trauma(s) to which a child has been exposed and remembers. This seems like a relatively straightforward requirement. However, especially in very young children, sexual abuse, for example, may be difficult to substantiate by child protective services, particularly if disclosures are variable and fragmented and there is no medical evidence. In these kinds of situations when it is not clear that maltreatment has occurred, it would not be clinically appropriate to implement TF-CBT. Moreover, trauma during infancy would be pre-verbal in nature and not be remembered by children. Accordingly, it would be impossible to deliver a "trauma-focused" approach when the child has no recall of what may have occurred.

TF-CBT would also be contraindicated if a youth is actively suicidal. Although some of the TF-CBT treatment components (e.g., relaxation; affective regulation) may be beneficial in the learning of more adaptive coping strategies, the trauma narrative and processing work would likely be overwhelming for actively suicidal youth and result in significant deterioration. Therefore, it would be wise to delay TF-CBT implementation until greater stabilization has occurred.

Changes in placement can be problematic when a child is participating in TF-CBT. This may occur if a child is being moved from one foster placement to another, from foster care back to the biological family, or from a residential program to placement in the community. Accordingly, TF-CBT therapists should try to insure that there is sufficient time to complete TF-CBT treatment prior to its initiation. Of greatest concern would be a youth who is unable to complete a trauma narrative because a placement change has interrupted treatment. The desired level of desensitization in this instance may not be achieved and potentially could result in significant feelings of vulnerability and distress. Often the youth does not know in advance that these placement changes will occur until the last minute; this is highly problematic for youth who have long histories of disrupted attachments as described earlier and does not allow the youth the opportunity to process these changes in treatment if therapy is also disrupted due to the placement change. Alternatively, if the youth knows about the placement change well in advance, the youth typically wants to vent about this crisis issue rather than continuing to progress in TF-CBT treatment. Although the disruption is typically related to previous traumas, making such connections in therapy requires time and consistent therapeutic progress.

When children and adolescents present with PTSD and/or other traumatic stress symptoms, co-morbidity is most often the rule, not the exception. For example, it is common for children exposed to trauma to have both traumatic stress symptoms and behavioral problems. If the behavioral difficulties are of a mild to moderate nature, TF-CBT would be clinically indicated, with a particular emphasis on parenting skills and behavior management (Deblinger et al., 2011). However, if a youth presents with serious behavior or conduct problems (e.g., fire setting; serious assaultive behaviors; delinquent activities), then it would be clinically appropriate to use a different evidence-based treatment with demonstrated efficacy for these difficulties. TF-CBT could be subsequently implemented if trauma symptoms persist after completion of the initial treatment. It should be noted that in some settings such as residential treatment, TF-CBT has been successfully implemented concurrently with behavioral interventions for such behavioral problems, but these are highly controlled environments. In outpatient settings, therapists typically need to prioritize the most pressing problems. If the therapist determines that he will likely be addressing "crisis" behavioral problems on a weekly or even daily basis due to the severity of the youth's behaviors, and that this would interfere with the therapist's ability to effectively deliver TF-CBT, it would make the most sense to start with an evidence-based treatment for the behavioral problems in these circumstances. In a parallel fashion, if the therapist were convinced that a traumatized youth had severe psychotic symptoms that would seriously impair reality contact and judgment, these would need to be treated and controlled first prior to the onset of trauma treatment. The therapist needs to carefully differentiate psychotic symptoms from traumatic re-experiencing or other trauma-related symptoms since 20 % of traumatized youth experience psychotic symptoms at some point and these would not necessarily preclude TF-CBT treatment.

TF-CBT Protocol

TF-CBT is implemented in parallel individual sessions with the child and caretaker (or other trusted adult, if a parent is not available) over the course of 8–16 weeks, although there may be as many as 25 treatment sessions in cases of complex trauma or when youth are placed in a residential program. The PRACTICE components are implemented sequentially, although there are instances when it would be clinically indicated to change the order. To illustrate, it would be appropriate to start TF-CBT with the Enhancing Safety component when there are acute threats to safety, such as in cases of domestic abuse where the child still resides with the perpetrating parent. This would provide the opportunity for the child, non-offending parent and therapist to develop a safety plan. Another example would be starting TF-CBT with In Vivo Exposure for a child who has been abused or bullied at school and is now refusing to attend school; as described earlier, developing and implementing exposure to a fear hierarchy would likely require several weeks. Also, the child would be missing school if this component were not begun early in treatment.

TF-CBT typically starts with Psychoeducation for both the child and parent and focuses on common psychological reactions to traumatic events and the physiological response to trauma, as well as providing information specific to the trauma that the child has experienced. Children and parents are also informed about the efficacy of TF-CBT so that they can have hope for recovery even early in treatment. The parenting component is conceptualized as critical to the child's recovery from trauma as described earlier and the parenting component is integrated throughout TF-CBT. From the outset of treatment, therapists help parents to make the connection between the child's trauma exposure and current behavior problems and to develop effective behavioral interventions to address these difficulties. Individual parent sessions are included throughout the skills and trauma narrative phases. During the skills building phase, the parent is learning the skills in parallel with the child and encouraging the child to implement these skills at home, particularly in response to trauma reminders that occur in the environment.

The skills-based components of TF-CBT consist of Relaxation, Affective Regulation, and Cognitive Coping. Relaxation is used to lower the hyperarousal associated with traumatic stress symptoms and may include progressive muscle relaxation, visual imagery, and deep breathing exercises. Relaxation strategies must be tailored, though, to meet the needs of individual children. Affective Regulation addresses feeling identification and expression but may also include other affective modulation strategies such as problem-solving and thought interruption procedures (Cohen et al., 2006). It should be noted that gradual exposure is incorporated into the Psychoeducation, Relaxation, and Affective Regulation components so that over time children gradually talk more about their traumatic experiences. For example, during the Relaxation component, children learn relaxation strategies that they can use when they have trauma reminders (e.g., male teacher reminds child of the sexual abuse perpetrator). With Cognitive Coping, children are taught about the connection between thoughts, feelings, and behaviors, automatic thoughts, and how changing their thoughts can have a positive impact on what they feel and do.

As children are progressing through these skills-based components, the parents are kept abreast of what the child is learning so that they can support the development and mastery of these skills. For example, if a child is learning to express anger directly with words, it is important that the parent learn to respond in helpful ways. Role-play exercises are often used to assist parents in this regard. Also, there can be joint sessions during this part of the treatment in which children teach parents what they have learned (e.g., relaxation strategies) so that these skills can be practiced and reinforced in the home setting.

The Trauma Narrative and Processing will typically take four to eight sessions, depending on the length of treatment. The therapist collaborates with the child to determine what trauma(s) will be focused on and what format will be used. The term "co-pilot" is sometimes used to describe the therapist's role as the trauma narrative is being developed (C. Grosso, personal communication, November 10, 2011). Although many children will write a "book", there are numerous other methods to develop trauma narratives, including poetry, talk show interviews, text messaging, and the use of play materials and drawings, especially with young children. The therapist encourages the child to add more and more details so that the process of desensitization can occur. Also, thoughts and feelings related to the trauma(s) are included in the narrative. If cognitive distortions and/or unhelpful thoughts are present, cognitive processing techniques such as Socratic questioning and the "Best Friend Role Play" (Cohen et al., 2006) are used to help children process their trauma in more accurate and/or helpful ways. A maladaptive cognition may be inaccurate or unhelpful. Either of these types of maladaptive thoughts may cause children (or parents) distress, and thus be a target for cognitive processing. An example of an inaccurate thought is "Every man will sexually abuse me". An example of an unhelpful thought is, "You can never tell who will sexually abuse you." A more accurate way of thinking about the first thought is, "Most men do not sexually abuse children". A more helpful way of thinking about the second thought is, "There are things I can do to keep myself safe." At the completion of the narrative, children are encouraged to "contextualize" their traumatic experiences in terms of what they have learned from therapy, how they have gotten stronger, and/or what they would tell other children who have gone through similar experiences.

The therapist typically shares the trauma narrative with the caretaker as it is being developed, although there may be confidentiality concerns that preclude sharing all or parts of the narrative. For example, a teenage girl may not want to share with a parent that she had been using drugs or drinking prior to being raped. Parents learn more about what actually happened to the child as they listen to the narrative and also undergo their own desensitization. If they have cognitive distortions and/or unhelpful thoughts of their own about the child's traumatic experiences, these will be addressed by the therapist.

After the trauma narrative has been completed, a child may continue to have trauma reminders to which they respond with fear and anxiety. Common triggers could be any innocuous stimuli that have become reminders because of their association with the trauma. In Vivo Exposure is used to address these trauma reminders so that the child can continue on a healthy developmental pathway. Common examples would be an in vivo plan for children who are afraid to attend a new school after being sexually abused at their old school or an in vivo plan for children who are reluctant to sleep alone in their own bedrooms. Strong support from the therapist is essential with In Vivo Exposure as both children and parents will likely be resistant to change.

Conjoint sessions with the child and parent can occur during different phases of TF-CBT, including near the beginning of treatment to address safety issues or behavioral problems. After the trauma narrative has been completed, a primary purpose of the conjoint sessions is for the child to share the narrative with the parent. This can be a very empowering experience for children to demonstrate how they have overcome their avoidance and learned to process the trauma in a healthier manner. Also, sharing of the narrative provides the opportunity for the parent to support the child and positively reinforce all of the hard work that has been accomplished. Other goals of conjoint sessions may include enhancing communication skills, planning for future trauma reminders, especially in cases of traumatic loss, additional psychoeducation; for example, providing more information about healthy sexuality if the child or parent appears to need such information, or starting joint work on safety skills such as practicing drug refusal or bullying skills.

The final component of TF-CBT is Enhancing Safety and Future Development. For children for whom there are ongoing concerns about violence, safety planning would be an important focus. Sexually abused children would learn about body safety skills and practice assertiveness so that they might be better able to deal with future situations that involve risk for revictimization. However, it is strongly emphasized to all children that if future abuse were to occur that it is not their fault and that the most important thing is to tell a trusted adult. For adolescents who have been sexually assaulted, information is provided about healthy sexuality. If appropriate, there would be education about bullying and conflict resolution.

Case Study

Jody is a 11 year-old girl who had been living with her mother, stepfather Bill, and 3 year-old half-brother Joey (child of mother and stepfather). The mother and father separated when Jody was 7, secondary to domestic violence perpetrated against the mother by the father. The mother remarried when Jody was 9. Jody had weekend visits with her father until he died in an automobile accident when she was 10. Jody and her father had had a reasonably close relationship but she displayed little emotion at the time of his death. After the father died, the stepfather began to lie down in bed with Jody at night, ostensibly to help her fall asleep. He eventually began to touch her genitals and then made her perform oral sex on him. The sexual abuse continued for about 1 year until the mother discovered Jody performing oral sex on Joey. When the mother asked her where she had learned this behavior, Jody disclosed that the stepfather forced her to do this to him.

The mother confronted the stepfather about Jody's allegation but he fervently denied that he had ever touched Jody inappropriately and claimed that he had been going into her bedroom only to help her fall asleep. The mother was unsure as to what to do. She consulted with a friend who was a teacher and had heard about a local child advocacy center. The friend also suggested that mother tell the stepfather to leave the house, at least until it became more clear as to what had happened. The forensic interview at the child advocacy center indicated that Jody was likely telling the truth about the abuse allegations and that there did not seem to be any reason for her to be lying. A mandated child abuse report was made to the local child protective services agency. The stepfather was not permitted to return to the home and was required to have no contact with Jody. The mother was devastated. Although she wanted to believe her daughter, the stepfather was the primary source of income for the family and otherwise a good husband. She was really scared about facing life without him.

The child advocacy center recommended that the mother seek treatment for Jody at a local child mental health program, which specializes in providing services for children who have experienced traumatic events. When Jody was evaluated, she was diagnosed with PTSD. She was also exhibiting behavior problems at home, sexualized behaviors, and sleep difficulties. School performance had declined. There were also concerns that the mother was under a great deal of stress and that her support for her daughter was considerably less than ideal. The evaluator mentioned that Jody continued to be sad about the death of her father but did not want to talk about this loss. Initial assessment included the following standardized instruments:

1. Child PTSD Symptom Scale (CPSS): score in the severe PTSD range
2. Child Behavior Checklist (CBCL): elevated scores in Total Behavior Problems, Internalizing Problems, and Externalizing Problems
3. Children's Depression Inventory (CDI): score in the moderately depressed range
4. Child Sexual Behavior Inventory (CSBI): score indicative of significant sexualized behaviors.

Although the mother had ambivalence about Jody being involved in therapy, she agreed to participate in TF-CBT with her daughter. Based on the above assessment, Jody's treatment goals included (1) resolving PTSD symptoms (decreasing intrusion, avoidance and arousal related to sexual abuse); (2) resolving aggressive and non-compliant behaviors at home; (3) resolving sexualized behaviors; and (4) resolving sleep problems and possible depressive symptoms related to sexual abuse.

TF-CBT treatment started with Psychoeducation about normal psychological and physiological responses to trauma. Additionally, both the mother and Jody were given information sheets about "myths and facts" related to sexual abuse. Jody felt relieved that she was not the only one who had ever been sexually abused while the mother began to see connections between Jody's abuse history and her behavioral difficulties. Jody responded well to both the Relaxation and Affective Regulation components, showing substantial improvement in arousal symptoms and behavioral problems during these components. She made a picture of a "safe place" which she carried in her backpack and began to use words to express her anger instead of not listening to her mother or hitting her brother.

It should be noted that the therapist was very empathic and validating with the mother, particularly the mother's feeling that she was "in the middle" and that she did not know what to believe. The therapist encouraged the mother to be more positive with Jody while she was working through these issues and this seemed to help Jody become more cooperative. Also, the therapist and mother collaboratively developed a behavioral plan to address Jody's sexualized behaviors with her brother. As these began to diminish, the mother became more hopeful, although she still found it shocking that Bill could have engaged her daughter in a sexual manner.

During Cognitive Coping, Jody learned the connection between thoughts, feelings, and behaviors and practiced this new set of skills in everyday situations. For example, she had a friend at school who sometimes did not talk with her when she said hello. Instead of thinking that this friend was upset with her, Jody began to substitute the thought that her friend was sad because her friend's mother had recently been diagnosed with cancer. Concurrently, Jody's mother began to discuss her own thoughts related to the abuse allegations, some of which were distortions such as "only strangers sexually abuse children" and "if this really happened, I would/should have known".

Jody decided that she wanted to write a "book" for her trauma narrative. She called it "My Life Up to Now." With the therapist's encouragement, she was able to describe her family and one time when her father had slapped her mother in the face.

There were two chapters on the sexual abuse. Jody wrote that she felt "sick to my stomach" when her stepfather touched her for the first time and "dirty" when he forced her to perform oral sex on him. When describing the latter, Jody became very anxious so the therapist suggested that she visualize her "safe place" for a few minutes prior to continuing the narrative. Jody indicated that she thought the abuse was her fault, in part, because if she had been able to sleep better after her father had died, her stepfather would not have had a reason to come into her bedroom.

The chapter on the death of her father was the most difficult for Jody. She was able to describe what she was doing when her mother told her about the father's accident and also described the funeral. She said that she sometimes still felt angry with her father because he had hit her mother and for his drinking. (The father had drunk excessively just prior to the accident.) At the end of the narrative, Jody wrote that she felt stronger for having participated in therapy and that she had some good memories of her Dad. In total, there were five trauma narrative sessions. Jody's only residual cognitive distortion was that she felt that she should have told sooner about the sexual abuse. The therapist used cognitive restructuring and Psychoeducation to help Jody understand that the stepfather had manipulated her to believe that if she had disclosed the abuse, the mother would have blamed her for breaking up the marriage.

With Jody's consent, the therapist had been sharing the trauma narrative with the mother as it was being developed. The mother was surprised that Jody had witnessed the mother being slapped by the father. Also, the details about the sexual abuse were very disturbing to her and reinforced her self-blame for not knowing this had been occurring. The therapist was able to use Psychoeducation and some cognitive restructuring to address this distortion. Regarding the death of the father, the mother acknowledged her own sadness about this loss and that perhaps she had been discouraging her daughter from talking about him.

In Vivo Exposure was used to help Jody to fall asleep more easily in her own room. She and her mother received education about trauma reminders. Also, they decided that they would re-arrange the furniture in Jody's bedroom to help her feel more comfortable. The therapist identified a relaxation tape that Jody could play at night when she was falling asleep. After Jody was able to sleep by herself for one night, she selected watching a movie with her mother as her reward. After 1 week of sleeping in her own room, Jody and her mother had a special dinner at Jody's favorite restaurant.

The major purpose of the conjoint session was to share the trauma narrative with the mother. The therapist initially met alone with Jody to review the narrative one final time and then with the mother alone. During the joint session, the mother cried but told Jody that she was proud of her and was sorry that Bill had hurt her. Additionally, Jody and her mother talked about how they might have a special remembrance for her father on his birthday and Father's Day.

During the final treatment session, there was a focus on safety education, and given Jody's age, on healthy sexuality. The mother participated in the latter discussion. Also, the therapist had made a certificate to give to Jody that reflected her successful completion of treatment. In total, there were 15 TF-CBT sessions. Jody was no longer engaging in any sexualized behaviors and her PTSD symptoms had markedly decreased. Although she continued to feel a great deal of sadness related to the loss of her father, she was no longer avoidant of talking about him. Instead she seemed to be engaged in a normal grieving process. At the end of treatment, assessment instruments were repeated. Scores were as follows:

1. CPSS: score in normal range
2. CBCL: no scores clinically elevated
3. CDI: score in non-depressed range
4. CSBI: score in non-clinical range

All of these scores were within normal limits. The mother was very relieved to see this substantial improvement in Jody's functioning and that her daughter was moving forward in a positive way.

Limitations of TF-CBT

As with all treatments for traumatized children and adolescents, TF-CBT is not the ideal treatment with all children and in all circumstances. In cases of sexual abuse, it is very important to include the non-offending caretaker in TF-CBT, but it would not be appropriate to include the sexual abuse perpetrator. Even if the perpetrator has acknowledged the abuse, it is highly likely that he would be a major trauma trigger for the child and that this would greatly interfere with the progress of treatment. As mentioned earlier, TF-CBT is also not appropriate for offending caretakers who have been physically abusive with a child. (AF-CBT or CPC-CBT would be better choices with physical abuse (Kolko & Swenson, 2002; Runyon & Deblinger, 2013).

The authors have been conducting ongoing TF-CBT consultation with therapists who provide services for adolescent sex offenders in residential treatment programs. Most of these offenders have their own history of sexual abuse. Historically, we have believed that these adolescents first need to receive treatment for their offending behaviors prior to any kind of trauma treatment. However, we have learned from these therapists that offender treatment (which is primarily provided in groups) and TF-CBT can be provided concurrently, without youths using the abuse as an "excuse" for their offending behaviors. For these treatments to be successful, it is essential that therapists have expertise in both interventions or that the treatments be delivered by different therapists each with expertise with one or the other model.

TF-CBT is not intended to be used immediately after a natural disaster, terrorist attack, or any other type of large-scale event. However, TF-CBT can be implemented for children who have been screened and have traumatic stress symptoms a couple of months or longer after a major disaster. For example, TF-CBT was effective in remediating PTSD symptoms in children exposed to the September 11 terrorist attack in New York City (Hoagwood & The CATS Consortium, 2007) and in children exposed to Hurricane Katrina in 2005 (Jaycox et al., 2010).

TF-CBT would also not be appropriate for infants and toddlers who have experienced traumatic life events, including sexual or physical abuse. Because the theoretical underpinnings of TF-CBT are cognitive-behavioral in nature, the interventions in this model would be beyond the developmental capabilities of this very young group. Another evidence-based treatment such as Child-parent Psychotherapy would be a good clinical fit for infants and toddlers who have experienced trauma (Lieberman & Van Horn, 2008). Additionally, for preschool children, it would not be expected that they would understand the cognitive triangle at an abstract level or some aspects of cognitive coping. However, it has been our experience that preschool children can comprehend some basic cognitive concepts, particularly when presented through Psychoeducation with children's books, such as the "The Little Engine that Could" (Piper, 1978), or with the use of concrete props to help them differentiate between thoughts, feelings, and behavior (Scheeringa, Weems, Cohen, Amaya-Jackson, & Guthrie, 2011).

Flexibility of TF-CBT

It is always a challenge to help therapists balance fidelity and flexibility. Of course, without a reasonable level of fidelity, therapists would not be implementing the model in a manner that would be consistent with the research base. On the other hand, without flexibility, therapists would perceive TF-CBT to be rigid and not appropriate for the children whom they serve. In fact, we have heard over and over at TF-CBT clinical trainings that it is the flexibility of TF-CBT that makes it an attractive model for many therapists.

Fidelity to the TF-CBT model is primarily achieved through the implementation of all of the TF-CBT components and generally in the order of the PRACTICE acronym. However, as mentioned earlier, it would be acceptable to revise the order of the components to address clinical needs such as starting TF-CBT with the Enhancing Safety component in situations when there is the threat of ongoing violence. Also, after the Trauma Narrative has been completed, the In Vivo Exposure component may not be required if there are no generalized trauma reminders interfering with a child's treatment progress or development.

Flexibility in the implementation of TF-CBT is primarily achieved through the large variety of treatment strategies that can be used for each of the PRACTICE components. This flexibility is based on numerous factors, including developmental issues and the unique qualities of every child. For young children, we strongly encourage the use of play materials, drawings, puppets, etc. to implement the TF-CBT components (Cavett & Drewes, 2012; Drewes & Cavett, 2012). Psychoeducation can be implemented through children's books, educational videos, information sheets, and psychoeducational games. Although deep breathing exercises and progressive muscle relaxation are often taught as part of the Relaxation component, there are numerous other strategies that can be used, including meditation, yoga, drawing, prayer, and listening to music.

Many therapists suggest that the Trauma Narrative component may be the most challenging to implement because of the avoidance that is present in the majority of children. To implement this component successfully, it is important to understand the abilities and interests of each child so that these may be used to facilitate the development of the narrative. For example, adolescents who enjoy poetry may write a poem for their trauma narrative. Or, text messaging may be used, given its popularity among adolescents in our culture. (For text messaging, these messages are not actually sent out electronically; this format is simply used to make it easier for clients to develop the narrative.) The guiding principle is to utilize a format for the trauma narrative with which the child is comfortable, as this will make it much easier for this component to be completed successfully.

Conclusion

TF-CBT has been rigorously studied over the past 20 years. The research base for this model is very strong. Additionally, the model has been widely disseminated across the United States, in Europe (e.g., Germany; Norway; Sweden; the Netherlands), and in some low resource countries such as Cambodia and Zambia. We anticipate that TF-CBT as a treatment approach will continue to evolve as additional research findings and dissemination projects provide new information on the best strategies to implement the model with children of different ages, clinical presentations, and cultural backgrounds.

References

American Psychiatric Association. (2000). *Diagnostic and statistical manual of mental disorders* (4th ed.). Washington, DC: American Psychiatric Association.

Beck, A. T., Steer, R. A., Ball, R., & Ranieri, W. (1996). Comparison of Beck Depression Inventories-IA and -II in psychiatric outpatients. *Journal of Personality Assessment, 67*, 588–597. doi:10.1207/s15327752jpa6703_13.

CATS Consortium. (2010). Implementation of CBT for youth affected by the World Trade Center disaster: Matching need to treatment intensity and reducing trauma symptoms. *Journal of Traumatic Stress, 23*, 699–707. doi:10.1002/jts.20594.

Cavett, A. M., & Drewes, A. A. (2012). Play applications and trauma-specific components. In J. A. Cohen, A. P. Mannarino, & E. Deblinger (Eds.), *Trauma-focused CBT for children and adolescents: Treatment applications* (pp. 124–148). New York: Guilford Press.

Cohen, J. A., Deblinger, E., Mannarino, A. P., & Steer, R. A. (2004). A multisite, randomized controlled trial for sexually abused children with PTSD symptoms. *Journal of the American Academy of Child and Adolescent Psychiatry, 43*, 393–402. doi:10.1097/01.chi.0000111364.94169.f9.

Cohen, J. A., & Mannarino, A. P. (1988). Psychological symptoms in sexually abused girls. *Child Abuse & Neglect, 12*, 571–577. doi:10.1016/0145-2134(88)90074-9.

Cohen, J. A., & Mannarino, A. P. (1996). A treatment outcome study for sexually abused preschool children: Initial findings. *Journal of the American Academy of Child and Adolescent Psychiatry, 35*, 42–50. doi:10.1097/00004583-199601000-00011.

Cohen, J. A., & Mannarino, A. P. (1998). Interventions for sexually abused children: Initial treatment outcome findings. *Child Maltreatment, 3*, 17–26. doi:10.1177/1077559598003001002.

Cohen, J. A., Mannarino, A. P., & Deblinger, E. (2006). *Treating trauma and traumatic grief in children and adolescents*. New York: Guildford Press.

Cohen, J. A., Mannarino, A. P., & Deblinger, E. (Eds.). (2012). *Trauma-focused CBT for children and adolescents: Treatment applications.* New York: Guilford.

Cohen, J. A., Mannarino, A. P., & Deblinger, E. (2010). Trauma-focused cognitive behavioral therapy for traumatized children. In J. A. Weiss & A. E. Kazdin (Eds.), *Evidence-based psychotherapies for children and adolescents* (pp. 295–311). New York: Guilford Press.

Cohen, J. A., Mannarino, A. P., & Iyengar, S. (2011). Community treatment of posttraumatic stress disorder for children exposed to intimate partner violence. *Archives of Pediatrics and Adolescent Medicine, 165,* 16–21. doi:10.1001/archpediatrics.2010.247.

Cohen, J. A., Mannarino, A. P., Kliethermes, M., & Murray, L. A. (2012). Trauma-focused CBT for youth with complex trauma. *Child Abuse & Neglect, 36,* 528–541. doi:10.1016/j.chiabu.2012.03.007.

Cohen, J. A., Mannarino, A. P., & Knudsen, K. (2004). Treating childhood traumatic grief: A pilot study. *Journal of the American Academy of Child and Adolescent Psychiatry, 43,* 1225–1233. doi:10.1097/01.chi.0000135620.15522.38.

Cohen, J. A., Mannarino, A. P., & Knudsen, K. (2005). Treating sexually abused children: 1 year follow-up of a randomized controlled trial. *Child Abuse and Neglect, 29,* 135–145.

Cohen, J. A., Mannarino, A. P., & Navarro, D. (2012). Residential treatment. In J. A. Cohen, A. P. Mannarino, & E. Deblinger (Eds.), *Trauma-focused CBT for children and adolescents: Treatment applications* (pp. 73–102). New York: Guilford Press.

Cohen, J. A., Mannarino, A. P., & Staron, V. (2006). A pilot study of modified cognitive-behavioral therapy for childhood traumatic grief (CBT-CTG). *Journal of the American Academy of Child and Adolescent Psychiatry, 45,* 1465–1473.

Cohen, J. A., Perel, J. M., DeBellis, M. D., Friedman, M. J., & Putnam, F. W. (2002). Treating traumatized children: Clinical implications of the psychobiology of posttraumatic stress disorder. *Trauma, Violence & Abuse, 3,* 91–108. doi:10.1177/15248380020032001.

Deblinger, E., Lippmann, J., & Steer, R. A. (1996). Sexually abused children suffering posttraumatic stress symptoms: Initial treatment outcome findings. *Child Maltreatment, 1,* 310–321. doi:10.1177/1077559596001004003.

Deblinger, E., Mannarino, A. P., Cohen, J., Runyon, M. K., & Steer, R. A. (2011). Trauma-focused cognitive-behavioral therapy for children: Impact of the trauma narrative and treatment length. *Depression and Anxiety, 28,* 67–75. doi:10.1002/da.20744.

Deblinger, E., Mannarino, A. P., Cohen, J. A., & Steer, R. A. (2006). Follow-up study of a multisite, randomized, controlled trial for children with sexual abuse-related PTSD symptoms: Examining predictors of treatment response. *Journal of the American Academy of Child and Adolescent Psychiatry, 45,* 1471–1484. doi:10.1097/01.chi.0000240839.56114.bb.

Deblinger, E., McLeer, S. V., Atkins, M., Ralph, D., & Foa, E. (1989). Post-traumatic stress in sexually abused children: Physically abused and non-abused children. *International Journal of Child Abuse and Neglect, 13,* 403–408. doi:10.1016/0145-2134(89)90080-X.

Deblinger, E., McLeer, S. V., & Henry, D. E. (1990). Cognitive/behavioral treatment for sexually abused children suffering post-traumatic stress: Preliminary findings. *Journal of the American Academy of Child and Adolescent Psychiatry, 29,* 747–752. doi:10.1097/00004583-199009000-00012.

Deblinger, E., Stauffer, L. B., & Steer, R. (2001). Comparative efficacies of supportive and cognitive-behavioral group therapies for young children who have been sexually abused and their non-offending mothers. *Child Maltreatment, 6,* 332–343. doi:10.1177/1077559501006004006.

Deblinger, E., Steer, R. A., & Lippmann, J. (1999). Two-year follow-up study of cognitive behavioral therapy for sexually abused children suffering post-traumatic stress symptoms. *Child Abuse & Neglect, 23,* 1371–1378. doi:10.1016/S0145-2134(99)00091-5.

Dorsey, S., Cox, J. R., Conover, K. L., & Berliner, L. (2011, Summer). Trauma-focused cognitive behavioral therapy for children and adolescents in foster care. *Children, Youth, and Family News.* Available at www.apa.org/pi/families/resources/newsletter/index.aspx

Drewes, A. A., & Cavett, A. M. (2012). Play applications and skills components. In J. A. Cohen, A. P. Mannarino, & E. Deblinger (Eds.), *Trauma-focused CBT for children and adolescents: Treatment applications* (pp. 105–123). New York: Guilford Press.

Foa, E. B., Cashman, L., Jaycox, L., & Perry, K. (1997). The validation of a self-report measure of posttraumatic stress disorder: The Posttraumatic Diagnostic Scale. *Psychological Assessment, 9,* 445–451. doi:10.1037//1040-3590.9.4.445.

Grosso, C. A. (2012). Children with developmental disabilities. In J. A. Cohen, A. P. Mannarino, & E. Deblinger (Eds.), *Trauma-focused CBT for children and adolescents: Treatment applications* (pp. 149–174). New York: Guilford Press.

Hoagwood, K. E., & The CATS Consortium. (2007). Implementing CBT for traumatized children and adolescents after September 11: Lessons learned from the Child and Adolescent Trauma Treatments and Services (CATS) Project. *Journal of Clinical Child and Adolescent Psychology, 36*, 581–592. doi:10.1080/15374410701662725.

Jaycox, L. H., Cohen, J. A., Mannarino, A. P., Walker, D. W., Langley, A. K., Gegenheimer, K. L., et al. (2010). Children's mental health care following Hurricane Katrina: A field trial of trauma-focused psychotherapies. *Journal of Traumatic Stress, 23*, 223–231. doi:10.1002/jts.20518.

King, N., Tonge, B. J., Mullen, P., Myerson, N., Heyne, D., Rollings, S., et al. (2000). Treating sexually abused children with post-traumatic stress symptoms: A randomized clinical trial. *Journal of the American Academy of Child and Adolescent Psychiatry, 59*(11), 1347–1355. doi:10.1097/00004583-200011000-00008.

Kliethermes, M., & Wamser, S. (2012). Adolescents with complex trauma. In J. A. Cohen, A. P. Mannarino, & E. Deblinger (Eds.), *Trauma-focused CBT for children and adolescents: Treatment applications* (pp. 175–196). New York: Guilford Press.

Kolko, D., & Swenson, C. C. (2002). *Assessing and treating physically abused children and their families*. Thousand Oaks, CA: Sage.

Konanur, S., & Muller, R. T. (2012). *A community-based study of the effectiveness of trauma-focused cognitive behavioural therapy with trauma-exposed school-aged children*. Paper presented at the annual Australian conference of child trauma, Gold Coast, Australia.

Lieberman, A. F., & Van Horn, P. (2008). *Psychotherapy with infants and young children: Repairing the effects of stress and trauma on early attachment*. New York: Guilford Press.

Lyons, J. S., Weiner, D. A., & Scheider, A. (2006). *A field trial of three evidence-based practices for trauma with children in state custody* (Report to the Illinois Department of Children and Family Services). Evanston, IL: Mental Health Resources Services and Policy Program, Northwestern University.

Mannarino, A. P., & Cohen, J. A. (1986). A clinical-demographic study of sexually abused children. *Child Abuse & Neglect, 10*, 17–28. doi:10.1016/0145-2134(86)90027-X.

Mannarino, A. P., Cohen, J. A., & Gregor, M. (1989). Emotional and behavioral difficulties in sexually abused girls. *Journal of Interpersonal Violence, 4*, 437–451. doi:10.1177/088626089004004004.

McLeer, S. V., Deblinger, E., Atkins, M., Foa, E., & Ralph, D. (1988). Post-traumatic stress disorder in sexually abused children: A prospective study. *Journal of the American Academy of Child and Adolescent Psychiatry, 27*(5), 650–654. doi:10.1097/00004583-98809000-00024.

O'Callaghan, P., & McMullen, J. (2012). *An RCT of trauma-focused cognitive behavioral therapy for sexually exploited, war affected girls in the DRC*. Unpublished manuscript submitted for publication, Queens College, Belfast, Ireland (Clinical Trials ID#NCT01483261).

Piper, W. (1978). *The little engine that could*. New York: Amazon.

Rivera, S. (2012). Schools. In J. A. Cohen, A. P. Mannarino, & E. Deblinger (Eds.), *Trauma-focused CBT for children and adolescents: Treatment applications* (pp. 29–48). New York: Guilford Press.

Runyon, M. K., & Deblinger, E. (2013). *Combined parent-child cognitive behavioral therapy (CPC-CBT): An approach to empower families at-risk for child physical abuse*. New York: Oxford University Press.

Scheeringa, M. S., Weems, C. F., Cohen, J. A., Amaya-Jackson, L., & Guthrie, D. (2011). Trauma-focused cognitive behavioral therapy for posttraumatic stress disorder in three through six year old children: A randomized controlled trial. *Journal of Child Psychology and Psychiatry, 52*, 853–860.

Silverman, W. K., Ortiz, C. D., Viswesvaran, C., Burns, B. J., Kolko, D., Putnam, F. W., et al. (2008). Evidence-based psychosocial treatments for children and adolescents exposed to traumatic events. *Journal of Clinical Child & Adolescent Psychology, 37*, 156–183. doi:10.1080/15374410701818293.

Stauffer, L., & Deblinger, E. (1996). Cognitive behavioral groups for nonoffending mothers and their young sexually abused children: A preliminary treatment outcome study. *Child Maltreatment, 1*(1), 65–76. doi:10.1177/1077559596001001007.

Chapter 11
Alternatives for Families: A Cognitive Behavioral Therapy: An Overview and a Case Example

David J. Kolko, Heather Simonich, and Anna Loiterstein

What Is AF-CBT?

Alternatives for Families: A Cognitive Behavioral Therapy, or AF-CBT, is an evidence-based intervention that targets the individual characteristics and family context associated with conflict or coercion in the home. Common manifestations of these circumstances include chronic levels of anger, hostility or verbal aggression, the use of physical force or corporal punishment, physical aggression, and/or child physical abuse (CPA; see Kolko & Kolko, 2010; Runyon & Urquiza, 2010). AF-CBT has also been used more recently as an intervention for children with behavioral problems (e.g., oppositional defiant disorder, conduct disorder). The intervention was recently expanded to accommodate children and adolescents with physical abuse or discipline-related trauma symptoms, such as posttraumatic stress disorder (PTSD).

Thus, the current AF-CBT curriculum (version 3.0, 11-1-2011) targets aggression or behavioral dysfunction, heightened anger and trauma-related emotional symptoms, poor social competence, cognitive attributional problems, and family relationship problems. For some problems, parallel content is delivered to both children and caregivers. Treatment includes separate individual sessions with the child and caregiver (most often the parent), and joint sessions with at least both of these participants.

D.J. Kolko, Ph.D., ABPP (✉)
Western Psychiatric Institute and Clinic, University of Pittsburgh, School of Medicine,
3811 O'Hara Street, Pittsburgh, PA 15213, USA
e-mail: kolkodj@upmc.edu

H. Simonich, MA, LPC
Neuropsychiatric Research Institute, 120 South 8th Street, Fargo, ND 58103, USA
e-mail: hsimonich@nrifargo.com

A. Loiterstein, BS
Department of Psychology, Carnegie Mellon University, CMU SMC 3092,
Pittsburgh, PA 15289, USA
e-mail: anna.loiterstein@gmail.com

S. Timmer and A. Urquiza (eds.), *Evidence-Based Approaches for the Treatment of Maltreated Children*, Child Maltreatment 3, DOI 10.1007/978-94-007-7404-9_11,
© Springer Science+Business Media Dordrecht 2014

Theoretical Background

The name and content of AF-CBT have evolved over the past few decades. Developed for child physical abuse and exposure to punitive discipline in 1985, the first edition was piloted with child inpatients by David Kolko and Sharon (Fishman) Hicks (1985–1989), evaluated in an initial outcome study (Kolko, 1996a, 1996b), and then outlined in a sourcebook (Kolko & Swenson, 2002). The early version of this intervention was described as "Abuse-Focused Cognitive-Behavioral Therapy" (Kolko, 2003a, 2003b) in an overview of early treatment programs for child maltreatment compendium of interventions (Saunders, Berliner, & Hanson, 2003).

In the second edition, AF-CBT was adapted and the name changed to "Alternatives for Families: A Cognitive-Behavior Therapy" (Kolko, Herschell, Baumann, & Shaver, 2007). We believed the new name more clearly reflected its focus on training in specific skills designed to provide both abusive and non-abusive families with alternative options for solving personal problems and interacting with others, and that it would be less likely to create treatment engagement obstacles by labeling clients' behavior as abusive, which elicits client defensiveness and self-perceptions of stigma. A related model called the PARTNERS CBT for Physical Abuse was developed in 2002 (Brown, 2005). In 2010, AF-CBT and the PARTNERS CBT were integrated into the current (third) edition of AF-CBT which was updated to address (1) the level of verbal and physical aggression found in non-abusive, but coercive families, (2) children's physical abuse or discipline related traumatic symptoms. This expanded clinical focus was also designed to enhance the scope, utility, and eventual dissemination of AF-CBT.

We review a few of the key historical developments in the articulation of the first edition of the AF-CBT approach. Based on an early review of the empirical literature, an initial logic model outlined some of the key clinical contributors to and consequences of a history of child physical abuse as well as exposure to physical coercion or aggression (see Fig. 11.1). The model highlights key child, parent, and family characteristics whose modification may bear treatment implications, many of which are still incorporated in the third edition of AF-CBT.

Based on this original logic model and the prevailing conceptual and clinical treatment approaches found in the child abuse and general child outcome research literatures, two complimentary approaches, Individual Child and Parent Physical Abuse-Focused Cognitive-Behavioral Treatment (CBT) and Physical Abuse-Informed Family Therapy (FT) were developed (see Saunders et al., 2003). When examined carefully, some of the treatment components were designed to reflect an "abuse-focus," whereas others reflected general psychosocial skills at both the individual and family levels. The CBT protocol administered parallel but separate procedures to children and their abusive caregivers, targeting characteristics related to abusive behavior, especially training and practice in specific intrapersonal (e.g., cognitive, affective) followed by interpersonal (e.g., behavioral) skills designed to enhance self-control. The FT protocol reflected a family therapy that included specific CBT methods and selected family techniques designed to alter the family's view of and

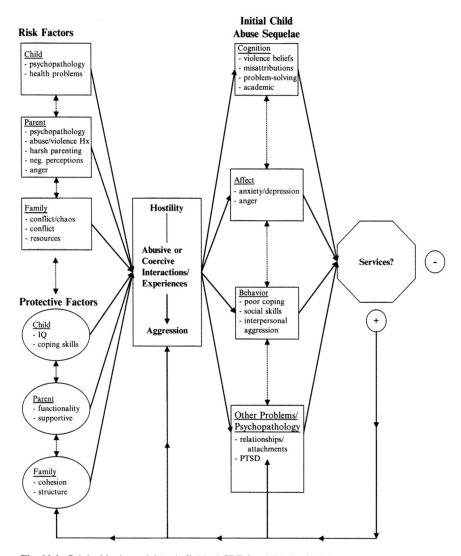

Fig. 11.1 Original logic model for individual CBT for child physical abuse

reliance upon aggression, interactional skills, and family routines. Both protocols were designed to alter the family context in which coercion occurs, albeit through alternative modalities and mechanisms, and to teach explicit skill alternatives.

Since the publication of the initial outcome study, several key developments have been made to this treatment model. Most notably, the content of AF-CBT was expanded and elaborated upon in a clinical sourcebook that included key conceptual and therapeutic principles from several areas that addressed many of the elements noted in the original logic model (see Kolko & Swenson, 2002). For example, AF-CBT incorporates concepts from family therapy, which examines patterns of interactions among family members in order to identify and alleviate problems, and develops strategies to help reframe how problems are viewed. The model also draws upon the methods used in cognitive therapy to identify alternative attributions. The psychology of aggression describes the processes by which aggression and coercion develop and are maintained. AF-CBT also draws on developmental victimology, which describes how the specific sequelae of exposure to traumatic or abusive experiences may vary for children at different developmental stages and across the lifespan. A feature of this updated material is that the core elements of the individual CBT and family treatment protocols that were separately found to be efficacious in the initial outcome study (Kolko, 1996a, 1996b) were integrated into one treatment approach. Other content updates were made to enhance the relevance of AF-CBT for families with clinically referred children who presented with verbal and/or physical aggression by including references to other types of referral incidents, including high conflict situations. And, material related to the use of imaginal exposure was included to help children who presented with traumatic reactions secondary to their exposure to child physical abuse or harsh punishment.

Purpose of Intervention

AF-CBT is designed to intervene with families referred for child physical abuse, verbal or physical aggression that includes use of excessive or threats of physical force, or conflict and coercion. The current edition of AF-CBT has been updated to accommodate children and adolescents with physical abuse or discipline related trauma symptoms, such as those associated with posttraumatic stress disorder (PTSD). Thus, AF-CBT is recommended for use with: (1) caregivers whose disciplinary or management strategies range from mild physical discipline to physically aggressive or abusive behaviors, or who exhibit heightened levels of anger, hostility or explosiveness; (2) children who exhibit significant externalizing or aggressive behavior (e.g., oppositionality, antisocial behavior), with or without significant physical abuse or discipline related trauma symptoms (e.g., anger, anxiety, PTSD); and, (3) families who exhibit heightened conflict or coercion or who pose threats to personal safety.

The intervention was designed to provide a comprehensive approach to addressing both the risks for and consequences of exposure to coercive behavior, especially aggression. Accordingly, it targets certain child, parent, and family characteristics (see Kolko & Kolko, 2010; Runyon & Urquiza, 2010). In particular, the approach focuses on reducing several risk factors, such as caregiver use of physical force (physical discipline or corporal punishment, aggression) and verbal aggression (anger, hostility), as well as negative child attributions and limited parenting skills. There are conceptual and empirical reasons to believe that controlling the severity of these problems may reduce the risk of re-abuse or additional aggressive incidents (see Kolko & Swenson, 2002; Runyon & Urquiza, 2010).

In addition to reducing the types of activities that support family conflict and violence, AF-CBT is designed to reduce or prevent some of the many effects of CPA and corporal punishment on the child and family system. For example, children and adolescents who have experienced CPA or corporal punishment may develop externalizing (aggression and antisocial behavior), and internalizing problems (depression and anxiety), and are at increased risk for engaging in abusive or aggressive behaviors with their children. Additionally, adults who report being physically abused during childhood are at significantly increased risk of having adult psychiatric disorders, especially attention-deficit hyperactivity disorder, post-traumatic stress disorder, and bipolar disorder (see Sugaya et al., 2012). Finally, AF-CBT also targets family contributors to coercion including poor communication and problem-solving skills.

In sum, AF-CBT aims to reduce conflict, use of coercion and physical force by the caregiver or child. Other goals of AF-CBT include promoting non-aggressive discipline and interactions, reducing child physical abuse risk or recidivism, and improving the level of child safety and family functioning. Overall, AF-CBT discourages coercive, aggressive, or violent behavior from caregivers as well as children, and promotes appropriate and prosocial behavior. AF-CBT attempts to reduce risk factors that contribute to physically aggressive or abusive incidents. These risk factors include negative perceptions of children, heightened anger or hostility, harsh parenting practices, coercive family interactions, and heightened stressful events.

Target Population

AF-CBT is appropriate for use with physically, emotionally, and verbally abusive or coercive parents and their school-aged children (Kolko, 1996a, 1996b). AF-CBT has also been adapted more recently (Kolko, Campo, Kelleher, & Cheng, 2010; Kolko et al., 2009) for use with children presenting with behavior problems or disorders, such as Oppositional Defiant Disorder (ODD) and Conduct Disorder (CD). These adaptations include changing the focus from an incident of abuse to another type of critical incident involving family conflict (e.g., heated argument) or that was initiated by the caregiver or child (e.g., physical discipline, child aggression), and allowing clinicians to skip over materials that are primarily "abuse-specific" in nature (e.g., discussion of child protection issues, use of clarification, imaginal exposure).

Treatment is not specifically designed for any one ethnic or racial group and AF-CBT has been delivered to families in multiple languages (e.g., English, Spanish, Japanese, Creole) and with different cultural backgrounds (e.g., European, African-American, African, Asian, Native American), with most work having been done with African-American families. Our materials frequently make reference to the need to address the backgrounds, values, and preferences of the family, including its cultural context, which often means learning more about their individual use of language and symbols, child rearing views, and norms governing how parents and children interact. Limited research has suggested comparable outcomes for different ethnic groups, which parallels our clinical experiences, but no systematic study of AF-CBT has been conducted to this end.

Screening and Assessment

Assessment is an integral part of AF-CBT. Clinicians who provide AF-CBT conduct an initial intake assessment that helps to guide treatment, collect ongoing information over the course of treatment to monitor treatment response on key clinical targets, and conduct a discharge assessment using some of the assessment measures collected at intake to provide information about treatment gains. The initial intake assessment uses information gathered from the referral record (e.g. CPS documents or casework reports, medical or health records), formal standardized instruments, clinical interviews, and observations made that help to better understand the case. When making an assessment, it is important to consider all of the potential sources of useful information because there are often discrepant views regarding the incident, family characteristics, and the perceptions of recent interactions. In addition, we recognize the importance of understanding the caregiver's and child's unique treatment goals, level of motivation, and clinical needs. This information can be specific to reducing the level of verbal and physical aggression, but it can also reflect more general targets to enhance personal competencies (e.g., teaching common social skills to children).

To help identify families who meet at least one of the three clinical problems noted earlier (caregiver aggressive/abuse, child behavior problems with possible PTSD symptoms secondary to exposure to physical force, family conflict), two screening tools have been designed to help identify appropriate cases for AF-CBT. The first tool is a brief checklist that outlines key eligibility criteria used to determine if a case is appropriate for this type of treatment. The primary items look for caregiver's physical abusiveness, high-risk behavior, or physical discipline, family conflict, and children's externalizing behavior, aggression, or trauma symptoms secondary to this family history. This information can be obtained by questioning a caregiver, by reviewing collateral informants, or from secondary materials and documents. The second tool is an algorithm that outlines a pathway for understanding how to integrate the answers to these screening questions with other information about a case that might be used to support or contraindicate the use of AF-CBT in that case. This algorithm is meant to guide a clinician's decision-making about the appropriateness of the case for AF-CBT. For example, these guidelines look for eligibility in terms of age (e.g., 5–17), primary clinical referral reason (e.g., physical abuse or child aggression), and participant availability (e.g., caregiver and child involvement), and suggest potential reasons for exclusion due to other treatment needs (e.g., emergent symptoms, active domestic violence with safety threats, recent sexual abuse).

There are several measures recommended for use in AF-CBT to help identify cases that exhibit some of the key clinical targets mentioned earlier. These include the Alabama Parenting Questionnaire (APQ; Shelton, Frick, & Wootton, 1996), the Brief Child Abuse Potential Inventory (B-CAP; Ondersma, Chaffin, Mullins, & LeBreton, 2005), the Child PTSD Symptom Scale (CPSS; Foa, Johnson, Feeny, & Treadwell, 2001), and the Strengths of Difficulties Questionnaire (SDQ; Goodman, Miltzer, & Bailey, 1998).

The APQ captures caregiver behavior and it is used in AF-CBT as a parent self-report, but it could also be completed by an older child or teenager. The 42-item scale includes six individual factors: Positive Parenting, Parental Involvement, Poor Parental Monitoring and Supervision, Inconsistent Discipline, Corporal Punishment, and Other Discipline. Cases that report modest levels of corporal punishment or low levels of positive parenting may be appropriate for AF-CBT.

The B-CAP is based on the full version of the Child Abuse Potential Inventory (Milner & Ayoub, 1980), because of its utility in helping to identify caregivers who may be at high risk for physical abuse or child maltreatment. The B-CAP has 24 items that form 9 factors, two of which are used to determine validity (e.g., random responses and lying), and seven others which are used to capture overall abuse risk potential. Caregivers who report heightened risk on the abuse scale or who report family conflict on a subset of three items within the abuse scale would seem appropriate for AF-CBT.

The SDQ measures child externalizing behavior (e.g. ODD/CD, aggression) and other relevant child problems. The SDQ is 25-item clinical rating scale, completed by caregivers on 3–16 year olds. The subscales include: Total Difficulties, Emotional symptoms, Conduct problems, Hyperactivity, Peer problems, and Prosocial Behavior. Children who fall above the clinical cutoff on the conduct problems scale are appropriate for AF-CBT.

The CPSS is a questionnaire designed to measure post traumatic stress disorder severity in children aged 8–18. It also contains questions about daily functioning and is designed to measure severity of impairment. It takes approximately 20 min to administer as an interview measure (by a clinician or a therapist) and 10 min to complete as a self-report. This 15 item questionnaire is designed to provide information on what specific events are underlying the PTSD symptoms the child is experiencing. The CPSS also assesses how the child felt while he or she was experiencing the traumatic event. Children who meet the clinical cutoff on the CPSS may benefit from the exposure to our recently incorporated imaginal exposure component. In addition to measuring PTS symptoms, we also encourage practitioners to consider using a specific set of items to identify the child's unique trauma history. This measure is suggested to determine the need to include imaginal exposure.

Description of Protocol

AF-CBT is a short-term treatment typically provided once or twice a week that may be delivered in 18–24 h of service over 6–12 months, although treatment may last shorter or longer as determined necessary to achieve key clinical goals. The revised and expanded curriculum for AF-CBT (version 3.0; 11-1-2011) includes an updated session guide with key fundamental skills and clinical examples, detailed presentations of the 17 content topics that help guide the administration of each session, supplemental worksheets/handouts designed to support instruction in each topic, and home practice assignments. Examples of the general application on these skills are provided in addition to specific suggestions for cases that may require adaptations or special circumstances. The content of AF-CBT is divided into three phases: Engagement and Psychoeducation, Individual Skill-Building, and Family Applications.

Phase I

Engagement and psychoeducation is the first phase of AF-CBT. The working relationship between the clinician and the family is crucial to the success of treatment. This relationship must be supportive, non-judgmental and trusting. Also, it is important that the clinician make the setting as comfortable, safe, and predictable as possible. In this stage, the clinician learns about the nature of the referral incident/conflict and the family's perspective on it. In the last component, psychoeducation, the primary caregiver and the clinician discuss physical discipline, as well as the caregiver's beliefs about it, followed by a short review of some of the common causes and consequences of exposure to physical force or punitive discipline. A similar but briefer discussion is held with the child.

Phase II

Phase II of AF-CBT focuses on individual skill building. The caregiver(s) learns to identify and control heightened anger and anxiety in a topic devoted to emotion regulation. It is common that children who were exposed to conflict, aggression, or abuse have seen adult models that are prone to anger. Because children often have the same reactions to frustration and stress as their caregivers do, the child also is taught self-regulation techniques that they can use to maintain self-control and appropriate behavior when they are frustrated or stressed. The emotion regulation content includes a review of the "ABC" model (A situation, Behavior, Consequences) for understanding behavior in context, a reaction triangle which depicts how thoughts, feelings, and behaviors are interrelated, triggers and cues related to anger and anxiety, and methods for controlling anger or anxiety, such as controlled breathing or progressive muscle relaxation.

An important aspect of this phase is for caregivers and children to learn to restructure negative thoughts and develop alternative thoughts. The caregiver learns to recognize, identify, and modify the types of unhelpful or critical thoughts that often arise in difficult experiences. The clinician uses cognitive coping with the child to teach new tools to address reactions and negative thoughts. Learning these coping skills helps the child handle common stressful situations as well as getting along with peers or family members.

Another critical component of skill building is training the caregiver in child behavior management techniques to promote desirable behavior. These techniques include the use of positive consequences, such as using praise, rewards, and differential reinforcement (i.e., giving attention to positive and ignoring negative behaviors).

An optional portion of phase two is imaginal exposure. This topic is designed for children who have symptoms of posttraumatic stress disorder or who are anxious when discussing or thinking about the referral incident or other experiences of abuse or conflict in the home. This allows the child to experience an emotional and cognitive process of the incident in a safe environment. Imaginal exposure results in a decrease of anxiety and anger when thinking about the abuse or conflict and helps the child make meaning out of the experience.

Phase III

In Phase III (Family Applications), the caregiver and child learn to apply the skills they have learned to their own family situation. The first component of this phase is to discuss how the caregiver and the child communicate with one another and ways to alter the kinds of verbal and non-verbal behaviors that they use. The goal of this work is to promote effective and mutually rewarding communication.

The clarification process is a culmination of all of the prior work with the caregiver. In this step, the caregiver writes a letter taking responsibility, apologizing, and describing how the home will be made safer and more comfortable. The child listens to the caregiver read this letter, and responds or asks questions in he or she chooses. This discussion of the referral incident or ongoing conflict helps to enhance communication about difficult topics and to set up a plan for how things will be different going forward.

Following the clarification letter, the family is taught six steps to solve problems in non-aggressive ways. The steps are designed to encourage them to patiently, thoughtfully, and clearly identify the problem and their goals, identify and evaluate potential solutions, and then apply and evaluate the solution they will choose to address the problem. The clinician reviews, illustrates, and discusses each step. The concluding sessions of AF-CBT focus on helping the family anticipate any future problems with the child's behavior and their responses, with the goal of preventing relapse.

In addition to these three phases, there are fundamental components of AF-CBT that should be routinely administered or kept in mind as they become relevant. The fundamental components of AF-CBT are: assessment and functional analysis, "CA$H" (defined below), alternatives for families plan, safety planning and other potential crises, addressing inconsistent attendance, managing escalation in session, and enhancing motivation. A Session Guide for AF-CBT has been developed that provides clinicians with a comprehensive, step-by-step approach that can be administered with this clinical population in a variety of practice settings. The techniques included in the Session Guide were selected because they have empirical support in the research literature and clinical utility.

AF-CBT is based on a cognitive behavioral therapy (CBT) framework. In CBT, assessment is central in that it yields clinically relevant information that helps to guide treatment. The underlying model of assessment in CBT is called Functional Analysis. The model is based on the idea that all behavior is functional and therefore, the key to assessment is to determine the function of the behavior. A functional analysis includes an assessment of what is occurring before the problem behavior and after the behavior, as well as a description of the actual behavior. Assessing frequency, duration, intensity, and pervasiveness of the behavior are all part of the functional analysis. Specifically, in AF-CBT, functional analysis includes assessment of problem behaviors exhibited by children (e.g., avoidance of trauma reminders, externalizing behaviors), caregivers (e.g., aggression), and families (e.g., conflict).

"CA$H" which stands for check-in on attendance, safety, and home practice is a brief weekly check-in that begins at the start of each session. The first component of the acronym is attendance check-in, which includes praising the caregiver and child for coming back for treatment. By supporting the caregiver's attendance, the clinician shows that he or she recognizes that treatment may require considerable sacrifice and resources. In some cases, the clinician addresses barriers to attendance proactively with the caregiver and child. The second component is the weekly safety check-in. This exercise has the caregiver and/or the child complete a handout about any recent conflicts, arguments, or physical force involving the caregiver and child. This provides information about the caregiver's use of various disciplinary strategies and is useful in reflecting on the family's progress during treatment. The last component is home practice check-in. Incorporated into each session are weekly home practice assignments. These assignments serve the important purpose of reminding the clients to use newly learned skills, to help clients apply the lessons learned in session are home or in the community, to help clients practice skills and report back to the clinician so that he or she can help problem-solve and refine the skills, and to prepare caregivers and children for the next session so that session time can be maximized.

The Alternatives for Families Plan (AFP) is a log and description of the client's personalized skills that the client has found to be useful or effective when applied to a current problem situation. The clients are encouraged to use these skills regularly. Throughout the course of treatment the AFP is expanded to include the skills that the caregiver and/or the child are using that they are finding helpful.

Establishing a safety plan is another fundamental component of AF-CBT. These plans are important if a family is "at risk" for physical abuse or unsafe family conflict. The first step in making the safety plan is to conduct a functional analysis of "at-risk" behaviors. The safety plan should incorporate three elements. The plan should involve immediate removal from the escalation or separation to keep the child safe. It should also include short-term de-escalation skills that help to keep oneself in control, such as emotional regulation skills. Lastly, it should include a plan to resolve the conflict (e.g., attain outside counseling).

There is also a routine for managing escalation that may occasionally be needed to maintain decorum during therapy sessions. This element is encouraged when the clinician recognizes that a client is becoming angry or challenging, and there is a need to keep everyone safe and calm in the session. It is very likely that many of the families being referred for services may be angry and frustrated. This structured routine guides the clinician to calmly acknowledge these feelings and address them appropriately through the use of questions for more information or suggesting about a reasonable course of action. The importance of maintaining such composure is to help the client incorporate self-control methods and to maintain the continuity of treatment. In addition, maintaining control may support efforts to demonstrate the client's appropriateness to maintain children in the home or get them back from placement. The last fundamental component of AF-CBT is enhancing motivation. Some AF-CBT clients either may not be interested in or actively try to avoid the content that is being discussed in a particular session. This can be a challenge with caregivers who are mandated to treatment or those who maintain strong beliefs that justify their behavior. It is likely that enhancing motivation to learn the content may be a critical contributor to retention during and achieving beneficial outcomes following treatment.

Research Evidence

In the initial outcome study with 55 referred families, the individual and family approaches in AF-CBT were evaluated separately and compared to a condition reflecting routine community services (RCS) in a clinical trial that evaluated key outcomes through a 1-year follow-up assessment. In terms of overall clinical outcomes through follow-up (Kolko, 1996a), both the individual CBT and family therapy conditions reported significantly greater improvements than RCS on certain child (i.e., less child-to-parent aggression, child externalizing behavior), parent (i.e., child abuse potential, individual treatment targets reflecting abusive behavior, psychological distress, drug use), and family outcomes (i.e., less conflict, more cohesion). The official recidivism rates for CBT and family were lower (5–6 %) than the rate for RCS (30 %), but did not reach statistical significance. Both CBT and family therapy had high consumer satisfaction ratings.

In a related analysis comparing the treatment course of the two randomized conditions (individual CBT vs. family therapy; see Kolko, 1996b), weekly ratings of parents' use of physical force and anger problems were found to decrease significantly faster among the individual child and parent CBT cases than those receiving family treatment, but both showed significant improvements over time.

Following this initial outcome study, the main elements of the individual CBT and family therapy conditions were integrated into a single AF-CBT treatment approach in the context of subsequent trainings and treatment applications (version 1.0). An uncontrolled study describes the long-term sustainability and outcome of AF-CBT as delivered by practitioners in a community-based child protection program who had received training in the model several years earlier (Kolko, Iselin, & Gully, 2011). In this study, practitioners were trained to administer these original methods in one of the first dissemination projects funded by the National Child

Traumatic Stress Network in 2002. Seven practitioners from the same community agency received a daylong training workshop, 12 monthly case consultation calls, and a follow-up booster workshop, to help them learn and apply basic AF-CBT content to their clients. The agency routinely collected intake and discharge data for program evaluation purposes, and these data were obtained to document the clinical and treatment outcomes of 52 families presenting with a physically abused child who received AF-CBT content between 2 and 5 years after training had ended.

In terms of the outcomes this study, measures of the use of AF-CBT and four other EBTs documented their frequency, internal consistency, intercorrelations, and relationship to several therapist- and parent-rated outcomes. The amount of AF-CBT General and Abuse-specific content delivered was found to predict several clinical and functional improvements in both children and caregivers, above and beyond the influence of the unique content of the other four EBTs. Specifically, the amount of AF-CBT abuse-specific content delivered was related to improvements on standardized parent rating scales (i.e., child externalizing behavior, anger, anxiety, social competence) and both parent and clinician ratings of the child's adjustment at discharge (i.e., child more safe, less scared, sad, more appropriate with peers). The amount of AF-CBT general content was related to a few discharge ratings (better child prognosis, helpfulness to parents). These novel naturalistic data document the sustainability and clinical benefits of AF-CBT in an existing community clinic serving physically abused children and their families, and are discussed in the context of key developments in the treatment model and dissemination literature.

PARTNERS, a CBT for child physical abuse that includes many of the components currently incorporated in the CBT and family therapy conditions found in AF-CBT, was piloted with physically-abused children and their caregivers by Brown (2005). The purpose of PARTNERS was to decrease children's internalizing symptoms (including posttraumatic stress disorder) and externalizing behavior problems, decrease caregivers' recidivism, improve children's cognitive processing of the abuse, and improve parenting practices. An open trial with pre-treatment, mid-treatment, post-treatment, and 3-month follow-up assessments was conducted to determine whether the mental health problems in children exposed to physical abuse would be reduced after completing a 16-week parent- and child-focused CBT. Eleven children (ages 6–12; 73 % boys; 82 % Latino and 18 % African American/ Black) and their primary caregivers participated. Children completed self-report measures of psychopathology, anger, and attributions about the abuse (e.g., shame, self-blame). Caregivers completed measures of parenting practice (including corporal punishment), child abuse potential, and psychopathology. At baseline, all of the children met criteria for a psychiatric disorder, with 45 % meeting criteria for two and 18 % meeting criteria for three disorders. The most common diagnoses were: posttraumatic stress disorder, separation anxiety disorder, and generalized anxiety disorder. Within-subjects repeated measures analyses indicated significant pre to post decreases in children's Conduct Problems and Anxiety (as measured by the Behavioral Assessment System for Children), and Shame. Both children and their caregivers reported significant decreases in caregivers' use of corporal punishment and physical abuse.

As mentioned earlier, AF-CBT was also adapted and expanded for use in treating children with Oppositional Defiant Disorder (ODD) or Conduct Disorder (CD) in a recent clinical trial that compared its delivery to children/families who were randomly assigned to receive the intervention either in the community or the clinic (Kolko et al., 2009). The adaptation of AF-CBT eliminated the materials related to language focusing on a history of physical abuse (e.g., discussion of referral incident, psychoeducation about abuse, clarification), but included other materials relevant for behavior disorders (e.g., modules to enhance peer/social, school, and community adjustment; ADHD medication protocol). This comprehensive program was organized into modules that were selected for administration by the clinician. Children in both conditions showed significant and comparable improvements in behavioral and emotional problems, psychopathic features, functional impairment, diagnosis status, and service involvement after the 6-month intervention period. Many of these improvements were maintained at 3-year follow-up. At the 3-year follow-up, 36 % of children in the community condition and 47 % of children in the clinic condition no longer met criteria for ODD or CD (Kolko et al.).

In another study, clinically referred children who were rated at or above the 75th percentile on an externalizing behavior scale were randomized to a protocol for on-site nurse-administered intervention (PONI) or to enhanced usual care (EUC) consisting of outside referral to a local provider (Kolko et al., 2010). PONI applied the AF-CBT and other treatment modules used in the aforementioned study (Kolko et al., 2009) which were adapted for delivery in busy primary care offices. EUC offered diagnostic assessment, recommendations, and facilitated referrals to a specialty mental health care provider in the community. Cases in the PONI (vs. EUC) condition were significantly more likely to receive and complete mental health services, reported fewer service barriers and more consumer satisfaction, and showed modest improvements on clinical outcomes 1 year later, such as remission for categorical behavior disorders. Both PONI and EUC conditions reported significant improvements on several clinical outcomes over time (Kolko et al., 2010).

While these findings support the notion that a more comprehensive psychosocial intervention for behavior problems can be delivered by nurses in a primary care setting, they also suggested the need to strengthen the effectiveness of this on-site treatment. Accordingly, PONI was expanded to include more on-site collaboration and coordination with the pediatrician (adaptation of chronic care model), an expanded clinical content curriculum to address ADHD and anxiety, and the use of technology, and was re-named as Doctor-Office Collaborative Care (DOCC; Kolko, Baumann, Herschell, Hart, & Wisniewski, 2012). DOCC continues to include the main clinical content of AF-CBT. In a second clinical trial, children with behavior problems were randomly assigned to DOCC or enhanced usual care (EUC) to evaluate the feasibility and clinical efficacy of this expanded integrated intervention. Using growth curve modeling, DOCC was associated with greater improvements in service use and completion, behavioral and emotional problems, individualized behavioral goals, and overall clinical response. This study provides support for the integration of AF-CBT and other collaborative mental health services to address common mental disorders in the primary-care setting (Kolko, Campo, Kilbourne, & Kelleher, 2012).

These few studies provide modest empirical support for the AF-CBT approach on a range of important clinical and safety outcomes. These outcomes extend across key domains (caregiver practices, child emotional and behavioral problems, family cohesion/conflict, etc.), among the many that might be targeted (see Kolko, 2002). In addition, many of the methods integrated in AF-CBT have been found efficacious in other outcome studies conducted with various populations of caregivers, children, and families over the past decade (see Kolko & Kolko, 2010; Kolko & Swenson, 2002). At the same time, there is a clear need for further controlled studies of AF-CBT that are based on the current curriculum and that can examine the relative contribution of some of its more novel intervention components. Further, research on applications of AF-CBT currently being conducted in alternative settings is needed, such in foster care placements, schools, child advocacy centers, domestic violence centers, and residential or day treatment programs (see Herschell, Kolko, Baumann, & Brown, 2012).

Case History

We report below a case history for a representative family referred for AF-CBT to address concerns regarding exposure to physical force/abuse and family conflict. All names have been changed to maintain confidentiality.

Child's History and Referral Reason

JR is an 11-year-old Caucasian male that is currently in the fifth grade. He was diagnosed with Attention Deficit/Hyperactivity Disorder (ADHD), Oppositional Defiant Disorder (ODD), and Major Depression about 1 year prior to beginning AF-CBT. He is currently prescribed Guanfacine for ADHD and Fluoxetine for depressive symptoms. Two months prior to starting AF-CBT, JR was hospitalized for 2 days due to suicidal ideation. Although JR has a long history of difficulty concentrating in class and completing his homework, these problems had worsened. Teachers reported that he generally appears detached and apathetic but that he occasionally acts extremely oppositional. Teachers also reported that he blurts out his opinions frequently in class and has difficulty getting along with his peers. In the clinical intake interview, the mother reported that JR recently had appeared depressed and was overly "emotional" when she corrected his behavior at home.

JR and his family were referred for mental health treatment by a local child protection caseworker. Treatment was strongly encouraged, but not required, due to a recent report of child physical abuse by the father. The abuse incident involved the father yelling, cursing, threatening, and repeatedly kicking JR as he lay on the living room floor of his father's apartment. As a result of this abuse, JR had significant bruising to his back and stomach. Additionally, JR's eyeglasses broke which resulted in several cuts to his face. JR's younger brother and only sibling (SR) witnessed the incident.

There had been no prior reports of physical abuse by the father toward the children. However, there was a history of domestic violence perpetrated by the father toward the mother during the time that they were married. Both children witnessed the domestic violence on multiple occasions. The mother and children also reported a long history of father being emotionally abusive to JR (e.g., name-calling, threatening, maintaining unreasonable expectations).

Family Demographics

JR's mother was 35 years old and single. She reported that she had been diagnosed with Bipolar Disorder and was participating in individual therapy to manage her depressive symptoms. She was prescribed Lithium, Neurontin and Seroquel to help regulate her anxiety and depression. Mother also reported a past history of alcohol dependence and post-traumatic stress disorder. She had been sober for 3 years and was unemployed at the time of the intake interview.

JR's father was 38 years old and lived with his girlfriend. He reported that he had been recently diagnosed with ADHD and Anxiety Disorder NOS because he had been experiencing muscle tension, restlessness, irritability, and difficulty sleeping. Father reported no other mental health problems and denied any substance use. He worked full-time as a welder for a manufacturing company at the time of the intake interview.

The parents had been divorced for 6 years and shared joint custody of their sons despite the recent episode of physical abuse; the mother had the children from 6 a.m. to 6 p.m. and the father had the two children from 6 p.m. to 6 a.m. with alternating weekend visitation. Mother did not have a vehicle so the father generally provided transportation.

The youngest child (SR) was an 8-year-old male. He had no history of mental health problems. The parents reported that he had always functioned well at home and at school.

Child Assessment and Diagnostic Impressions

In addition to a general clinical interview, JR completed a brief trauma history interview, the Alabama Parenting Questionnaire (APQ), and the UCLA PTSD Reaction Index. In the trauma history interview, JR disclosed physical and emotional abuse by his father, witnessing domestic violence between his father and mother, and being in a car accident that left both his brother and mother severely injured. The APQ (parent and child versions) revealed concerns on the following subscales: Positive Parenting Practices, Inconsistent Discipline, Corporal Punishment and Parental

Involvement. JR had a total score of 34 on the UCLA PTSD Reaction Index, which is the suggestive of a "partial diagnosis" of PTSD (Pynoos & Em, 1986).

In the clinical interview, JR endorsed several symptoms of depression, including feeling sad, feeling like no one likes him, crying easily and sleeping less than usual. JR also reported that he has always had difficulty paying attention in school and following directions but that recently school was more difficult than usual. Based on the clinical interview and assessment results, AF-CBT appeared to be an appropriate intervention to decrease anger and aggression in the home, promote alternative discipline strategies, and reduce the trauma-related symptoms experienced by JR.

Treatment Procedures

AF-CBT (2nd edition, 7/2009) was delivered in 17 sessions over the course of 22 weeks. Sessions were typically 60–75 min in length and the time was occasionally split in half between child and parent. See Table 11.1 below for a summary of treatment format, session-by-session key interventions, and commentary.

Phase I: Engagement and Psychoeducation

Although Mom and JR easily engaged in treatment, it was critical that Dad participate given he was the perpetrator of the emotional and physical abuse that recently occurred in the home. Furthermore, dad continued to share equal custody of the children despite the abuse incident. Mom clearly understood why he needed to be involved in treatment but she was reluctant to participate with him. Utilization of the decisional balance worksheet helped mom explore and evaluate the benefits and consequences of encouraging JR's father to participate fully in treatment.

The father attended the third session with JR and remained the primary participant throughout the course of treatment. The mother decided it was in the best interest of the two children for her ex-husband to be in this role. Maintaining a nonjudgmental, validating, and normalizing stance with JR's father was the key to gaining his trust and increasing his motivation to participate. Offering hope and focusing on strengths seemed to give him the courage to try something new even though he admitted to feeling very uncomfortable. He reported at the end of the third session that he was too ashamed to show up for the first two sessions but now understood how this treatment might really improve his relationship with his son. The father was nervous but motivated to make change and outlined realistic goals for treatment. The Weekly Safety Check-In (formerly called the Weekly Report of Discipline Practices) was a key intervention throughout the course of treatment as it provided many opportunities to examine disciplinary interactions that occurred at home and apply the CBT model in session. This in depth examination of disciplinary consequences helped dad recognize the discipline strategies that weren't working well and increased his motivation to learn and implement more effective discipline

Table 11.1 Summary of AF-CBT session content, clients, topics, and comments on the case

Phase	Session	Client	Topic and key interventions	Comments
I	1	Mom, JR, SR	Orientation Discussed confidentiality limitations Provided treatment overview Created safety plan	Mom and children extremely receptive to treatment but waiting for Dad to commit. Dad refused to attend and Mom reluctant to be in same room with him
		JR	Orientation/build rapport Completed goal setting form Getting to know you activity	JR quiet initially but engaged in getting to know you activity pretty easily. Goal for treatment is to get along better with Dad
I	2	Mom	Engagement Completed and reviewed stressful life experiences worksheet Utilized decisional balance worksheet Outlined treatment goals Discussed involving ex-husband in treatment	Mom was grateful for reviewing stressful events and listening to her story – states that no one usually cares. Utilized decisional balance sheet to discuss involving ex-husband in treatment – Mom cautiously decides to invite him to our next session
I	3	Dad	Orientation/engagement Discussed confidentiality limitations Normalized and instilled hope Provided treatment overview Completed decisional balance worksheet and established goals	Dad unexpectedly attended session and responded surprisingly well. He agreed to participate in the treatment. Importantly, he expressed feeling too embarrassed and ashamed of his recent behavior to engage in family treatment
		Dad, JR	Psychoeducation Reviewed CBT model Discussed less force agreement Introduced weekly report of discipline practices	Review of CBT model well received – both generated relevant examples. Dad agreed to less force but reluctant about ability to complete WRDP each week. He agreed to try the WRDP form one time
I	4	JR	Discussion of upsetting experiences Introduced emotion identification and expression skills Read books about physical abuse Discussed referral incident	Normalization of physically abusive experiences helped JR discuss referral incident. Focused on emotions behind anger. JR stated that referral incident was not his fault
I	5	Dad	Abuse discussion and clarification Discussed use of physical force/hurtful words Explained clarification process	Dad noticeably anxious but able to discuss referral incident and purpose of clarification. Described what he wants to say to his son and was right on target

(continued)

Table 11.1 (continued)

Phase	Session	Client	Topic and key interventions	Comments
I	6	JR	Discussed clarification process	JR appears comfortable with clarification
		Dad, JR	Clarification Dad read note to JR JR expressed feelings and thoughts about Dad's note	Dad displayed appropriate emotion as he read note. JR avoids looking at Dad until he is quiet then looks up and says he is glad Dad is working on getting better
I	7	SR, Mom	Discussion of clarification Prepared Mom and SR for clarification	Ex-wife and SR were willing to hear Dad's note. Mom reported improvement in relationship with ex-husband
		SR, Mom, Dad	Clarification Dad read note to SR and ex-wife	Mom and youngest son both emotional and grateful for discussion with Dad
II	8	JR	Cognitive processing Completed ABC worksheet Discussed thinking errors Identified alternative coping strategies	JR acknowledged several thinking errors and developed list of alternative coping strategies for negative mood. JR reported that Dad is less angry at home
II	9	Dad	Maintaining positivity Reviewed CBT model Discussed thinking errors Discussed child development and reasonable expectations	Dad successfully generated several examples using the CBT model. Applied model to automatic thoughts associated with JR. Dad expressed continued frustration with JR's impulsive behaviors
II	10	JR	Emotion regulation Psychoeducation about our body's response to stress Identified and practiced relaxation strategies	JR reported that he rarely feels relaxed. JR responded positively to deep breathing and progressive muscle relaxation. JR reported that Dad got upset last week but didn't explode
		Dad	Emotion regulation Reviewed skills from mandated anger management course Practiced deep breathing and progressive muscle relaxation	Dad reluctantly practiced deep breathing and progressive muscle relaxation in session. Identified music and a few minutes alone as essential relaxation skills. Dad admits to "losing it" last week
II	11	JR	Social skills Practiced with role plays	Role plays were critical for JR to receive necessary constructive feedback
		Dad	Behavior management Discussed consistency, attending/ignoring, and praise Practiced with role plays	Dad surprised by suggestion to increase praise – admits that will feel very "weird" for him but willing to try and report back next week

(continued)

Table 11.1 (continued)

Phase	Session	Client	Topic and key interventions	Comments
II	12	Dad, Mom	Behavior management Reviewed previous session material Introduced rewards and discussed giving effective instructions Introduced discipline strategies	Mom and Dad acknowledged they have very different strategies – Mom more passive and Dad more controlling. Both agreed to try strategies presented in session
II	13	Dad, Mom	Behavior management – discipline Reviewed effective discipline strategies Role plays and completed what would you do scenarios	Dad reported that increased praise is making a dramatic difference. Mom admits that she struggles to follow through with consequences
III	14	Dad, JR	Communication skills Identify patterns/preferences In session practice	Dad and JR shared communication preferences and acknowledged differences. Practiced skills in session
III	15	Dad, JR	Communication and problem-solving skills Reviewed problem-solving model Psychoeducation about ADHD diagnosis	Dad reported improved communication with JR but blurting out still a problem for JR. Dad tells JR that he also has ADHD
III	16	Dad, JR	Problem-solving skills Reviewed model and "real life" problem solving examples	Good discussion regarding at home problem solving – Dad and JR effectively implement problem solving model
III	17	Dad, JR	Termination Reviewed and celebrated progress	Dad reported significant skill learning. JR reports mixed feelings about termination
		All	Termination celebration	Family pleasantly interacts

Key: *I* engagement and psychoeducation, *II* individual skill-building, *III* family application

strategies. Although JR and his father rarely completed the Weekly Report of Discipline Practices form at home, they were both very good at verbally describing any discipline interaction from the previous week.

JR had not discussed the referral incident with his father prior to the clarification process. The father reported that he initially thought it was best to avoid the topic with JR but quickly realized in treatment that it might be beneficial to discuss the abuse incident. In session five, the father spontaneously recited what he wanted to say to his son about the referral incident. He explained that he needed to take responsibility for what occurred, apologize to JR, and tell him that it was not his fault. He also wanted to tell his son that he was working hard to make sure it didn't happen again (for example, taking medication for anxiety, completing anger management course and attending therapy with JR). After a lengthy discussion about including the long-standing emotional abuse that had occurred over the previous years, the father agreed to create a bulleted list to share with JR the following session.

The following week, the father read the bulleted list he had created to JR. The list had been reviewed with the clinician prior to sharing it with JR and included all the essential elements of a clarification letter. JR was extremely quiet but attentive as Dad read aloud in session. JR avoided eye contact with Dad initially but when Dad stopped talking he immediately looked at him and quietly said "I am glad you are working hard because I like being with you. It is getting better." Dad was appropriately touched emotionally in session and later reported that reading his note to JR was the most difficult but rewarding thing he had ever done.

Phase II: Individual Skill Building

Phase II began with a review of the CBT model with both JR and his father. Understanding the connection between thoughts, feelings, and behaviors helped them to identify thinking patterns that interfered in their relationship. The father realized that his interactions with JR often began with negative automatic thoughts about JR (e.g., "he is so annoying" or "he never learns"). Once these types of thoughts were identified, he began noticing how often they occurred, and how they contributed to escalating his anger and consequently his negative behavior. Interestingly, the father even shared the CBT model with his girlfriend in an attempt to work on their relationship issues.

Emotion regulation strategies were also helpful to both JR and his father. Although they were very self-conscious as they practiced deep breathing and progressive muscle relaxation in session, both JR and his father fully participated and acknowledged that they felt relaxed. JR explained that he rarely feels relaxed at home or school so identifying several effective relaxation strategies for JR was a priority. The father reported that the anger management skills he learned in his mandated anger management course, and reviewed again in AF-CBT, had been very helpful in reducing his anger with his sons. He also admitted that he wasn't always successful in using the skills, which led to an important conversation about maintaining realistic expectations for himself as he attempted to change long-standing behavior.

Given that JR had a long history of problems getting along with his peers at school and inappropriately intervening in adult conversations that did not involve him, it was essential to provide him social skills training. Although JR could verbally explain proper social skills when presented with varying social situations, he struggled to act appropriately when role-plays were conducted in session. JR was more receptive to and successful with the role-plays when instructed to pretend that he was at an audition for a guest appearance on one of his favorite shows. This active in-session practice provided opportunity for constructive feedback balanced with abundant praise.

The last three sessions of Phase II focused on behavior management strategies and both parents were encouraged to attend these sessions together. Early in treatment it was clear that each parent had substantially different parenting strategies. In general, JR's mother tended to be overly permissive with discipline in the home and his father overly controlling. Sessions with both parents occasionally got mildly contentious but were crucial to establishing consistency and similar expectations in each setting. It was apparent that neither parent had been taught effective discipline strategies, so providing instruction regarding effective behavior management skills was enlightening for them. For example, the father had been taking away JR's iPod for a month anytime his behavior warranted a removal of privilege. He agreed to try removing the iPod for a day at a time and reported that it was much more effective. Finally, both parents realized that their homes were lacking positive attention and praise and were shocked at how much increasing praise improved JR's behavior. The father also stated that he also felt much better about himself when he began to increase praise with JR.

Phase III: Family Applications

JR and his father participated well together in the Phase III sessions. Interactions between the two of them had noticeably improved since the start of treatment, providing a more relaxed session tone to begin working on communication and problem solving skills. Recognizing communication patterns and preferences was helpful to both JR and his father. The father reported that he continued to be very frustrated with JR's blurting out and interrupting adult conversations that did not involve JR. JR was not aware of the behavior so Dad agreed to gently but directly point out the behavior when it occurred. Additionally, the father agreed to provide reinforcement when JR was successfully redirected or avoided the behavior entirely. JR responded well but admitted that it was difficult for him to slow down before blurting out – a common difficulty for children with ADHD. Psychoeducation about ADHD appeared to help the father become more tolerant of his son's "blurting out" and impulsiveness. Furthermore, JR's lack of knowledge about ADHD had left him feeling like he was just a "dumb kid". The psychoeducation on ADHD provided him with a new understanding of his diagnosis and behavioral difficulties. Importantly, Dad spontaneously disclosed his own ADHD diagnosis to JR in that same session, which was validating for JR. JR and his father successfully applied problem-solving skills to several hypothetical situations in session but most importantly reported that they used the skills to solve a problem in between sessions, showing that they were able to generalize the skills to their home lives.

Assessment Outcomes

JR completed the Alabama Parenting Questionnaire and the UCLA Reaction Index at intake and at session 16. The Alabama Parenting Questionnaire was also administered with each parent at the beginning and end of treatment.

As treatment came to end, progress was reviewed and celebrated with JR and his father. JR expressed mixed feelings counseling coming to an end and his father responded appropriately, supporting him in session. JR requested that his younger brother and mother join them for the termination celebration and his father agreed. JR and his father reported that there had been no serious physical discipline since treatment began and that name-calling and threatening were virtually non-existent. Scores on the Alabama Parenting Questionnaire also supported these observations. Both JR and his father showed substantial improvement on the following subscales from pre-treatment to post-treatment, respectively, Positive Parenting (JR's scores were 12 and 22; Dad's scores were 13 and 20), Parental Involvement (JR's scores were 21 and 25; Dad's scores were 19 and 28), Inconsistent Discipline (JR's scores were 18 and 14; Dad's scores were 16 and 9), and Corporal Punishment (JR's scores were 8 and 3; Dad's scores were 7 and 3). The father also reported that there had been substantial improvement in communication with JR over the course of treatment. His mother reported noticeable improvement in JR's mood and behavior. PTSD symptoms also appeared to improve for JR as his scores on the UCLA PTSD Reaction Index severity score dropped from 34 to 18, indicating that JR no longer met criteria for a partial PTSD diagnosis.

Overcoming Barriers and Challenges

Although this family responded well to AF-CBT overall, there were several challenges to successfully delivering the service. The first challenge was to get the father engaged in treatment with his son. Not only was the mother reluctant to participate in treatment with the father, but the father refused to participate in treatment. However, after orienting Mom to the treatment model and using the decisional balance sheet to help her understand the components of the decision, the mother realized that it would be most beneficial to JR if her ex-husband attended the sessions and she were less involved. Fortunately, encouragement by the father's caseworker and his ex-wife seemed to be enough to get him to attend session three. Interestingly, over the course of treatment JR's parents appeared to get along much better. They even attended several sessions together.

The second challenge was scheduling regular sessions with JR and his father. The daily visitation schedule made it difficult to schedule sessions with the father and intensified the need for effective communication with both parents. The father eventually agreed to pick up JR on his day off so they could attend sessions regularly. Additionally, regular phone calls from clinician to the mother were critical to keeping her engaged in the process and supportive of JR.

The third challenge was to coordinate information among the family's service providers. There was very little communication among the family's support team, which contributed to confusion and service overload. For example, this family was involved with six different mental health providers at the outset of AF-CBT, many of which were initiated at the suggestion of separate team members. We believed that the family's mental health services could be better coordinated to reduce burden, increase effectiveness, and make regular attendance feasible. After consultation with the family, a team meeting was organized to prioritize treatment goals and reduce the number of interventions that were recommended for the family.

Training and Dissemination

A recent randomized trial provides some unique information about the dissemination of AF-CBT to eight diverse community agencies serving the child welfare and mental health systems (Kolko, Baumann, et al., 2012). A sample of 182 practitioners was randomized to receive AF-CBT training or routine training as usual in the agency (TAU). The training consisted of 4 days of a didactic/experiential workshop and ten consult calls in 6 months, with a few supplemental (2–4) advanced training ("booster") sessions over the next few months. Growth model analyses revealed significant initial improvements for those in the AF-CBT training condition (vs. TAU) in knowledge about AF-CBT and its targeted population, and the use of AF-CBT teaching processes, abuse-specific skills, and general psychological skills. The training program also was associated with high rates of consumer satisfaction. These findings lend support to the training model, but the level of overall improvement by the end of follow-up was modest. Further, there was a steady decline in the level of morale found among the practitioners in both conditions. Of course, additional studies are needed to better understand what background characteristics or program elements contribute to AF-CBT use and improvements in family status, and how we can maximize the sustainability of training in a given agency, especially when training involves practitioners with diverse backgrounds, professional experiences, client populations, and service settings. Such work should help us understand the role of various treatment training, research, and work force issues in promoting treatment sustainability, which would then be used to refine our training program methods and structures.

Efforts to disseminate AF-CBT have expanded to include training programs for practitioners working in alternative service delivery settings affiliated with the mental health and child welfare systems. These diverse practitioners include psychiatrists, psychologists, social workers, marriage and family therapists, and case managers with varied clinical responsibilities primarily in outpatient and in-home settings. More recently, we have conducted trainings for those working in residential treatment centers, and those who work with families involved with foster care, the military, and domestic violence. Reports from trained practitioners generally indicate positive results in terms of clinical improvements (e.g., reductions in parental use of force/abusive behavior, improved parent–child relationships) and child protective services system outcomes (e.g., successful case closures or reunification), though more standardized and objective measures are being developed to more fully evaluate these benefits. Our training program methods are also being adapted for use in different countries (e.g., Canada, Germany, Holland, Israel, Japan, Singapore).

Our latest training programs are described on the AF-CBT website (www.afcbt.org). Interested professionals can request a training program through an on online request form. Proposed eligibility requirements are as follows: (1) Master's degree or higher in MH field (e.g., clinical/counseling psychology, social work, or related field of counseling); (2) Licensed in MH profession or supervised by licensed MH professional by the time AF-CBT training begins (with expectation that this continues throughout the training); and (3) Access to appropriate AF-CBT cases for ongoing consultation. Briefly, a typical training program is provided in the context of a year-long learning community which includes a 3-day intensive skills training workshop (didactics and experiential exercises), followed by monthly case consultation calls (often with two presenter/call), audio file reviews with feedback for fidelity monitoring, a booster training/seminar, supervisor consultation calls, program metrics, and a year end summary/progress report.

Conclusions and Directions

It is important to mention some of the challenges to delivering effective treatment to angry, aggressive, and abusive families using AF-CBT. These include the difficulty of working with caregivers or children who are challenging with one another at home and in session (e.g., dismissive, defiant, angry/hostile, aggressive), families who may not be living together or who spend little time with one another (e.g., separation, protection from abuse orders), and families who are involved with other services, providers, and systems. Current efforts are underway to help clinicians tailor the material to the needs of these and other clients, which requires that clinicians engage in frequent decision-making about what content should be emphasized. In addition, the treatment can at times be lengthy, may involve working with difficult to engage families, and requires that practitioners draw upon considerable personal and professional resources. There is also a need to develop more cost-effective training programs that promote efficient methods to enhance the sustainability of AF-CBT in a given agency, once the training and consultation program has ended. Current efforts to finalize proposed credentialing criteria for clinician, supervisor, and trainer are intended to address this important need.

In recognition of these and other clinical challenges, we have updated and adapted the content of AF-CBT to maximize its relevance to and utility with families of school-aged children who are referred for physically coercive/abusive behavior, verbal and physical aggression by caregiver or children, and/or heightened family conflict placing families at risk for safety concerns. AF-CBT has been used primarily in outpatient and in-home settings, but is now being extended to other settings (e.g., residential) and populations (e.g., foster care, military), especially if there is some ongoing contact between caregiver and child. AF-CBT is directed towards specific targets related to caregivers (e.g., negative child perceptions, heightened anger or hostility, harsh/punitive/ineffective parenting practices), children (e.g., externalizing behavior problems, poor social competence), and families (e.g., heightened conflict/coercion, poor problem solving, communication, concerns about safety).

The few outcome studies reviewed herein have provided empirical support for the utility of AF-CBT with families referred for caregiver coercion/abusive behavior and child externalizing problems and who present with diverse child and caregiver demographic background variables (e.g., age, gender, ethnicity, intellectual functioning and family constellation). However, applications to specific cultural groups or settings have not been formally reported and additional outcome studies are needed to extend the evaluation of the current version of AF-CBT. Other developments are underway to simplify the content of the intervention, maximize training efficiency and benefit, provide support to clinicians and supervisors trained in the model, and conduct additional empirical evaluations of its outcomes and cost-effectiveness. These refinements will hopefully enable any clinician to address the broad and challenging clinical concerns often associated with heightened levels of anger and aggression among individuals and/or their families.

Acknowledgements Preparation of this chapter was supported, in part, by grants from the NIMH (074737) and SAMHSA (SM54319). We acknowledge our AF-CBT team colleagues, Barbara Baumann, Elissa Brown, Amy Herschel, Kevin Rumbarger, Komol Sharma-Patel, and Megan Shaver.

References

Brown, E. J. (2005, June). *Efficacy of a parent-child intervention for physically abused children and their caregivers.* Paper presented at the annual colloquium of the American Professional Society on the Abuse of Children, New Orleans, LA.

Foa, E. B., Johnson, K. M., Feeny, N. C., & Treadwell, K. R. H. (2001). The child PTSD symptom scale: A preliminary examination of its psychometric properties. *Journal of Clinical Child and Adolescent Psychology, 30*(3), 376–384.

Goodman, R., Meltzer, H., & Bailey, V. (1998). The strengths and difficulties questionnaire: A pilot study on the validity of the self-report version. *European Child & Adolescent Psychiatry, 7*(3), 125–130.

Herschell, A. D., Kolko, D. J., Baumann, B. L., & Brown, E. J. (2012). Application of alternatives for families: A cognitive behavioral therapy to school settings. *Journal of Applied School Psychology, 28,* 270–293.

Kolko, D. J. (1996a). Clinical monitoring of treatment course in child physical abuse: Psychometric characteristics and treatment comparisons. *Child Abuse & Neglect, 20*(1), 23–43.

Kolko, D. J. (1996b). Individual cognitive-behavioral treatment and family therapy for physically abused children and their offending parents: A comparison of clinical outcomes. *Child Maltreatment, 1,* 322–342.

Kolko, D. J. (2002). Child physical abuse. In J. E. B. Myers, L. Berliner, J. Briere, C. T. Hendrix, C. Jenny, & T. Reid (Eds.), *APSAC handbook of child maltreatment* (2nd ed., pp. 21–55). Thousand Oaks, CA: Sage.

Kolko, D. J. (2003a). Individual child and parent physical abuse-focused cognitive-behavioral treatment. In B. E. Saunders, L. Berliner, & R. F. Hanson (Eds.), *Child physical and sexual abuse: Guidelines for treatment* (Final report: January 15, 2003, pp. 43–44). Charleston, SC: National Crime Victims Research and Treatment Center.

Kolko, D. J. (2003b). Physical abuse informed family therapy. In B. E. Saunders, L. Berliner, & R. F. Hanson (Eds.), *Child physical and sexual abuse: Guidelines for treatment* (Final report: January 15, 2003, pp. 84–85). Charleston, SC: National Crime Victims Research and Treatment Center.

Kolko, D. J., Baumann, B. L., Herschell, A. D., Hart, J. A., & Wisniewski, S. (2012). Implementation of AF-CBT by community practitioners serving mental health and child welfare: A randomized trial. *Child Maltreatment, 17*, 32–46.

Kolko, D. J., Brown, E. J., Shaver, M. E., Baumann, B. L., & Herschell, A. D. (2011, November 1). *Alternatives for families: A cognitive-behavioral therapy: Session guide* (3rd ed.). Pittsburgh, PA: University of Pittsburgh Medical Center.

Kolko, D. J., Campo, J. V., Kelleher, K., & Cheng, Y. (2010). Improving access to care and clinical outcome for pediatric behavioral problems: A randomized trial of a nurse-administered intervention in primary care. *Journal of Behavioral and Developmental Pediatrics, 31*, 393–404.

Kolko, D. J., Campo, J. V., Kilbourne, A., & Kelleher, K. (2012). Doctor-office collaborative care for pediatric behavior problems: A preliminary clinical trial. *Archives of Pediatrics & Adolescent Medicine, 166*, 224–231.

Kolko, D. J., Dorn, L. D., Bukstein, O. G., Pardini, D. A., Holden, E. A., & Hart, J. D. (2009). Community vs. clinic-based modular treatment of children with early-onset ODD or CD: A clinical trial with three-year follow-up. *Journal of Abnormal Child Psychology, 37*, 591–609.

Kolko, D. J., Herschell, A. D., Baumann, B. L., & Shaver, M. E. (2007). *Abuse-focused cognitive-behavioral therapy: Session guide* (2nd ed.). Pittsburgh, PA: University of Pittsburgh School of Medicine.

Kolko, D. J., Iselin, A. M., & Gully, K. (2011). Evaluation of the sustainability and clinical outcome of Alternatives for Families: A Cognitive-Behavioral Therapy (AF-CBT) in a child protection center. *Child Abuse & Neglect, 35*, 105–116.

Kolko, D. J., & Kolko, R. P. (2010). Psychological impact and treatment of child physical abuse. In C. Jenny (Ed.), *Child abuse and neglect: Diagnosis, treatment and evidence* (pp. 476–489). New York: Elsevier.

Kolko, D. J., & Swenson, C. C. (2002). *Assessing and treating physically abused children and their families: A cognitive behavioral approach*. Thousand Oaks, CA: Sage.

Milner, J. S., & Ayoub, C. (1980). Evaluation of "At Risk" parents using the child abuse potential inventory. *Journal of Clinical Psychology, 36*(4), 945–948.

Ondersma, S. J., Chaffin, M., Mullins, S., & LeBreton, J. (2005). The brief child abuse potential inventory: Development and validation. *Journal of Clinical Child and Adolescent Psychology, 34*, 301–311.

Pynoos, R. S., & Em, S. (1986). Witness to violence: The child interview. *Journal of the American Academy of Child Psychiatry, 25*, 306–319.

Runyon, M., & Urquiza, A. J. (2010). Treatment of physically abused children and their families. In J. E. B. Myers, L. Berliner, J. Briere, C. T. Hendrix, C. Jenny, & T. Reid (Eds.), *The APSAC handbook of child maltreatment* (3rd ed.). Thousand Oaks, CA: Sage.

Saunders, B. E., Berliner, L., & Hanson, R. F. (2003). *Child physical and sexual abuse: Guidelines for treatment* (Final report: January 15, 2003). Charleston, SC: National Crime Victims Research and Treatment Center.

Shelton, K. K., Frick, P. J., & Wootton, J. (1996). Assessment of parenting practices in families of elementary school-age children. *Journal of Clinical Child Psychology, 25*(3), 317–329.

Sugaya, L., Hasin, D. S., Olfson, M., Lin, K., Grant, B. F., & Blanco, C. (2012). Child physical abuse and adult mental health: A national Study. *Journal of Traumatic Stress, 25*(4), 384–392.

Part V
Interventions for Adolescents

The developmental neurological research paints a picture of adolescence as a unique developmental period, where the brain transforms into a new dimension of functioning. While adolescents can use reasoning skills as well as adults, when aroused by emotions or the presence of others, their decision-making supports more impulsive and risky behavior. We also know that although emotions are involved in much of adolescents' decision-making, their ability to perceive and understand others' emotions is still developing. Parents' roles appear to continue to play an important role in supporting healthy development for adolescents. We argue that the research findings support the idea that effective interventions should include strategies for managing negative emotions, supporting healthy decision-making and impulse control, and involve parents, helping them to support and monitor their adolescents.

In the following two chapters, we examine very different multi-modal intervention approaches for difficult-to-treat adolescents that similarly combine cognitive-behavioral strategies, family support, case management to reduce their clients' risk of self-destructive behavior: Multisystemic Therapy – Child Abuse and Neglect (MST-CAN), and Dialectical Behavior Therapy (DBT). Swenson and Schaeffer describe MST-CAN in Chap. 12; and Berk and her colleagues present DBT in Chap. 13. We asked the authors to be more exhaustive about their descriptions of their interventions than is typical, laying a strong theoretical groundwork, and adding details about decisions they made about the suitability of their intervention for different aged children, cultural implications, and information about the systematic use of assessment.

Chapter 12
Dialectical Behavior Therapy for Suicidal and Self-Harming Adolescents with Trauma Symptoms

Michele S. Berk, Janine Shelby, Claudia Avina, and Keegan R. Tangeman

Suicide is a significant public health concern for adolescents. In 2010, suicide was the third leading cause of death among 10–14 year-olds and 15–19 year-olds in the United States (Centers for Disease Control and Prevention [CDC], 2013). Recent statistics from the Youth Risk Behavior Survey, a nationally based, yearly survey of high-school students in the United States, showed that 13.8 % had seriously considered attempting suicide in the past year, 10.9 % had made a plan about how they would attempt suicide, and 6.3 % had attempted suicide one or more times (Eaton et al., 2010). Suicides are less common in young children and it has been speculated that suicide rates increase in adolescence due to the emergence of psychiatric disorders that increase the risk of suicide during this phase of development (Gould, Greenberg, Velting, & Shaffer, 2003; Shaffer, Gould, Fisher, & Trautman, 1996). Risk factors for suicide in adolescence are similar to those in adulthood and include severe psychopathology (e.g., depressive disorders, substance abuse, disruptive behavior disorders, and Borderline Personality Disorder), a family history of

M.S. Berk, Ph.D. (✉)
Harbor-UCLA Medical Center, Torrance, CA, USA

Los Angeles Biomedical Research Institute, Torrance, CA, USA

David Geffen School of Medicine, University of California, Los Angeles, CA, USA
e-mail: mberk@labiomed.org

J. Shelby, Ph.D.
Harbor-UCLA Medical Center, Torrance, CA, USA

David Geffen School of Medicine, University of California, Los Angeles, CA, USA
e-mail: jshelby@dmh.lacounty.gov

C. Avina, Ph.D. • K.R. Tangeman, Psy.D.
Harbor-UCLA Medical Center, Torrance, CA, USA

Los Angeles Biomedical Research Institute, Torrance, CA, USA
e-mail: cavina@labiomed.org; ktangeman@labiomed.org

S. Timmer and A. Urquiza (eds.), *Evidence-Based Approaches for the Treatment of Maltreated Children*, Child Maltreatment 3, DOI 10.1007/978-94-007-7404-9_12,
© Springer Science+Business Media Dordrecht 2014

suicide, and access to lethal means (Brent et al., 1994; Lewinsohn, Rohde, & Seeley, 1993; Shaffer et al., 1996). A history of prior suicide attempts is one of the strongest predictors of subsequent suicide attempts and suicide deaths in both adolescents and adults (e.g., Harris & Barraclough, 1997; Lewinsohn, Rohde, & Seely, 1994; Shaffer et al. 1996). Nonfatal suicidal behaviors (e.g., suicide attempts) are also a problem in their own right, with approximately 100–200 attempts for every completed suicide among youth ages 15–24 (Goldsmith, Pellmar, Kleinman, & Bunney, 2002). It is clear that adolescent suicide attempters constitute a high risk population in need of intensive suicide prevention efforts.

Youth who have experienced child maltreatment are also at increased risk for self-harm and suicidal behaviors. There is a great deal of support for the association between childhood sexual abuse and suicidal behaviors (Briere & Runtz, 1987; Briere & Zaidi, 1989; Lanktree, Briere, & Zaidi, 1991; Saunders, Villeponteaux, Lipovsky, & Kilpatrick, 1992) and some evidence for the link between childhood physical abuse and suicidality (Riggs, Alario, & McHorney, 1990). Unfortunately, the association between child abuse victimization and suicidality can persist into the long term. For example, a community sample of abused children showed increased suicidal ideation and suicide attempts compared to nonabused youth in a 17-year longitudinal study (Silverman, Reinherz, & Giaconia, 1996).

Given that suicidal and self-harm behaviors and trauma-related symptoms frequently co-occur, there is a need for treatments that target both problems. Across both child and adult treatments for PTSD symptoms, exposure and the emotional processing that occurs during exposure are considered to be the key components leading to symptom reduction (Cohen, Mannarino, & Deblinger, 2006; Foa & Rothbaum, 1998; Ford & Cloitre, 2009). In most trauma treatment protocols, cognitive-behavioral coping skills are taught for both symptom management and to make the exposure more palatable (i.e., to help the youth to tolerate the exposure tasks). Treatments for child and adolescent trauma have tended to exclude or delay the treatment of suicidal youth, given that the strong negative thoughts and feelings evoked during exposure tasks may subsequently increase suicide risk (Ford & Cloitre, 2009). In fact, recent practice guidelines from the International Society for Traumatic Stress Studies (ISTSS) recommend that exposure-based treatment be delayed until the individual is no longer suicidal (Foa, Keane, Friedman, & Cohen, 2009).

While this approach to treatment makes intuitive sense in terms of safety, trauma symptoms are often intertwined with suicidal behavior (e.g., nightmares or intrusive memories may precipitate suicidal and self-harm behaviors), which makes it difficult to adequately treat one condition without also addressing the other. Moreover, allowing traumatized youth to endure acute and uncomfortable trauma-related symptoms for extended periods of time may increase suicidal thoughts and feelings. At present, there are a small number of treatments available for adolescents with both trauma symptoms and suicidal/self-harm behaviors. These treatments (e.g., Structured Psychotherapy for Adolescents Responding to Chronic Stress [SPARCS], DeRosa & Pelcovitz, 2008, TARGET, Ford & Russo, 2006; Life Skills/Life Story, Cloitre, Cohen, & Koenen, 2006; and Seeking Safety, Najavits,

2006) emphasize the development of coping skills but do not include a formal exposure component.

It is also the case that relatively little empirical research has been conducted on the treatment of adolescent suicidal and self-injurious behavior in general. At present, there are no treatments that have been proven effective in randomized trials at preventing suicide attempts by teens. Fewer than 10 randomized trials have been conducted to date, and among those trials, only two yielded significant effects showing an impact on decreasing suicidal behavior (Huey et al., 2004; Wood, Trainor, Rothwell, Moore, & Harrington, 2001). Neither of these studies has been replicated.

The adult literature on the treatment of suicidal behavior has yielded better results. In particular, Dialectical Behavior Therapy (DBT; Linehan, 1993) has been shown to decrease suicidal and self-harm behaviors in multiple randomized, clinical trials with adults with Borderline Personality Disorder (BPD; e.g., Linehan, Armstrong, Suarez, & Allmon, 1991; Linehan et al., 2006; Linehan, Heard, & Armstrong, 1993). BPD is a severe and debilitating psychiatric disorder that is characterized by repetitive suicidal and self-harm behaviors, as well as extreme mood lability and disturbed interpersonal relationships. BPD is associated with high rates of completed suicide (American Psychiatric Association, 2001). As documented in the most recent version of the *Diagnostic and Statistical Manual for Mental Disorders*, it is the only disorder other than major depression to include suicidal behavior as one of its diagnostic criteria (4th ed., text rev.; *DSM–IV–TR*; American Psychiatric Association [APA], 2000). It has been found that patients with BPD, including those with comorbid major depression, reported greater lethality for their most serious lifetime suicide attempt than those with depression alone (Soloff, Lynch, Kelly, Malone, & Mann, 2000). Although estimates vary across studies, BPD is strongly associated with a history of childhood sexual abuse, as well as other forms of child abuse and neglect (e.g., Soloff, Lynch, & Kelly, 2002; Zanarini et al., 1997), and symptoms overlap with depictions of complex trauma (see Resick et al., 2012). Accordingly, DBT targets both PTSD symptoms and suicidal and self-harm behaviors (Linehan, 1993; see also Harned, Korslund, Foa, & Linehan, 2012), given that these symptoms are frequently comorbid in this patient population.

As noted above, because of the lack of empirically-supported treatments for adolescent suicide attempters and the strong support for the effectiveness of DBT with suicidal adults, a logical next step in the field is to determine if DBT is an effective treatment for suicidal adolescents. In doing so, it makes sense to consider if a treatment targeting BPD is appropriate to use with adolescents. Clinicians are often reluctant to diagnose adolescents with Axis II disorders, given that their personality traits may still be in the process of development. However, recent research supports the position that BPD can be diagnosed in adolescence with reliability and validity, and that the disorder may persist into adulthood for a subset of these youth with more severe symptoms (for a review, see Miller, Muehlenkamp, & Jacobson, 2008). Because treatments for Axis I and Axis II disorders associated with suicidal and self-harm behaviors may differ, accurate diagnosis is essential in providing effective treatment (Miller et al., 2007). Apart from diagnostic issues, adolescents who engage in suicidal and/or self-harm behaviors frequently display difficulty with affect regulation and impulsivity, which are core features of BPD (Miller, Rathus, & Linehan, 2007). In fact, DBT was initially developed to treat suicidal and self-harming behaviors and only later developed into a treatment targeting BPD, due to the considerable overlap between the two (Miller et al., 2007). In sum, the use of DBT with adolescents appears warranted. In the remainder of this chapter, we will review the DBT approach and its application to suicidal, traumatized adolescents, and provide a case study.

Theory Underlying DBT

The DBT approach is based on Linehan's (1993) biosocial theory. In the theory, persistent and severe difficulty regulating emotions (i.e., "emotion dysregulation") is seen as the primary dysfunction contributing to suicidal and self-harm behaviors, as well as other features of Borderline Personality Disorder. Difficulty regulating emotion is thought to develop in childhood based on the transaction between: (a) a biological predisposition to emotional vulnerability on the part of the child, and (b) an invalidating environment. The model is transactional in that both factors need to be present beginning early in development for pervasive emotional dysregulation to develop.

According to the theory, emotional vulnerability is described as biologically-based and present from birth. It is characterized by the child's heightened sensitivity to emotional stimuli (e.g., a low threshold for an emotional reaction to an event), increased emotional intensity (e.g., emotions are experienced as stronger and more intense than in an individual without this vulnerability), and a slow return to emotional baseline (e.g., emotional states dissipate slowly, leaving the individual vulnerable to additional triggering of negative emotions). The invalidating environment is defined as one in which communication of emotion is met with caregiver responses that are inconsistent, inappropriate to the emotion expressed, and/or trivializing of the emotional experience. As a result, "the child does not learn how to adequately label or control emotional reactions" (Linehan, 1993, p. 51). An invalidating environment is seen as particularly problematic early in development because young children rely heavily on caregivers to regulate their emotions and help them alleviate distress (Calkins & Hill, 2007). Hence, it is proposed that repeated, unsuccessful child-caregiver transactions may lead to deficits in the child's emotion regulation skills, which persist into adulthood (Crowell, Beauchaine, & Linehan, 2009). Consequently, suicide attempts and non-suicidal self-injurious behaviors are developed as means to manage severe emotion dysregulation in the absence of more constructive coping strategies. For example, individuals with BPD or BPD traits frequently experience intensely painful negative mood states (e.g., depression, anger, anxiety, guilt, or shame), which can feel unbearable and/or intolerable. At the same time, they have not developed adequate coping skills to alleviate this pain and resort to self-harm and/or suicidal behavior as a means of terminating, avoiding, and/or escaping from these negative emotional experiences. In the model, sexual abuse is considered to be one of the most extreme forms of invalidation in which the individual's power, agency, and emotional experience are negated. Hence, sexual abuse is seen as a risk factor for the development of self-harm behaviors and BPD.

Overview of the DBT Approach

Based on the biosocial theory described above, DBT focuses on eliminating self-injurious behaviors by teaching more adaptive coping skills to decrease emotion dysregulation. DBT is a principle-based treatment and incorporates a range of behavioral strategies, as well as practices derived from philosophy and Eastern religion (e.g., mindfulness, radical acceptance, and dialectics), aimed at teaching clients emotion regulation skills.

DBT begins with a "pre-treatment" stage, in which the client is oriented to the treatment and asked to commit to working on eliminating suicidal/self-harm behaviors and to participating in all components of the treatment for a specified period of time. DBT focuses on commitment at the outset of treatment in order to increase the likelihood that the client is motivated to work toward treatment goals and to decrease premature termination. Given the life-threatening nature of the behaviors targeted by DBT, obtaining commitment to decrease these behaviors is critical. Stage 1 of treatment typically lasts 1 year and focuses on stabilization of the client, and in particular, on eliminating suicidal and self-harm behaviors and other potentially dangerous behaviors (e.g., substance use, delinquent/criminal behaviors, high risk sexual behavior), as well as reducing symptoms of acute, comorbid Axis I disorders, such substance abuse, eating-disordered behaviors, mood disorders, anxiety disorders, and PTSD symptoms. Research on DBT has focused on Stage 1 treatment, which is the only stage that has been formally outlined and tested in randomized clinical trials. Adolescent adaptations of DBT have shortened the length of Stage 1 treatment, ranging from 12 weeks (Rathus & Miller, 2002) to 6 months (Goldstein, Axelson, Birmaher, & Brent, 2007), in order to increase adolescents' willingness to commit to a course of treatment. However, additional research is needed to determine the optimal treatment length for adolescents. Stage 2 of treatment focuses on decreasing PTSD and trauma symptoms (when applicable) as well as other Axis I conditions; and subsequent phases focus on increasing self-respect, continuing to pursue individual goals, and self-actualization. The length of the later stages of treatment is not pre-determined and is based on the client's needs.

Although the stages of treatment were designed to be completed in chronological order, it is often the case that earlier stages need to be re-visited or that topics related to later stages need to be addressed sooner in the treatment. For example, exposure-based treatment generally is not implemented until suicidal and self-injurious behaviors have ceased for a period of time and the client has sufficient coping skills to tolerate the distress commonly associated with exposure to traumatic material. However, in a case of a client with severe trauma symptoms where the client becomes suicidal while completing trauma-focused treatment in Stage 2, the therapist may stop and return to Stage 1 interventions to stabilize him or her prior to resuming trauma work. Alternatively, if trauma symptoms (e.g., nightmares, flashbacks, or other intrusive experiences) are a frequent trigger for suicidal/self-harm behaviors, then the therapist may need to target them in Stage 1 using DBT coping skills in order to sufficiently reduce suicidal behaviors.

DBT is comprised of four mandatory modes including individual therapy, group skills training, telephone-based skills coaching between sessions, and a weekly consultation team meeting for therapists. For adolescents, family sessions are also conducted as needed and group skills training is conducted in a multi-family format (Miller et al., 2007). The client is considered to have dropped out of treatment if he or she misses 4 sessions in a row of either individual or group therapy.

Because clients with suicidal and self-harm behaviors and/or BPD symptoms often present in therapy with multiple crises and problems that can make therapy sessions chaotic and derail progress, DBT follows a hierarchy of behavioral treatment targets to set the agenda for the session. Life-threatening behaviors are always targeted first, therapy-interfering behaviors are targeted second, and quality of life interfering behaviors are targeted third. Life-threatening behaviors include suicide attempts, non-suicidal self-injury, and suicidal ideation, as well as another other behaviors that are potentially life-threatening (e.g., potentially life-threatening use of drugs and alcohol, severe symptoms of an eating disorder, high risk sexual behaviors). Therapy-interfering behaviors include all behaviors on the part of both the client and the therapist that impede treatment (e.g., not completing therapy homework, coming late to sessions, negative feelings about the therapist or client). Finally, quality of life interfering behaviors include all other problems that decrease the client's quality of life (e.g., comorbid Axis I conditions, interpersonal problems, family conflict, school/work problems). Clients complete a weekly "diary card," which is a daily self-monitoring form on which they rate their urges to engage in suicidal and self-harm behaviors, use substances, and to quit therapy, as well as their level of emotional misery and use of DBT skills. The diary card is reviewed at the beginning of the session and used to structure the session according to the hierarchy of treatment targets.

Individual therapy sessions utilize a range of cognitive-behavioral interventions to address treatment targets and improve emotion regulation abilities. DBT is a behaviorally based therapy, and hence, contingency management is a central intervention. The therapist conducts a detailed behavioral analysis of each episode of self-injurious behavior that occurs during treatment in order to determine which coping skills are needed to prevent the behavior from occurring in the future as well as the triggers and reinforcers of the behavior. The therapist is careful to avoid inadvertently reinforcing suicidal/self-harm behaviors and other dysfunctional behaviors in his or her behavior toward the client. With adolescents, the therapist also works with family members to ensure that they are not reinforcing the adolescent's problem behaviors and that positive behaviors are being rewarded (Miller et al., 2007). For example, if a parent increases nurturing and validation following a suicide attempt, and the youth finds these things rewarding, the therapist would work with the parent to instead keep his or her affect and behavior neutral following self-harm behaviors (i.e., the use of extinction) and to increase positive responses following adaptive behaviors (i.e., provide reinforcement for positive versus negative behaviors).

Another hallmark of DBT is that the therapist takes a dialectical approach to working with the client and promotes the notion that opposite viewpoints may exist (i.e., both between self and another person and conflicting viewpoints about oneself), helping the client to reach a synthesis of viewpoints. The central dialectic in DBT is acceptance and change. The therapist accepts and validates the client's thoughts, feelings, and behaviors, while at the same time, working for change in these areas. For example, the therapist may convey understanding that the client engaged in self-harm behavior because he or she was experiencing unbearable emotional pain and desperately wanted to stop that pain. At the same time, the therapist also conveys that self-harm was not an effective way to manage feelings and that new coping skills must be learned. Stylistically, the therapist may also use irreverent responses, as well as stories, analogies, and metaphors, in order to communicate information to the client in novel, unexpected ways, which increase the likelihood of his or her paying attention to what the therapist is saying (Linehan, 1993).

Including validation as well as change-focused interventions is seen as an essential component of DBT. Validation differs from agreement in that validation communicates that one understands the other person's perspective, whereas agreement indicates that one approves of the other's thoughts, feelings, or behaviors (Linehan, 1993). Given the hypothesized connection between invalidation in childhood and later self-harm behaviors, clients may experience the therapist's attempts to change their behaviors as extremely invalidating, which can lead to ruptures in the therapeutic relationship and premature treatment termination (Linehan, 1993). Hence, validation typically precedes change-based interventions. An overall goal of the DBT therapist is to assist the client in "building a life worth living" as an antidote to suicidal behavior.

In addition to a weekly individual therapy session, adolescents also participate in a multi-family skills training group. In the DBT approach, therapists teach skills in the group sessions in order to maximize the amount of time devoted to therapeutic work during the individual therapy time. The group is run in a didactic format, in which adolescents and parents are taught a new skill each week and complete homework on that skill. The individual therapist then works with the client to select which skills are relevant to their particular difficulties, to engage in in-depth practice of skills, and trouble-shoot his or her difficulties using skills. DBT includes four domains of skills, including mindfulness skills, interpersonal effectiveness skills, distress tolerance skills, and emotion regulation skills (Linehan, 1993).

Mindfulness skills are used to help clients increase attention, awareness, and acceptance of emotional responses, which may decrease impulsively acting upon emotions in a destructive manner. Mindfulness practice typically involves focusing one's attention on a particular task or body sensation for a brief period of time, while training the mind to continually return to the point of focus when distractions occur. With adolescents, concrete, engaging tasks are typically used (Miller et al., 2007), such as mindful eating or playing a game requiring concentration (e.g., "last-letter/ first letter", in which the teen must say a word that begins with the last letter of the word said by the prior teen). The interpersonal effectiveness module teaches clients adaptive ways to communicate their needs to others and cope with interpersonal problems that lead to strong negative emotions. For example, clients are taught social skills and assertiveness skills, as well as how to prioritize their goals in a given inter- action (e.g., to get what they want, to maintain a relationship, or to maintain their self-respect) and behave accordingly. Distress tolerance skills are taught to help cli- ents tolerate crises and intense negative emotions in the short term without engaging in self-harm or other destructive behaviors. These skills include multiple methods of distraction (e.g., counting backwards from 100, going for a walk, watching a funny movie), as well as self-soothing using each of the five senses (e.g., listening to music, looking at a pleasing photograph, eating a favorite food, smelling scented candles or other favorite scents, and feeling something soft and soothing, such as petting their cat). Finally, the emotion regulation module teaches ways to decrease emotion dys- regulation in the long term by reducing vulnerabilities (e.g., attending to physical illnesses, proper nutrition, adequate sleep), teaching clients how to identify and label emotions, and increasing behaviors likely to elicit positive affect and decrease nega- tive affect (e.g., pleasant activity scheduling, exposure, problem-solving).

Additional skills training on dialectics, validation, and behaviorism/contingency management and how they can be applied to the parent-child relationship has also been recommended for use with adolescents and families (i.e., "Middle Path" skills; Miller et al., 2007). For instance, the concept of dialectics is applied to parent-teen conflict by encouraging the parents and teens to recognize the "truth" in the others' viewpoints and to seek resolutions that honor both perspectives. For example, a parent and teen may be in conflict about the teen's curfew and, upon discussion, the parent's primary concern may be about safety, whereas the teen's may be that miss- ing certain social events that occur late at night will make it hard for him or her to be "popular." In this case, the parent and teen would be coached to practice acknowl- edging the validity of both viewpoints and to brainstorm solutions that address both concerns, such as allowing the teen to attend some events later in the evening if they occur in another teen's home where there is parental supervision, or to maintain an early curfew, but to allow the teen to attend additional after school activities that increase access to desired peers.

As described earlier, it is hypothesized that invalidation plays a key role in the development of severe emotion dysregulation and therefore reducing invalida- tion in the teen's environment is a critical component of the treatment. The parent is coached to validate the teen by communicating that his or her feelings, thoughts, and actions make sense given the current situation or past experiences, even if the parent does not "agree" with the feelings or associated behaviors. In the same manner, the teen is also encouraged to validate his or her parent. Finally, as DBT is a behavioral treatment approach, parents and teens are taught standard principles of contingency management (e.g., positive reinforcement, extinction) as a means of increasing desired behaviors in each other and decreasing negative behaviors.

Additional modes of treatment include telephone coaching and the consultation team for therapists. In standard DBT, the therapist is continually available to the client for skills coaching by telephone. Clients are instructed to call their therapists when they are experiencing a crisis so that the therapists can assist them implement DBT skills instead of self-harm or other destructive behaviors. Phone coaching is considered to be essential for generalizing the skills learned in therapy to real life problems. In order to ensure that phone contacts with the therapist are not reinforcing suicidal/self-harm behaviors, a "24-hour rule" is used in which the client is not allowed to call the therapist after he or she has engaged in self-harm behaviors (unless the behavior is life-threatening, in which case the therapist initiates needed emergency services). Use of the 24-hour rule prevents the development of an association between increased therapist contact and self-harm behavior. Instead, the client is encouraged to call the therapist before engaging in self-harm, when skills coaching is still applicable and the client has not already "solved the problem" by using self-harm. Further research is needed to determine if the 24-hour rule is appropriate for adolescents and more flexibility may be needed (Miller et al., 2007). In DBT with adolescents, the parent is also offered telephone coaching by the multi-family skills group leader (Miller et al., 2007).

Finally, therapists delivering DBT to clients are required to take part in a weekly consultation team meeting. In this meeting, therapists provide support and guidance to each other using the principles of DBT (e.g., validation, contingency management, problem solving), in order to manage the stress of working with highly suicidal clients and to maintain treatment fidelity.

Research on DBT with Adolescents

As noted above, DBT has been adapted for use with suicidal and self-harming adolescents (Miller et al., 2007). Initial research has yielded promising results. In one quasi-experimental trial, 111 adolescents were assigned to either DBT or treatment as usual (TAU) based on the degree of fit with the DBT approach. Adolescents with a history of a suicide attempt within the past 16 weeks or current suicidal ideation and at least three BPD features were assigned to DBT. Adolescents meeting either the suicidality or the BPD criteria, but not both, were assigned to TAU. The treatment was modified from the adult version to be more developmentally appropriate using the following adaptations: shortening the length of treatment; including parents in family sessions, collateral sessions, and telephone coaching; including additional emphasis on dialectics, validation, and contingency management; simplifying the language and materials from the adult versions; and using examples relevant to adolescents when teaching DBT skills. Although the overall number of suicide attempts in this study was too small to permit meaningful between-group comparisons, results indicated that adolescents who received DBT-A showed a significant pre- to post-treatment decrease in suicidal ideation, as well as significantly fewer hospitalizations than those youth receiving treatment as usual (Rathus & Miller, 2002).

Additional small studies of DBT with suicidal adolescents have been conducted with some encouraging results. Katz and colleagues (Katz, Cox, Gunasekara, & Miller, 2004) conducted a quasi-experimental trial comparing a 2-week long adaptation of adolescent DBT to treatment as usual with a sample of adolescent inpatients. Although the DBT group had fewer behavioral problems while on the ward, no differences in suicide attempts were found between the two groups at 1-year follow-up. Woodberry and Popenoe (2008) conducted a small open trial using Miller and colleagues' model with suicidal adolescents in an outpatient clinic. Pre- to post-treatment comparisons showed significant decreases in suicidal ideation and psychopathology. Adaptations of DBT for bipolar adolescents (Goldstein et al., 2007) and adolescents with Oppositional Defiant Disorder (Nelson-Gray et al., 2006) have also been tested in small open trials, with positive results regarding feasibility and decreases in psychopathology. Taken together, these results suggest that DBT is a promising treatment for suicidal adolescents. A randomized trial is needed to definitively determine the effectiveness of DBT with adolescents.

DBT Approach to Treating PTSD/Trauma

DBT includes general guidelines for addressing PTSD/trauma symptoms. In Stage 1 DBT, trauma symptoms are targeted via the application of DBT skills as they occur in relation to life-threatening behavior, therapy-interfering behavior, and quality of life interfering behaviors. Exposure treatments are not recommended until the patient is stable and non-suicidal, and has mastered the coping skills needed to tolerate the strong negative affect associated with exposure to traumatic material. However, given that clients may experience a great deal of suffering due to PTSD symptoms, and that these symptoms may also be related to suicidal and self-harm behaviors, postponing exposure-based treatment is also problematic.

Recent work with adults has focused on developing and testing a protocol for delivering exposure treatment to Stage 1 DBT clients who are experiencing PTSD symptoms (Harned et al., 2012; Harned & Linehan, 2008). DBT supports the use of evidence-based ancillary treatments (when available) to target specific problems (Linehan, 1993). In particular, a DBT Prolonged Exposure (DBT PE) protocol was created for use in Stage 1 DBT. Prolonged Exposure was chosen because it has the largest evidence-base for PTSD treatments with adults (Powers, Halpern, Ferenschak, Gillihan, & Foa, 2010). In order to maximize safety, the following criteria were required for the client to begin the DBT PE protocol: (1) no risk of imminent suicide, (2) no suicidal or self-harm behavior for the past 2 months, (3) ability to control life-threatening behaviors when in the presence of triggers of these behaviors, (4) no serious therapy interfering behaviors, (5) PTSD is the highest priority quality of life target for the patient, and (6) ability to experience strong emotions without engaging in maladaptive behaviors (Harned et al.). The protocol was designed to be implemented concurrently with Stage 1 DBT, by the DBT therapist, either in a combined individual therapy session or a second individual session per week.

In order to address the needs of DBT clients, the DBT PE protocol was modified from standard PE in several ways, including: obtaining commitment to participate in PE, obtaining commitment to not engaging in self-harm or suicidal behaviors during PE, conducting pre and post-session (as well as before and after each exposure task within the session) assessments of suicidal and self-harm urges, creating a safety plan of DBT skills to be used if suicidal/self-harm urges occur during PE, and progressing more slowly and gradually with exposure tasks (Harned & Linehan, 2008). Several aspects of the exposure protocol were modified. For instance, in-vivo exposure tasks (i.e., approaching excessively or inappropriately avoided stimuli associated with the traumatic event) were first conducted in the presence of the therapist rather than as a homework assignment. Imaginal exposure (i.e., detailed discussion of the traumatic event), which is typically conducted in the third PE session, was delayed until the client had successfully managed items at lower levels of the fear hierarchy (i.e., had successfully completed exposure to stimuli associated with lower levels of anxiety prior to those likely to induce greater anxiety). These decisions to modify the protocol were based upon clients' reports that directly talking about and remembering the traumatic event were the most distressing tasks on the exposure hierarchy (Harned & Linehan). If life-threatening or therapy-interfering behaviors re-emerged during implementation of the DBT PE protocol, the trauma treatment was temporarily suspended in order for these higher priority targets to be addressed.

Results of a small open trial of DBT plus the DBT PE protocol with adult women with BPD, PTSD, and recent suicidal/self-harm behavior showed that the approach is feasible, acceptable to clients, and can be delivered safely (Harned et al., 2012). Dropout rates from the DBT PE protocol were low and clients reported high treatment satisfaction. The average intensity of pre- and post-session urges to engage in suicidal/self-harm behavior did not differ between DBT and DBT PE sessions and suicidal/self-harm urges were more likely to decrease pre- to post-session in DBT PE versus DBT sessions. In contrast to earlier work showing that the rate of PTSD remission in Stage 1 DBT was low (i.e., approximately 35 %; Harned et al., 2008), use of DBT plus the DBT PE protocol led to a remission rate of 71.4 % for those who completed the protocol and 60 % in the intent-to-treat sample (Harned et al., 2012). Clients who received the DBT PE protocol also reported significant pre- to post-treatment decreases in dissociation, trauma-related guilt cognitions, shame, anxiety, depression and global adjustment (Harned et al., 2012). As clients reported being highly motivated to obtain relief from trauma symptoms, the authors speculated that the low incidence of suicidal/self-harm urges and behaviors seen in the DBT PE protocol may have been because clients had to agree to stop these behaviors in order to receive DBT PE.

DBT and Trauma-Focused Treatment with Adolescents

At present, an adolescent-specific protocol for conducting exposure-based treatment in Stage 1 DBT has not been delineated; and research in this area is urgently needed. Because it is common when treating children and adolescents to involve the parent/family in the treatment, and parents have been included in evidence-based treatments for child trauma (e.g., Cohen, Mannarino, Berliner, & Deblinger, 2000), it would make sense for any trauma protocol conducted as part of DBT with adolescents to also include the caregiver. In addition, at the outset of treatment with an adolescent who has experienced child abuse, the physical safety of the youth's current environment should be addressed, to ensure that he or she is not currently at risk for further victimization. More work is needed to determine the most appropriate and effective point to offer DBT exposure-based interventions to adolescents and whether or not they should be conducted concurrently, as in the DBT PE protocol, or sequentially when Stage 1 is completed. On average, adult clients receiving the DBT PE protocol met criteria to begin the protocol at week 18.5 of Stage 1 DBT treatment (e.g., in months 4 to 5 of a year long program; Harned et al., 2012). As adolescent DBT programs are typically shorter in length (i.e., 12 weeks to 6 months), the question of whether or not to conduct exposure treatment during or after Stage 1 may not be relevant, as adolescents are likely to be at or near completion of Stage 1 at the point when the adult clients met criteria for beginning exposure.

In our DBT program, we have treated traumatized, suicidal adolescents using the standard DBT protocol. That is, we completed Stage 1 treatment (which in our clinic is 6-months long), in which the client was stabilized and suicidal/self-harm behaviors were eliminated, and then offered an evidence-based exposure protocol, using the procedures delineated in Trauma-Focused CBT (TF-CBT, Cohen et al., 2006; see Chap. 9 of this book). Because TF-CBT (Cohen et al.) has received the most empirical attention and support among child trauma treatments, it is a counterpart to PE with adults and appeared to be the most appropriate approach to use with adolescents. TF-CBT contains multiple components including: psychoeducation; relaxation; affect regulation; cognitive coping; construction of a trauma narrative (i.e., imaginal exposure) and cognitive restructuring; in vivo exposure; and enhancement of future safety. Throughout the treatment, the non-offending caregiver participates in collateral sessions that focus on enhancing parenting skills, participating in conjoint therapy session(s) in which the caregiver hears the adolescent's trauma narrative, and learning the same coping and psychoeducational information as the youth (Cohen et al., 2006).

Because many of the cognitive-behavioral coping skills taught in TF-CBT overlap with those taught in Stage 1 DBT, as will be detailed below, we used only the components of TF-CBT that were not already covered. If needed, trauma-specific coping skills not included in DBT (e.g., grounding techniques, nightmare and other intrusive re-experiencing management strategies) were taught during Stage 1. In this case, these skills were reviewed again as needed during the trauma-focused portion of the treatment. The exposure protocol was conducted using standard TF-CBT procedures. More specifically, adolescents were led through graduated exposure in various formats such as drawing, story-writing, or simply recounting the narrative of the traumatic event. During the exposure protocol, both DBT and trauma-specific coping interventions were used, along with subjective units of distress and cognitive reprocessing interventions, as outlined in the TF-CBT protocol. Finally, the completed trauma narrative was shared with the parent. Throughout the treatment, the therapist (who was typically the same therapist who provided the DBT) regularly assessed suicidality and self-harm urges using the weekly DBT diary card and stopped the trauma work and returned to DBT interventions if the client displayed an increased risk of self-harm. A case study illustrating our approach is provided below.

Case Study

"Anna" was a 16 year-old Caucasian female who presented to our outpatient clinic after making a suicide attempt 1 month earlier, after which she had been hospitalized for 1 week. She also reported a history of non-suicidal self-injury behaviors in which she cut herself on her arms, stomach, and legs approximately three times per month for the past year. Anna had been sexually abused on multiple occasions by her god-father when she was 12-years old. Following the abuse, she developed symptoms consistent with PTSD including intrusive re-experiencing of thoughts and memories about the abuse, feeling disconnected and detached from friends, significantly decreased in interest in activities such as dance and school clubs, and anger outbursts that had resulted in disciplinary actions at school. Anna had a history of poor school performance and had failed several classes. She also had a history of troubled relationships with peers. She also reported conflict with her mother and stated that they engaged in verbal arguments approximately twice a week. Her parents were aware of Anna's allegations of sexual abuse, but continued to allow her godfather to visit their home occasionally, and admitted they were not sure Anna was telling the truth as she often "manipulates" them. The abuse had been reported to local child protection services and law enforcement, but there had not been enough evidence to prosecute her godfather and the allegations were determined to be unsubstantiated.

Based on this information obtained at intake, Anna was referred to our adolescent DBT program. In order to determine if DBT was in fact the most appropriate form of treatment for her, a detailed history of her past suicide attempts and self-harm behaviors was obtained and she was administered the Borderline Personality Disorder Section of the Structured Clinical Interview for DSM IV Axis II Personality Disorders (SCID-II; First, Gibbon, Spitzer, Williams, & Benjamin, 1997). As noted above, Anna reported a history of one lifetime suicide attempt and having engaged in non-suicidal self-injury approximately 36 times in the past year. Anna also met criteria for a diagnosis of BPD, due to endorsing five of the nine criteria for the disorder, including difficulties in interpersonal relationships, impulsivity, recurrent suicidal or self-harm behaviors, affective instability, difficulty controlling anger, and dissociation. Based on this information, DBT appeared to be an appropriate treatment approach for Anna and she was assigned to a therapist in our DBT program in order to begin the pre-treatment process.

Pre-treatment Sessions

At her first DBT session, Anna presented as irritable and defiant. She stated, "I don't like therapy and I am only here because my mother made me come." She reported being seen by two different therapists in the past and felt neither had been helpful. The first four pre-treatment sessions focused on obtaining Anna's commitment to stop engaging in suicidal and self-harm behavior and to participating in 6 months of DBT, including individual therapy, multifamily group therapy, and telephone coaching. Anna's parents were also asked to commit to participating in the weekly multifamily skills group and in collateral and family sessions as needed. Although the focus was on individual therapy with Anna, the therapist included both parents for portions of the initial sessions as described below.

Anna stated that she wanted to stop engaging in self-harm and to not attempt suicide again, as she did not like having scars and did not want to return to the hospital. The therapist asked Anna to commit to using DBT skills instead of self-harm and/or suicidal behaviors for the next 6 months of treatment. In order to ensure the strength of Anna's commitment to stopping self-harm, the therapist engaged in her in a detailed discussion of the pros and cons of giving up self-harm. The therapist also used the "devil's advocate" technique to strengthen Anna's commitment by pointing out potential roadblocks (e.g., "It's going to be really hard to stop something that you are so used to doing. Can you really do this?") and asking Anna to describe how she would handle them. The therapist addressed Anna's resistance to taking part in therapy by having her describe difficulties in her life and illustrating specifically how the DBT approach would address each of these issues. Anna agreed that she wanted to "build a life worth living," as long as this was defined by her and not by her parents. In order to decrease future therapy-interfering behaviors (on the part of both Anna and the therapist), the therapist also addressed Anna's negative prior experiences in therapy and asked Anna to immediately notify her she was experiencing difficulty with the current therapy or with the therapist.

In the first session, the therapist gathered information about Anna's most recent suicide attempt to better assess her current safety and identify key treatment targets needed to prevent future self-harm behaviors. The therapist conducted a chain analysis, in which she obtained a detailed description from the client of the pre-existing vulnerability factors, proximal triggers, thoughts, and emotions that occurred prior to engaging in suicidal behavior, as well as potential reinforcers that occurred after the behavior. In Anna's case, her suicide attempt was triggered by a nightmare about being abused. She awoke in the middle of the night experiencing intense fear and had the thought, "I can't tolerate the pain." She also indicated that she thought her emotional distress would "last forever," and that killing herself was the only way to stop the pain. This information was used to develop a safety plan of skills Anna could use to avoid attempting suicide in the future. For example, the therapist taught Anna the "crisis survival" skills from the Distress Tolerance module (e.g., distraction, self-soothing), which she could use to tolerate episodes of severe emotion dysregulation without attempting suicide.

The therapist included Anna's parents in the first session, oriented them to the DBT approach, and discussed the biosocial theory by explaining that the transaction between a biological predisposition to experiencing intense emotions and an invalidating environment (especially one that includes abuse) underlies problems with emotion dysregulation and self-harm behaviors. This provided Anna and her parents with an explanation for her behaviors that was non-judgmental and helped to decrease their criticism of her and belief that she was "manipulative," underscoring the importance of validation. Given Anna's history of sexual abuse by her godfather, the therapist also spoke with Anna and her parents about insuring her physical safety and preventing an increase in PTSD symptoms by not allowing him to have any contact with her. The therapist also instructed Anna and her parents to remove any lethal means or implements that could be used for self-harm from their home and from Anna's belongings, in order to decrease her ability to impulsively harm herself. At the end of the pre-treatment sessions, the therapist introduced the diary card to Anna and had her complete it weekly as homework, as is standard in DBT, enabling the therapist to monitor her suicidal thoughts and behaviors, self-harm urges and behaviors, emotional misery, and skill use between sessions. A sample of the diary card that we use in our clinical program is provided in Fig. 12.1. The reader is referred to Linehan (1993) and Miller et al. (2007), for published examples of DBT diary cards.

Stage 1 DBT Treatment

During the first 2 months of treatment, Anna reported on her diary card having engaged in self-harm and suicidal ideation following intrusive thoughts about the abuse or arguments with her mother. Accordingly, the initial phase of treatment focused primarily on teaching Anna distress tolerance skills, with the goal of decreasing the chances she would harm herself. Each time Anna engaged in self-harm behavior, the therapist conducted a chain analysis of that behavior, to better understand its triggers and functions. In a chain analysis conducted in her second month of treatment, it became clear that Anna's mother negatively reinforced her self-harm behaviors, as her mother ceased arguing with her and became nurturing after Anna cut herself. The therapist worked with Anna and her mother to remove this reinforcer by having them engage in planned pleasant activities together in which her mother could be nurturing (e.g., taking Anna shopping for clothing) prior to Anna engaging in self-harm and by agreeing that immediately following a cutting episode, her mother would insure Anna's safety and would then stop interacting with her (e.g., use extinction). Although multiple chain analyses indicated that intrusive thoughts about the sexual abuse preceded the cutting behavior, no attempt was made to reprocess or restructure these thoughts, given that Anna was still engaging in self-harm behaviors and experiencing suicidal ideation, and thus it did not appear safe to being the exposure process at this time. Instead, the therapist used distraction and self-soothing skills from the Distress Tolerance module in order to help Anna cope with these experiences.

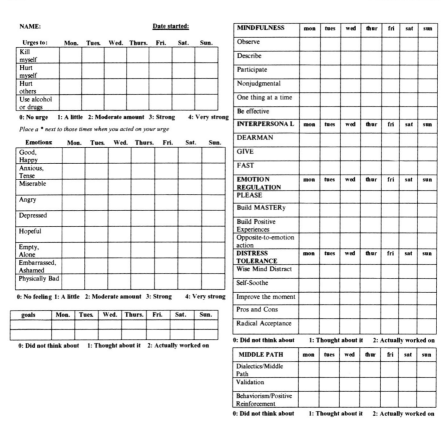

Fig. 12.1 Diary card for Dialectical Behavior Therapy clients, Harbor-UCLA Child and Adolescent Program

Early in treatment, Anna displayed therapy-interfering behavior by not completing the Diary Card between sessions. The therapist used several strategies to deal with this, such as providing reinforcement (e.g., praise, candy) when Anna did complete the diary card, psychoeducation about the purpose of the diary card, making sure Anna understood how to complete it correctly, and reviewing her level of commitment to her treatment goals. The therapist also worked with Anna to determine the function of her behavior of not completing the diary card. Anna indicated that she "didn't want to think about negative thoughts and feelings" during the week. The therapist then targeted Anna's difficulty tolerating negative emotions by outlining specific distress tolerance skills she could use when completing the diary card.

Additionally, Anna was reluctant to call the therapist for telephone coaching, stating that when in the midst of a crisis, "I really can't think straight anymore." In order to target this, the therapist had Anna create written reminders to call her (including her telephone number) and place them in places around her home and belongings where she could easily find them. The therapist also assigned telephone coaching "practices," in which Anna called weekly at an agreed upon time for a brief check-in with the therapist, in order to make calling the therapist a habitual response that she could easily execute in a crisis.

The next treatment target aimed at increasing Anna's mother's ability to validate Anna's emotions and experiences. Anna's mother believed that Anna exaggerated her distress in order to get attention and to get her parents to agree to her demands (e.g., to stay out past her curfew). Consequently, Anna's mother frequently ignored her when she was in emotional distress or became angry and yelled at her. Both of these types of responses served as triggers for Anna's cutting. In order to address this, the therapist continued to discuss the biosocial theory with Anna and her mother and emphasized that a propensity to experience strong negative emotions is biological and is not Anna's choice or an attempt to "manipulate" her. The importance of validation in reducing emotional distress was also discussed. Accordingly, the therapist worked with Anna and her mother on the skill of validation, in which they were taught to communicate an understanding of the others' feelings and behaviors, even if they did not agree with each other. Anna and her mother also practiced validation skills in the multifamily skills group. Anna reported that when her mother validated her feelings, such as letting her know that she understood how disappointing and frustrating it was to have an earlier curfew than some of her friends, she was able to manage her reactions without engaging in self-harm. The therapist also practiced mindfulness with Anna and her mother, in order to help each of them have greater awareness of their own and each other's emotional experiences and perspectives. Interpersonal Effectiveness skills were also utilized, helping Anna and her mother to balance their demands of one another with the need to maintain the quality of their relationship and their self-respect.

At approximately three-and-a-half months into treatment, with her greater use of distress tolerance skills to manage PTSD symptoms and an improved relationship with her mother, Anna's cutting and suicidality reduced significantly. Hence, her treatment shifted to focusing primarily on qual-ty of life issues. Problems with peers were targeted using Interpersonal Effectiveness skills and therapy continued to focus on improving the relationship between Anna and her parents. Time was also spent reviewing Emotion Regulation skills, in which Anna learned how to identify and label her emotions, plan pleasant activities, and to work toward long-term goals in order to "build a life worth living." Anna indicated that she wanted to improve her performance at school and that being able to go to college was an important future goal. The therapist coached Anna to use assertiveness skills from the Interpersonal Effectiveness module to request extra help from teachers and to obtain tutoring. She was also able to effectively use Distress Tolerance skills to manage emotion dysregulation that occurred at school and interfered with her learning. Anna ceased engaging in self-harm behaviors during the fourth month of treatment. However, given that she continued to experience PTSD symptoms, the therapist and Anna collaboratively agreed to start a trauma focused therapy at the conclusion of the 6 months of Stage 1 DBT treatment.

Exposure-Based Treatment

Anna continued to complete the weekly DBT Diary Card so that the therapist could monitor any urges to engage in suicidal or self-harm behavior that occurred during the trauma work. Given that Anna had established fundamental affect regulation, relaxation, and behavioral coping skills for managing intense negative emotions during the prior 6 months of Stage 1 DBT, the overlapping coping, affect regulation, and relaxation skills modules of TF-CBT were not taught. In addition, as parent skills (e.g., validation, contingency management) were also earlier addressed in DBT, this module was also excluded. The trauma-focused treatment was conducted over 16 additional sessions with Anna. Although several TF-CBT modules were eliminated, the length of the treatment remained at 16 sessions (i.e., the typical length of TF-CBT) in order to carefully titrate the exposure. The components of TF-CBT that were administered included psychoeducation about the effects of sexual trauma, trauma-specific coping skills that were not taught in Stage 1 DBT, construction of a trauma narrative and cognitive restructuring, in vivo exposure to excessively or inappropriately avoided stimuli associated with the traumatic event, a conjoint exposure session, and enhancement of Anna's future safety related to victimization.

Initial sessions focused on providing psychoeducation about common trauma reactions. These sessions helped Anna to identify and normalize the trauma symptoms she was experiencing. In collateral sessions with Anna's mother, the typical psychoeducation module of TF-CBT was blended with the DBT concept of validation in order to enhance the mother's ability to validate Anna's trauma-related reactions and experiences. Next, the therapist reviewed the affect regulation, relaxation, and behavioral coping skills learned in DBT in order to specifically target distressing reactions to trauma-related cues and to prepare Anna for the upcoming exposure-focused sessions. In collateral sessions, Anna's mother practiced mindfulness skills, distraction and paced breathing techniques learned in Stage 1 DBT to help her manage her own reactions to her daughter's traumatic experiences. Next, the therapist reviewed the cognitive model (e.g., the connection between thoughts, feelings, and behaviors) and taught Anna how to use additional cognitive coping strategies to both address ongoing symptoms and to use during future exposure sessions. The therapist also taught Anna's mother about the cognitive model.

Trauma exposure was conducted over multiple sessions by having Anna write an autobiographical book in which she described various chapters of her life in each session, starting with benign material (e.g., her early life experiences, likes and dislikes, and friendships) and later including a detailed narrative of the traumatic event. Following completion of the trauma narrative, maladaptive cognitions that occurred during the exposure tasks were addressed using cognitive restructuring techniques. In particular, Anna experienced a great deal of guilt that she did not tell her godfather to stop abusing her and believed, "it is all my fault." The therapist worked with Anna to contrast what the 12 year-old Anna knew about the trauma while it was occurring, with what the present-life Anna new to be "right or wrong."

As a result, Anna was able to restructure her beliefs about her own victimization with more relevant and helpful attributions.

While Anna constructed her trauma narrative, the therapist also worked with Anna's mother to respond in a supportive, validating manner and to manage her emotional reactions to when hearing about Anna's descriptions of the abuse. As the trauma narrative was being constructed, the therapist shared portions of it with Anna's mother in collateral session, in preparation for Anna to share this material with her herself. As the therapist and Anna's mother discussed the trauma narrative, the therapist assisted her with restructuring maladaptive cognitions about the abuse, such as "I don't believe her godfather would do something like this." After hearing the details of the abuse, her mother began to believe that he had actually perpetrated this crime and felt a great deal of guilt for not realizing this sooner. At the end of treatment, a conjoint session occurred in which Anna described the abuse incidents to her mother. Her mother was able to provide Anna with support and validation during this session and Anna indicated a great deal of relief that "my mother finally understands me." With her newly gained understanding of the details of the abuse, Anna's mother was better able to ensure safety by not only discontinuing contact between Anna and her godfather, but also eliminating contact between him and the entire family. Finally, the therapist worked with Anna and her mother on how to enhance safety in the future.

At the conclusion of treatment, Anna's functioning had improved significantly. Post-treatment assessments indicated that she had not engaged in suicidal or self-harm behaviors since the fourth month of treatment and she no longer met criteria for BPD. She was able to regulate her emotions effectively, reported many positive experiences and affect, and had reduced conflict with her mother and with peers. She was attending school regularly, however, would graduate 1 year behind her peers. Her PTSD symptoms had also markedly improved. She reported less difficulty concentrating and did not display the anger outbursts. She continued to have thoughts and memories about the abuse, but she was able to adequately manage negative resulting emotions. She had a few significant peer relationships and was hopeful about her future.

Conclusion

Suicidal behavior is a significant problem among teens. Indeed, the loss or serious injury of a young person due to a potentially preventable cause such as suicidal behavior is a tragic outcome. Youth who have experienced maltreatment are at increased risk for suicidal behavior (Briere & Runtz, 1987; Briere & Zaidi, 1989; Lanktree et al., 1991; Riggs et al., 1990; Saunders et al., 1992). At present, there are no evidence-based treatments for suicidal youth with PTSD symptoms, and the treatments that exist often exclude or significantly delay exposure-based treatments. DBT is a treatment approach that targets both suicidal and self-harm behaviors and PTSD symptoms, and has a great deal of evidence of its effectiveness with adults (e.g., Linehan et al., 1991, 1993, 2006). It has been adapted to be developmentally-appropriate for use with adolescents by including parents in the treatment, tailoring the language and examples used to teach skills to be appropriate to the adolescent age group, and shortening the length of treatment. Preliminary studies with adolescents have yielded promising results (Rathus & Miller, 2002), however, it has not yet been tested in a randomized trial with this population. DBT for adults has recently been expanded to include a formal exposure protocol (Harned et al., 2012). We have utilized the DBT approach with suicidal, traumatized adolescents in our clinic with positive outcomes. Further research on the effectiveness of DBT with adolescents with comorbid suicidal behavior and trauma symptoms is urgently needed.

References

American Psychiatric Association [APA]. (2000). *Diagnostic and statistical manual of mental disorders* (4th ed., text rev.). Washington, DC: Author.

American Psychiatric Association [APA]. (2001). *Practice guideline for the treatment of patients with borderline personality disorder*. Washington, DC: APA.

Brent, D. A., Johnson, B. A., Perper, J., Connolly, J., Bridge, J., Bartle, S., et al. (1994). Personality disorder, personality traits, impulsive violence, and completed suicide in adolescents. *Journal of the American Academy of Child and Adolescent Psychiatry, 33*, 1080–1086.

Briere, J., & Runtz, M. (1987). Post sexual abuse trauma: Data and implications for clinical practice. *Journal of Interpersonal Violence, 2*(4), 367–379.

Briere, J., & Zaidi, L. Y. (1989). Sexual abuse histories and sequelae in female psychiatric emergency room patients. *American Journal of Psychiatry, 146*(12), 1602–1606.

Calkins, S. D., & Hill, A. (2007). Caregiver influences on emerging emotion regulation: Biological and environmental transactions in early development. In J. J. Gross (Ed.), *Handbook of emotion regulation* (pp. 229–248). New York: Guilford Press.

Centers for Disease Control and Prevention [CDC]. (2013). *Web-Based Injury Statistics Query and Reporting System (WISQARS)*. Retrieved from http://www.cdc.gov/injury/wisqars/index.html

Cloitre, M., Cohen, L. R., & Koenen, K. C. (2006). *Treating survivors of childhood abuse: Psychotherapy for the interrupted life*. New York: Guilford Press.

Cohen, J. A., Mannarino, A. P., Berliner, L., & Deblinger, E. (2000). Trauma-focused cognitive behavioral therapy for children and adolescents: An empirical update. *Journal of Interpersonal Violence, 15*(11), 1202–1223.

Cohen, J. A., Mannarino, A. P., & Deblinger, E. (2006). *Treating trauma and traumatic grief in children and adolescents*. New York: Guilford Press.

Crowell, S. E., Beauchaine, T. P., & Linehan, M. M. (2009). A biosocial developmental model of borderline personality: Elaborating and extending Linehan's theory. *Psychological Bulletin, 135*(3), 495–510.

DeRosa, R., & Pelcovitz, D. (2008). Group treatment for chronically traumatized adolescents: Igniting SPARCS of change. In D. Brom, R. Pat-Horenczyk, & J. D. Ford (Eds.), *Treating traumatized children: Risk, resilience, and recovery* (pp. 225–239). London: Routledge.

Eaton, D.K., Kann, L., Kinchen, S., Shanklin, S., Ross, J., Hawkins, J., et al. (2010, June 4). Youth Risk Behavior Surveillance—United States, 2009. *Morbidity and Mortality Weekly Report (MMWR)*. Retrieved from http://www.cdc.gov/MMWR/preview/mmwrhtml/ss5905a1.htm

First, M. B., Gibbon, M., Spitzer, R. L., Williams, J. B. W., & Benjamin, L. S. (1997). *Structured clinical interview for DSM-IV for Axis II personality disorders (SCID-II) interview and questionnaire*. Washington, DC: American Psychiatric Press.

Foa, E. B., Keane, T. M., Friedman, M. J., & Cohen, J. A. (2009). *Effective treatments for PTSD: Practice guidelines from the International Society for Traumatic Stress Studies* (2nd ed.). New York: Guilford Press.

Foa, E. B., & Rothbaum, B. (1998). *Treating the trauma of rape: Cognitive-behavioral therapy for PTSD*. New York: Guilford Press.

Ford, J. D., & Cloitre, M. (2009). Best practices in psychotherapy for children and adolescents. In C. A. Courtois & J. D. Ford (Eds.), *Treating complex traumatic stress disorders: An evidence-based guide* (pp. 59–81). New York: Guilford Press.

Ford, J. D., & Russo, E. (2006). Trauma-focused, present-centered, emotional self-regulation approach to integrated treatment for posttraumatic stress and addiction: Trauma Adaptive Recovery Group Education and Therapy (TARGET). *American Journal of Psychotherapy, 60*(4), 335–355.

Goldsmith, S. K., Pellmar, T. C., Kleinman, A. M., & Bunney, W. E. (2002). *Reducing suicide: A national imperative*. Washington, DC: National Academies Press.

Goldstein, T. R., Axelson, D. A., Birmaher, B., & Brent, D. A. (2007). Dialectical behavior therapy for adolescents with bipolar disorder: A 1-years open trial. *Journal of the American Academy of Child and Adolescent Psychiatry, 46*(7), 820–830.

Gould, M. S., Greenberg, T., Velting, D. M., & Shaffer, D. (2003). Youth suicide risk and preventive interventions: A review of the past 10 years. *Journal of the American Academy of Child and Adolescent Psychiatry, 42*, 386–405.

Harned, M. S., Chapman, A. L., Dexter-Mazza, E. T., Murray, A., Comtois, K. A., & Linehan, M. M. (2008). Treating co-occurring Axis I disorders in recurrently suicidal women with borderline personality disorder: A 2-year randomized trial of dialectical behavior therapy versus community treatment by experts. *Journal of Consulting and Clinical Psychology, 76*(6), 1068–1075.

Harned, M. S., Korslund, K. E., Foa, E. B., & Linehan, M. M. (2012). Treating PTSD in suicidal and self-injuring women with borderline personality disorder: Development and preliminary evaluation of a dialectical behavior therapy prolonged exposure protocol. *Behaviour Research and Therapy, 50*(6), 381–386.

Harned, M. S., & Linehan, M. M. (2008). Integrating dialectical behavior therapy and prolonged exposure to treat co-occurring borderline personality disorder and PTSD: Two case studies. *Cognitive and Behavioral Practice, 15*(3), 263–276.

Harris, E. C., & Barraclough, B. (1997). Suicide as an outcome for mental disorders: A meta-analysis. *British Journal of Psychiatry, 170*, 205–228.

Huey, S. R., Henggeler, S. W., Rowland, M. D., Halliday-Boykins, C. A., Cunningham, P. B., Pickrel, S. G., et al. (2004). Multisystemic therapy effects on attempted suicide by youths presenting psychiatric emergencies. *Journal of the American Academy of Child and Adolescent Psychiatry, 43*(2), 183–190.

Katz, L. Y., Cox, B. J., Gunasekara, S., & Miller, A. L. (2004). Feasibility of dialectical behavior therapy for suicidal adolescent inpatients. *Journal of the American Academy of Child and Adolescent Psychiatry, 43*(3), 276–282.

Lanktree, C., Briere, J., & Zaidi, L. (1991). Incidence and impact of sexual abuse in a child outpatient sample: The role of direct inquiry. *Child Abuse & Neglect, 15*(4), 447–453.

Lewinsohn, P. M., Rohde, P., & Seeley, J. R. (1993). Psychosocial characteristics of adolescents with a history of suicide attempt. *Journal of the American Academy of Child and Adolescent Psychiatry, 32*, 60–68.

Lewinsohn, P. M., Rohde, P., & Seely, J. R. (1994). Psychosocial risk factors for future adolescent suicide attempts. *Journal of Consulting and Clinical Psychology, 62*, 297–305.

Linehan, M. M. (1993). *Cognitive-behavioral treatment of borderline personality disorder* New York: Guildford Press.

Linehan, M. M., Armstrong, H. E., Suarez, A., & Allmon, D. (1991). Cognitive-behavioral treatment of chronically parasuicidal borderline patients. *Archives of General Psychiatry, 48*(12), 1060–1064.

Linehan, M. M., Comtois, K., Murray, A. M., Brown, M. Z., Gallop, R. J., Heard, H. L., et al. (2006). Two-year randomized controlled trial and follow-up of dialectical behavior therapy vs therapy by experts for suicidal behaviors and borderline personality disorder. *Archives of General Psychiatry, 63*(7), 757–766.

Linehan, M. M., Heard, H. L., & Armstrong, H. E. (1993). Naturalistic follow-up of a behavioral treatment for chronically parasuicidal borderline patients. *Archives of General Psychiatry, 50*(12), 971–974.

Miller, A. L., Muehlenkamp, J. J., & Jacobson, C. M. (2008). Fact or fiction: Diagnosing borderline personality disorder in adolescents. *Clinical Psychology Review, 28,* 969–981.

Miller, A. L., Rathus, J. H., & Linehan, M. M. (2007). *Dialectical behavior therapy with suicidal adolescents.* New York: Guilford Press.

Najavits, L. M. (2006). Seeking safety: Therapy for posttraumatic stress disorder and substance use disorder. In V. M. Follette & J. I. Ruzek (Eds.), *Cognitive-behavioral therapies for trauma* (2nd ed., pp. 228–257). New York: Guilford Press.

Nelson-Gray, R. O., Keane, S. P., Hurst, R. M., Mitchell, J. T., Warburton, J. B., Chok, J. T., et al. (2006). A modified DBT skills training program for oppositional defiant adolescents: Promising preliminary findings. *Behaviour Research and Therapy, 44*(12), 1811–1820.

Powers, M. B., Halpern, J. M., Ferenschak, M. P., Gillihan, S. J., & Foa, E. B. (2010). A meta-analytic review of prolonged exposure for posttraumatic stress disorder. *Clinical Psychology Review, 30,* 635–641.

Rathus, J. H., & Miller, A. L. (2002). Dialectical behavior therapy adapted for suicidal adolescents. *Suicide and Life-Threatening Behavior, 32*(2), 146–157.

Resick, P. A., Bovin, M. J., Calloway, A. L., Dick, A. M., King, M. W., Mitchell, K. S., et al. (2012). A critical evaluation of the complex PTSD literature: Implications for DSM-5. *Journal of Traumatic Stress, 25,* 241–251.

Riggs, S., Alario, A. J., & McHorney, C. (1990). Health risk behaviors and attempted suicide in adolescents who report prior maltreatment. *Journal of Pediatrics, 116*(5), 815–821.

Saunders, B. E., Villeponteaux, L. A., Lipovsky, J. A., & Kilpatrick, D. G. (1992). Child sexual assault as a risk factor for mental disorders among women: A community survey. *Journal of Interpersonal Violence, 7*(2), 189–204.

Shaffer, D., Gould, M. S., Fisher, P., & Trautman, P. (1996). Psychiatric diagnosis in child and adolescent suicide. *Archives of General Psychiatry, 53*(4), 339–348.

Silverman, A. B., Reinherz, H. Z., & Giaconia, R. M. (1996). The long-term sequelae of child and adolescent abuse: A longitudinal community study. *Child Abuse & Neglect, 20*(8), 709–723.

Soloff, P. H., Lynch, K. G., & Kelly, T. M. (2002). Childhood abuse as a risk factor for suicidal behavior in borderline personality disorder. *Journal of Personality Disorders, 16,* 201–214.

Soloff, P. H., Lynch, K. G., Kelly, T. M., Malone, K. M., & Mann, J. J. (2000). Characteristics of suicide attempts of patients with major depressive episode and borderline personality disorder: A comparative study. *American Journal of Psychiatry, 157,* 601–608.

Wood, A., Trainor, G., Rothwell, J., Moore, A., & Harrington, R. (2001). Randomized trial of group therapy for repeated deliberate self-harm in adolescents. *Journal of the American Academy of Child and Adolescent Psychiatry, 40*(11), 1246–1253.

Woodberry, K. A., & Popenoe, E. J. (2008). Implementing dialectical behavior therapy with adolescents and their families in a community outpatient clinic. *Cognitive and Behavioral Practice, 15*(3), 277–286.

Zanarini, M. C., Williams, A. A., Lewis, R. E., Reich, R. B., Vera, S. C., Marino, M. F., et al. (1997). Reported pathological childhood experiences associated with the development of borderline personality disorder. *American Journal of Psychiatry, 154,* 1101–1106.

Chapter 13
MST-CAN: An Ecological Treatment for Families Experiencing Physical Abuse and Neglect

Cynthia Cupit Swenson and Cindy M. Schaeffer

Physical abuse and neglect place children at risk of mental health difficulties that can remain present through their developmental lifespan (Cyr, Euser, Bakermans-Kranenburg, & Van Ijzendoorn, 2010; Kim, Cicchetti, Rogosch, & Manly, 2009). In addition, child maltreatment and other stressors combined are related to serious life threatening health problems (Felitti & Anda, 2009; Felitti et al., 1998). Moreover, the impact of maltreatment can become part of an individual's way of parenting and affect the well-being of future generations (Sidebotham & Heron, 2006; Springer, Sheridan, Kuo, & Carnes, 2007). The problem of maltreatment is found globally and is so serious that strong measures are needed to help parents put in place peaceful solutions and positive problem-solving and reduce the mental health problems that they and their children may be experiencing.

Multisystemic Therapy for Child Abuse and Neglect (MST-CAN; Schaeffer, Swenson, Tuerk, & Henggeler, 2013) is an evidence-based treatment for families with serious clinical needs who come to the attention of Child Protective Services due to physical abuse and/or neglect. Importantly, MST-CAN addresses the referral behaviors plus key risk factors that keep families coming through the revolving door of child protection.

In this chapter we present the MST-CAN treatment model. First, we discuss the theoretical foundation of the MST-CAN model. Second, we present the target population for whom this treatment is intended and populations for whom the treatment is not intended. Third, we delineate the treatment model and requirements to implement an MST-CAN program. Fourth, we provide the research findings that are the evidence base for MST-CAN. Finally, we present a case study to show the reader how the model is applied clinically.

C.C. Swenson, Ph.D. (✉) • C.M. Schaeffer, Ph.D.
Department of Psychiatry and Behavioral Sciences, Family Services Research Center,
Medical University of South Carolina, 176 Croghan Spur Rd., Suite 104,
Charleston, SC 29407, USA
e-mail: swensocc@musc.edu; schaeffc@musc.edu

S. Timmer and A. Urquiza (eds.), *Evidence-Based Approaches for the Treatment of Maltreated Children*, Child Maltreatment 3, DOI 10.1007/978-94-007-7404-9_13,
© Springer Science+Business Media Dordrecht 2014

Theoretical Foundation for MST-CAN

Theoretically, MST-CAN is based on a social-ecological model (Bronfenbrenner, 1979). This model holds that children are surrounded by various systems (e.g., family, parents) that they influence and that influence them. Because MST-CAN is a strengths-based model, protective factors across these systems are given first consideration as they can be built upon and used as leverage for change. Likewise, when maltreatment occurs risk factors across these systems need to be assessed and those that are pertinent to the family should be targeted for change. The literature on protective factors and causes and correlates of physical abuse and neglect provide a basis for understanding strengths and potential risk factors. Importantly, this body of literature shows that physical abuse and neglect are highly overlapping events that are determined by multiple factors (Chaffin, Silovsky, Hecht, & Bonner, 2001).

Protective Factors

Among the factors that protect children from being abused and parents from abusing, social support is paramount. According to Egeland (1988), the availability of supportive individuals is a factor that distinguishes women who are able to break the cycle of abuse from those who are not. A supportive relationship with a spouse or significant other appears to reduce the risk of maltreatment (Crouch, Milner, & Thomsen, 2001). In general, appraisal support (i.e., having someone to talk to) relates to more positive mental health among adults who were sexually abused as children (Hyman, Gold, & Cott, 2003). Among children, those who are blamed by others for the maltreatment, indicating low support from the family for abuse disclosure, tend to blame themselves and, perhaps as a result, have higher post-traumatic stress symptoms (Chaffin, Wherry, & Dykman, 1997).

Risk Factors

Regardless of the continent on which the research is conducted, risk factors for physical abuse and neglect are highly consistent and evident across multiple systems including child, parent, family, and social network (Sidebotham & Heron, 2006). For example, youth with behavioral difficulties such as aggression and noncompliance (Black, Heyman, & Slep, 2001) are at an increased risk for abuse. Similarly, abuse and neglect have been linked with parental mental health problems (Sidebotham & Heron) and certain parenting characteristics such as low involvement with the child (see Kolko & Swenson, 2002). In addition, parents who abuse or neglect their children have been shown to experience low social support and tend to be socially isolated (Crouch et al., 2001).

Recent studies that have evaluated maltreatment risk within ecological and biopsychosocial frameworks indicate that risk factors have differing levels of influence and there are factors that are more proximal to abuse occurrence. In a prospective study of comprehensive risk factors conducted in England, Sidebotham and Heron (2006) found that parents who were younger, had histories of mental health difficulties and maltreatment, and had low educational attainment were more likely to have been investigated for abuse and to have a child who is the subject of a child protection plan. In addition, having a poor social network doubled the risk of maltreatment. Slep and O'Leary (2007) found that attitudes approving of parental aggression, parental attribution of child responsibility for misbehaviour, overreactive discipline and anger expression were predictors of parents' aggression toward their child. These important multivariate studies show that factors from differing systems come together to heighten the risk of abuse and neglect.

The implication of risk factors in multiple systems is that to be effective treatment must address pertinent factors from each of the systems (youth, parent, family, school, social network). Furthermore, risk factors must be individualized by family indicating that one size fits all treatments will not be sufficient and will not take into account important cultural and developmental characteristics of individual families with complex situations. An example of addressing multiple risk factors and individualizing treatment is a 2-parent family referred for treatment due to neglect, characterized by the children not attending school and the parents not monitoring the children. At first glance it appears that treatment will involve parent interventions to help them monitor their children. However, when a thorough assessment of strengths and needs is completed the complexity of the case becomes apparent. The factors that are driving the neglect include low parenting skills (parents), heroin use (parents), post-traumatic stress disorder (PTSD) symptoms due to a history of sexual abuse (mother), economic distress due to unemployment (parents), the youth associating with youth who regularly skip school (youth), and the parents being unaware their son is leaving school due to a low home-school link (school and parents). Given that multiple risk factors are present, the clinical team must determine which risk factors are the primary drivers of the neglect and which factors create a safety risk. Interventions for these drivers are prioritized. However, all major risk factors must be addressed to help the family prevent re-abuse. A single intervention treatment would not be sufficient to prevent re-abuse with such a complex case. Next we discuss the purpose of MST-CAN interventions and further delineate the model.

Purpose of the Interventions

The overarching goals for MST-CAN are to keep families together safely by applying research based interventions to prevent placement out of the home, eliminate further incidents of physical abuse and/or neglect, and alter key factors that heighten the risk for abuse or neglect. Examples of factors that heighten the probability of maltreatment are child and parent mental health difficulties, low social support, parenting with force, neglectful parenting, substance misuse, parental relationship issues, school difficulties, housing and employment problems (Kolko & Swenson, 2002). Importantly, risk factors targeted are specific to the needs of each specific family. All interventions applied are those with research support and are implemented in a context of treatment engagement and cultural respect. As noted earlier, MST-CAN addresses the referral problems targeted by the family and Child Protective Services along with key risk factors.

MST-CAN Target Population

The inclusion referral criteria for the MST-CAN program are based on the characteristics of families that were a part of the efficacy and effectiveness trials. The families are those with multiple, serious clinical problems who come to the attention of Child Protective Services (CPS) due to their recent history of physical abuse and/or neglect. Participants must have a child in the family who has been physically abused or neglected (i.e., target child) and who is within the 6–17 year-old age range. As described subsequently in the clinical treatment section, MST-CAN interventions are tailored to the developmental needs of the children in a given family.

Typically, families will have had multiple contacts with CPS. However, the report of physical abuse and/or neglect of the target child must be within the last 180 days. Children in the family will typically be at heightened risk of removal from the home and placement in out-of-home care. Some children will have been in out-of-home care for a short period with the expectation of a rapid return and appropriate safety and monitoring plans in place.

Families who are not appropriate for MST-CAN are families who have experienced one-time maltreatment and are having mild problems for which a short stint of less intensive outpatient therapy will suffice. As our clinical trials have not included active sexual abuse or active partner violence, in the absence of child maltreatment, we do not include families with these experiences currently going on. MST-CAN is not a program that provides sex offender treatment. One caveat is that we often have families referred who have historically experienced sexual abuse or partner violence and MST-CAN is well equipped to treat the impact of traumatic events. In addition, given that MST-CAN uses evidence-based interventions, many of which are from a cognitive behavioral framework and that our clinical trials have not included children on the autistic spectrum, we do not take cases of children with autism. Finally, it is important to be clear that while MST-CAN works with families who have the most serious and complex needs and often does work with youth and parents who have had a suicide attempt, MST-CAN is not a replacement for hospitalization or other programs for youth or parents who are actively suicidal.

Implementing the MST-CAN Model

Implementation Guidelines

MST-CAN is licensed through the Medical University of South Carolina (MUSC). A company called MST Group LLC, doing business as MST Services, has an exclusive licensing agreement through MUSC for the dissemination of MST-CAN technology and intellectual property. Under their licensing agreement MST Group is also authorized to grant sublicenses, provide program support and training in the model to organizations that implement MST-CAN. MST-CAN has very strict requirements for implementation so that it can be delivered with fidelity (i.e., the way it was conducted in research trials where outcomes were attained). Agencies interested in implementing MST-CAN must complete a site assessment with an MST-CAN program developer. To be a licensed program, they must complete goals and guidelines and a feasibility checklist and agree to the terms of MST-CAN implementation such as collaborative relationships, established referral criteria, established program clinical goals, a team structure, and an agreement to implement the program fidelity requirements. Importantly, there must be evidence of a working relationship and buy-in from key stakeholders such as Child Protective Services.

The Core Model

MST-CAN is based on standard Multisystemic Therapy (MST: Henggeler, Schoenwald, Borduin, Rowland, & Cunningham, 2009) that was originally developed to meet the clinical needs of youth experiencing serious antisocial behavior and their families. Rather than using a scripted treatment manual, standard MST interventions are guided by nine treatment principles (see Table 13.1). The core structure of MST (nine principles, analytic process, home-based service delivery, flexible hours, ecological focus, and quality assurance system) is also the core of MST-CAN. The clinical service and service delivery are slightly different from Standard MST given that the population is different. Table 13.2 shows the key differences between MST-CAN and standard MST.

The Clinical Team

MST-CAN is operated as a distinct clinical team that does not take cases outside those referred to the team (i.e., does not serve families referred to other programs in the agency). A full-time supervisor oversees the work of 3–4 masters-level therapists and a bachelor-level case manager. Approximately 20 % psychiatrist protected time is reserved for youth and parents in the project.

Table 13.1 Multisystemic therapy nine treatment principles

1.	The primary purpose of assessment is to understand the "fit" between the identified problems and their broader systemic context.
2.	Therapeutic contacts should emphasize the positive and use systemic strengths as levers for change.
3.	Interventions should be designed to promote responsible behavior and decrease irresponsible behavior among family members.
4.	Interventions should be present-focused and action-oriented, targeting specific and well-defined problems.
5.	Interventions should target sequences of behavior within and between multiple systems.
6.	Interventions should be developmentally appropriate and fit the developmental needs of the youth.
7.	Interventions should be designed to require daily or weekly effort by family members.
8.	Intervention efficacy should be evaluated continuously from multiple perspectives.
9.	Interventions should be designed to promote treatment generalization and long-term maintenance of therapeutic change.

Table 13.2 Differences between standard MST and MST-CAN

Standard MST	MST-CAN
Core model	
Theoretical basis is a social ecological model	Theoretical basis is a social ecological model
All aspects of the treatment are conducted in a context of family engagement for which the therapist and team is responsible	All aspects of the treatment are conducted in a context of family engagement for which the therapist and team is responsible
Uses MST analytic process (do-loop)	Uses MST analytic process (do-loop)
Follows nine principles	Follows nine principles
Ecology is the client	Ecology is the client
Uses research supported treatments targeting fit factors related to youth antisocial behavior	Uses research supported treatments but the treatments may differ
Addresses risk factors for antisocial behavior across multiple systems	Addresses risk factors for physical abuse and/or neglect across multiple systems. Risk factors differ from antisocial youth behavior
Prevents model drift through a structured quality assurance system	Prevents model drift through a structured quality assurance system
Population	
Antisocial youth and their families	Families who are being followed by Child Protective Services due to physical abuse and/or neglect for whom a new report of abuse or neglect has been made in the last 180 days
Target Youth ages 13–18	Target Youth ages 6–17
Serious, deep-end, complex cases	Serious, deep-end, complex cases

(continued)

Table 13.2 (continued)

Standard MST	MST-CAN
Team	
Supervisor – full-time with a case load or part-time with no caseload	Supervisor – full-time with no caseload
Three therapists	Three therapists
	Full-time crisis caseworker
	20 % dedicated psychiatrist time
Services	
Caseload of four to six families	Maximum caseload of four families
Focus on behavior of youth	Focus on behavior of parent and youth if indicated
Treatment is of youth through the parents	Treatment is of the entire family averaging 5 people per family
Treatment length 4–6 months	Treatment length 6–9 months
Delivered in the home, community, places convenient to families	Delivered in the home, community, places convenient to families
Delivered at times convenient to the family	Delivered at times convenient to the family
Availability of 24 h a day, 7 days a week crisis on-call service	Availability of 24 h a day, 7 days a week crisis on-call service
Supports families through court processes	Supports families through court processes
Quality assurance	
5-day MST orientation training	5-day MST orientation training
	4-day MST-CAN training
	4-day booster on treatment of child and adult trauma
Quarterly booster training	Quarterly booster training
Weekly supervisor development phone conference	Weekly supervisor development phone conference
Weekly group supervision	Weekly group supervision
Monthly telephone interviews with families to assess adherence to the model	Monthly telephone interviews with families to assess adherence to the model

Services Structure

MST CAN treatment sessions are primarily conducted in the family's home. However, some work is carried out in the youth's school and elsewhere in the community. Each therapist carries a maximum caseload of four families and although each therapist is the lead clinician for four families, the caseworker may conduct case management with all families served by the team if needed. Because parents' actions of abusing or neglecting their children result in a referral to MST-CAN, to a great extent the focus of treatment is with the adults in the family. On average, five people per family are treated. For example, the parent may be treated for substance abuse, the grandmother for depression, and the child for behavioral problems at school. The team works a flexible schedule seeing families at times that are convenient for them. Sessions may be during traditional work hours, at night or on the weekend. The team operates a 24-h per day, 7 days per week on-call rotation service to help families manage crises that arise outside of general working hours.

Clinical Treatment

Engagement

A key factor supporting the capacity of the family to achieve treatment milestones is engagement with the therapist and clinical team. When a family has had multiple or long-term contacts with Child Protective Services, they may fear losing their children and have little trust for professionals overall. Low levels of trust may lead them to avoid treatment providers. Some families may show highly negative and verbally aggressive behaviors towards providers that actually lead the providers to avoid the family. All of these experiences make engagement with the family challenging for an MST-CAN therapist. To overcome the challenges to engagement, the MST-CAN therapist must always keep a strengths-focus and take a one-down approach, allowing the family to "teach" the therapist about themselves. Listening to the family's past experiences is key to understanding, even when the telling of those experiences is done with high emotion. Given that the problems associated with abuse and neglect are highly treatable and that families can resolve their conflict through strong evidence-based treatments, the MST-CAN therapist can bring a great deal of hope to the family. For avoidant families, positive persistence can result in strong engagement. Families are often surprised to find that the therapist has enough confidence in the family to keep trying to engage them in treatment even when the family will not answer the door. Engagement is an ongoing process throughout treatment. In some cases families making strides in treatment experience an unexpected stressor and disengage from the team when they are well into treatment. When a family disengages, the focus of treatment becomes re-engaging. MST-CAN therapists are known for doing "whatever it takes" to help families. As such, regardless of the reason for disengagement, the therapist and team maintain a very positive stance about the family and the progress they have made.

Treatment Principles

MST-CAN follows the Standard MST nine principles (Henggeler et al., 2009). When these principles are followed with fidelity, clinical outcomes are better for families (Schoenwald, Sheidow, Letourneau, & Liao, 2003). These nine principles serve to keep the clinical team on track with regard to keeping a family and ecology focus, staying goal oriented, delivering evidence-based interventions in ways that meet the developmental needs of families, continuously assessing progress or barriers to progress, and keeping a focus on sustainability of outcomes.

Analytic Process

The MST analytic process, also called the "do loop" is a tool for outlining the structure of the MST-CAN treatment process. The process begins with a thorough assessment of the referral behaviors and family history and the development of an extensive genogram to understand the ecology and family structure. The strengths of the family and ecology across multiple systems (e.g., child, parent, social network) are determined. The initial contacts with the family include an assessment of child and adult traumatic events and the impact of these events on current functioning. The next step in the process includes interviewing all key people in the family's ecology (e.g., parents, children, grandparents, teachers, CPS staff) to understand their desired outcomes. The desired outcomes are combined into the family's overarching goals for treatment.

Once the clinical team has an understanding of the family's strengths and referral behavior and the overarching goals have been set, the "do loop" guides intervention development and implementation. To determine what interventions are pertinent to helping the family meet their goals, the team must understand the "fit" of the target problems. That is, the team must determine which factors are driving the target problems. For example, a family was referred to MST-CAN because the children were not being supervised (i.e., neglect) and because they were aggressive towards their mother and peers at school. On the face, the problem appeared to be inadequate parenting skills. An assessment of the "fit" (i.e., driving factors) of the neglect revealed that the parent had good knowledge of parenting but was unable to access these skills because she was often high from cocaine use. This understanding of fit of the neglect led the team to implement a research-supported treatment for substance misuse instead of engaging in parent training with the mother.

Each week, the MST-CAN therapist sets intermediary goals related to the treatments being implemented and reports to the supervisor, team, and consultant on a family's progress towards achieving these goals. If goals are not met, the team (including the parent) works together to understand barriers to progress and how the intervention might need to be altered to help the family achieve their goals. If an intervention continues to be largely unsuccessful, the team reexamines the "fit factor," acknowledging that they may not have understood the dynamic correctly, and further exploration of a new understanding of "fit" is taken.

Evidence-Based Interventions

All interventions used in the context of MST-CAN are research based. Though families by and large receive different interventions depending on their strengths and the "fit" of their target problems, some interventions are provided to all families for the purposes of safety and sustainability of progress. Early in treatment, each family completes a safety plan that is specific to the risks that are understood early in the case. Weekly in-depth safety assessments are conducted to enable the team and family to understand any change in safety needs that will result in a revision of the plan. Importantly, in cases where parents are misusing illegal drugs or alcohol and a relapse occurs, a plan specific to safety from substance use and associated activities is used. Second, critical to a good relationship between the family and Child Protection, MST-CAN works closely with caseworkers, often including them in family sessions and considering them a valuable part of the team. Third, each family completes a clarification process (Lipovsky, Swenson, Ralston, & Saunders, 1998) through which the parent addresses cognitions about the abuse or neglect incident and takes responsibility for all actions that had a negative impact on the child or family. This work is done by the parent drafting a letter of apology and responsibility to the child and family, editing it with the therapist multiple times to remove words that might hurt the parent-child relationship and to think through how to take responsibility for his or her actions in writing, and reading it aloud to the family in a session.

Other research-supported interventions approved for use in MST-CAN are applied only in situations where these particular treatments are needed to address drivers of key problems. For example, functional analysis is used in cases of physical abuse or ongoing family conflict to understand the sequences of events and where the interactions take a turn towards physical or verbal aggression. The functional analysis helps identify when and where in the sequence to put in place interventions that will de-escalate a family conflict. Many of the research supported treatments applied in the MST-CAN model are behavioral or cognitive behavioral in nature. When youth or parents exhibit difficulty in managing anger, cognitive behavioral treatments for anger management are used (e.g., Feindler, 2006; Feindler, Ecton, Kingsley, & Dubey, 1986). A behavioral family treatment (Robin, Bedway, & Gilroy, 1994) is used when families have difficulty with communication and problem-solving. For families who are experiencing PTSD symptoms, cognitive behavioral treatments are used for adults (Foa, Hembree, & Rothbaum, 2007; Foa, & Rothbaum, 1998; Kilpatrick, Veronen, & Resick, 1982) and children (Cohen, Mannarino, & Deblinger, 2006, 2012) Finally, for adults experiencing substance misuse, Reinforcement-Based Treatment (RBT; Tuten, Jones, Schaeffer, Wong, & Stitzer, 2012) is provided.

The developmental level of the children in the family is a key consideration in selecting and implementing interventions (MST Principle 6; see Table 13.1). For example, in a given family, child noncompliance and low parenting skill may be prioritized drivers of abusive family interactions. To address these drivers, the MST-CAN therapist would select an evidence-based parent training protocol (i.e., the Incredible Years Training for Parents; Webster-Stratton et al., 2001) if the children in the family were school-aged, but use a family communication/problem-solving approach (using protocols from Standard MST) when pre-teens and adolescents are involved. In families with multiple children of various developmental levels, both approaches would be delivered simultaneously, with an explicit treatment focus on helping parents tailor their parent management approach to the child's developmental level. Implementation of interventions also is tailored to the developmental needs of children. For example, parents are coached to use developmentally-appropriate language when writing clarification letters.

Maintaining Treatment Fidelity: The MST-CAN Quality Assurance Process

The purpose of the MST-CAN quality assurance program is to deliver MST-CAN with fidelity (as it was delivered in research trials) and prevent drift from the model protocols. The quality assurance program includes training and measures of model adherence.

Training

Each member of the clinical team completes a 5-day orientation to the Standard MST model to gain an understanding of how to conceptualize cases from a social ecological perspective and provide targeted interventions. Next, each team member completes 4 days of training in MST-CAN, with two of those days focusing on training in RBT for adult substance misuse. Child Protective Services caseworkers who will be interacting with the team are invited to as much of the MST and MST-CAN training as they are able to attend. Child Protection supervisors are strongly encouraged to attend day one of the 5-day MST orientation and all 4 days of MST-CAN.

In addition to the initial trainings, quarterly booster trainings are held to address clinical issues and treatments that the team needs additional expertise on. The first booster is a 4-day training on treatment of trauma for adults and children from a cognitive behavioral perspective. Child Protection workers who interact closely with the team are invited to attend booster trainings as well.

Once per week the supervisor of the team convenes a 1–2 h supervision session to discuss each case, crises that have occurred, success of current interventions, and next steps. Each team is assigned an MST-CAN expert (called a consultant) whose role is to help the team maintain fidelity to the model. Weekly, the team completes a goals and progress report that is sent to the consultant for review prior to telephone consultation. On a weekly basis, following the supervision session, the MST-CAN expert meets by telephone with the MST CAN team to review cases and problem solve particularly challenging issues. Each clinician may also participate in individual supervision with the MST-CAN supervisor on an as needed basis.

Measuring Adherence

As with Standard MST, MST-CAN utilizes two measures of adherence. The MST-CAN Therapist Adherence Measure (CAN-TAM) is a Likert-format interview that is conducted with the parent by an independent interviewer who does not provide clinical services. The measure is scored to provide therapists feedback regarding whether the treatment is being delivered with fidelity. Therapists complete a Supervisor Adherence Measure (SAM) to rate the supervisor's adherence to the model. Adherence scores are discussed in consultation and during booster trainings.

Research Findings

MST-CAN is an evidence-based treatment model with 15 years of clinical and research piloting, efficacy and effectiveness studies, and transportability piloting to its history. Two randomized clinical trials (RCT) form the current evidence base supporting MST-CAN. The first RCT for MST-CAN was an efficacy study implemented by Brunk, Henggeler, and Whalen (1987). Forty-three families with children from age 6 to 9 who had indicated cases of either abuse or neglect were randomized to MST or Behavioral Parent Training. Findings indicated that families who received standard MST showed more favorable pre- to post-treatment changes on amelioration of family problems, restructuring parent-child relations, and increased effectiveness at key parenting behaviors than did families that received group-based parent training. Parent training, however, was superior to MST in decreasing social problems, perhaps because it was implemented as a group program and by definition established a temporary social support network. This study was critical to establishing feasibility and efficacy of applying the MST model to physical abuse and/or neglect. However, follow-up was not conducted, and placement and re-abuse were not measured. In addition, mental health functioning of the parent and child were not assessed. These are areas that were addressed in the effectiveness study.

A randomized clinical effectiveness study (Swenson, Schaeffer, Henggeler, Faldowski, & Mayhew, 2010) funded by the National Institute of Mental Health was conducted through a county mental health center in Charleston, South Carolina. Eighty-six families who had substantiated cases of physical abuse and in which the target child was in the age range of 10–17 were randomized to either MST-CAN or Enhanced Outpatient Therapy (EOT). The latter involved all parents attending a parenting group called Systematic Training for Effective Parenting of Teens (STEP-TEEN; Dinkmeyer, McKay, McKay, & Dinkmeyer, 1998; Gibson, 1999) plus extra efforts on the part of the EOT therapist to engage the family in treatment, assist them with transportation and assure that they connected with referrals for treatments that they needed (e.g., individual child, family, substance abuse, anger management) for the problems they were experiencing. The confidence in the study outcomes were boosted by the occurrence of a 98 % recruitment rate and high treatment retention rates for both groups (98 % for MST-CAN; 83 % for EOT).

Intent-to-treat analyses across 16 months post-baseline indicated that MST-CAN was more effective than EOT in reducing adolescent internalizing problems (dissociation, PTSD, internalizing and total symptoms of the Child Behavior Checklist), out-of-home placements, and number of placement changes, for those who were placed out-of-home (e.g., foster care, residential). With regard to caregivers, MST-CAN was more effective than EOT in reducing caregiver psychiatric distress and parenting associated with maltreatment (i.e., minor assault, severe assault, neglect, psychological aggression). MST-CAN parents were more likely to use non-violent discipline. MST-CAN was significantly more effective at increasing caregivers' perceived social support (i.e., ratings on the Interpersonal Support Evaluation List; Cohen, Mermelstein, Kamarck, & Hoberman, 1985) from natural ecology members and caregivers indicated greater treatment satisfaction. Fewer MST-CAN youth experienced an incident of re-abuse but base rates were low and the difference was not statistically significant.

These two randomized trials established MST-CAN as an evidence based intervention for families where physical abuse and neglect is occurring and where families are experiencing multiple and serious clinical needs. MST-CAN is cited as an evidence-based program by the California Evidence-Based Clearinghouse for Child Welfare and as a promising program by the Office of Justice Programs. Following the MST-CAN RCTs, transportability research pilots have evaluated the feasibility, acceptability and preliminary outcomes of applying MST-CAN to the context of Denver, Colorado, Eastern Australia, Holland, Switzerland, and England. Positive outcomes have been shown for families in all transportability pilot programs.

Other research that includes MST-CAN is taking place in Connecticut. To address the serious clinical needs of families who experience physical abuse and neglect plus serious parental substance misuse, the Family Services Research Center of the Medical University of South Carolina, the Connecticut Department of Children and Families, and Wheeler Clinic, with consultation from Michelle Tuten from Johns Hopkins University, combined MST-CAN with a treatment for adult substance abuse called Reinforcement Based Treatment (RBT; Tuten et al., 2012) to develop the MST-Building Stronger Families model (MST-BSF). This is a program to help parents in maltreating families stabilize recovery and reduce risk of harm to their children. MST-BSF has been implemented in Connecticut for 7 years. Preliminary outcomes from a matched-cases pilot funded by the Annie E. Casey Foundation showed that MST-BSF was more effective than the comprehensive community treatment (CCT) provided in Connecticut at reducing out-of-home placements for the children (13 % vs. 39 %) and preventing re-abuse (CCT families had, on average, four times the number of substantiated reports as MST-BSF families) at 24 months post referral (Schaeffer, Swenson, Tuerk, & Henggeler, 2013). The MST-BSF program in Connecticut is currently the subject of an RCT funded by the National Institute on Drug Abuse (NIDA).

The case example that follows represents a typical family referred to an MST-CAN program, one with multiple prior maltreatment incidents. It illustrates how the 9 MST-CAN treatment principles (see Table 13.1) and analytic process guide treatment conceptualization and implementation, as well as how evidence-based interventions are selected and administered within the MST-CAN framework.

Case Example

Lucy, age 34, was referred to MST-CAN by her caseworker at the Department of Social Services (DSS) soon after receiving a hotline call alleging Lucy's educational and medical neglect of her two children, ages 11 and 13. Personnel at the children's school reported that the children had missed 35 days of school in 6 months and were at risk of not advancing to the next grade. They also reported that Lucy's son Carlos, a 6th grader, suffered from severe asthma that was poorly managed (e.g., he reported not owning an inhaler), and that both children urgently needed dental care. Lucy's daughter, Shayla, in 7th grade, had also been suspended twice during the school year for fighting. The school's attempts to address the issue with Lucy had been unsuccessful, with Lucy not returning the school's calls and missing meetings. Lucy had a history of DSS involvement, with 3 previous neglect reports in the past 4 years for similar issues.

Lucy had lived with the children's father since she was 19 until he was imprisoned in another state 3 years earlier for assault and drug charges. Lucy described her ex-boyfriend as extremely violent and controlling, and although he sent frequent letters to her and the children from prison, she had no desire to resume their relationship. Lucy was unemployed with a limited work history, and received social security disability benefits for a diagnosis of bipolar disorder. The family lived in a small home in a neighborhood characterized by crime and drug violence. Although Lucy's mother lived in a nearby community 10 miles away, they were estranged and had not spoken in over 5 years.

As specified in MST-CAN clinical procedures, the therapist's initial assessment of the family was multifaceted and strove to identify systemic strengths, treatment outcomes desired by all stakeholders, and the fit between identified problems and their broader systemic context (MST Treatment Principle 1; see Table 13.1). Through initial conversations with Lucy, her children, school personnel, and the DSS caseworker, the therapist identified many strengths and needs across Lucy's key ecological systems (see Table 13.3). Systemic strengths included Lucy's sophistication in accessing public resources (e.g., public housing assistance); warm, loving family relations; concerned teachers to whom the children were bonded; and the children's prosocial interests (e.g., in art and sports). Ecological needs included the family's history of traumatic experiences; Lucy's low parenting skills and social isolation; and a potentially dangerous housing environment. Lucy's desired outcomes were to "take better care of my kids," for Carlos' "asthma to get better," and "to worry less about stuff I can't control." Shayla reported a desire for "the kids at school to leave her alone" and "to go visit my father." Carlos' desired outcomes were "to not be held back a grade" and for his mother to "do more stuff with us, like take us to the mall." DSS and school personnel shared several desired outcomes for the family in common, including "improved school attendance for the children and promotion to the next grade" and "family medical needs addressed." In addition, DSS expressed a desire that "Lucy address her mental health needs," and that the family "have no additional reports to DSS in the future."

With these strengths, needs, and desired outcomes in mind, the MST-CAN therapist gained a consensus among all stakeholders on several overarching treatment goals, including (a) improved school attendance and grade promotion, (b) all child medical and dental needs addressed, (c) improved mental health for Lucy, Shayla, and Carlos, (d) no additional school fights for Shayla, and (e) children to have a say in family decisions, such as weekend activities.

Table 13.3 Lucy case example: strengths and needs

System	Strengths	Needs
Individual	Lucy intelligent, has high school diploma and a year of community college credit Lucy values school and wants her children to go to college Lucy personable, giving, "a caretaker" Shayla artistic ability Carlos has interests in sports	Lucy unemployed Lucy avoids leaving house Lucy trauma history – domestic violence Children's trauma history – witness to domestic violence, police raid Unmet child medical and dental needs – Carlos' asthma Lucy not taking psychiatric medication previously prescribed Carlos trouble sleeping, worries Shayla irritability, "on edge"
Family	Warm, loving relationship between Lucy and children, enjoy being together Siblings get along Some income (disability checks) Lucy savvy in getting family services (e.g., housing support, food stamps)	Lenient parenting, few skills for getting children to school Very low finances Poor financial management – e.g., electricity turned off last year Estranged from extended family Father's letters disruptive – children often ask to see him
Peer	Both Carlos and Shayla have friends in neighborhood Lucy friendly with next door neighbor, an elderly woman	Lucy socially isolated – no same-age friends Shayla fights at school Neither child in prosocial activities
School	Carlos likes school Concerned and interested teachers – "they are not bad kids" Shayla bonded to her art teacher Both children of at least average intelligence – capable of A and B work	High absences Both children may be held back a grade Shayla disengaged, disinterested in class, "spaced out" Poor parent-school link
Community	Friendly next door neighbor Boys and girls club within walking distance Several churches nearby Grocery store in walking distance On a central bus route, well-connected	No medical or dental providers in immediate neighborhood Few structured prosocial activities for youth Lots of crime and drug activity Father's family lives nearby, harass family House is site of domestic violence

The MST-CAN therapist combined information across sources and identified the most likely drivers for the issues that led to referral, namely, the children's poor school attendance and unmet medical needs. As illustrated in Fig. 13.1, the main drivers for medical neglect were that Lucy avoids leaving her house, has had negative experiences with doctors, and is not engaged with a primary care physician.

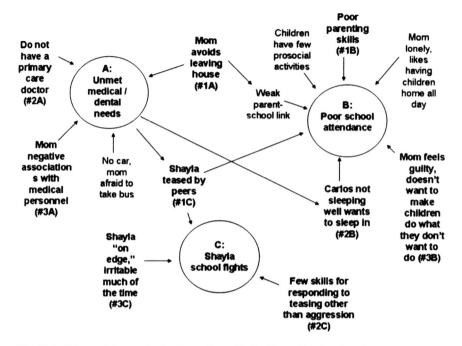

Fig. 13.1 Drivers of three main family problems (A, B, C) resulting in referral

The children's poor school attendance was related mainly to Lucy's low skills for responding when the children overslept or protested going to school, her guilt about requiring them to do something they don't want to do, Carlos' insomnia (oversleeps), and the fact that Shayla gets teased by peers at school (about having a chipped tooth and a father in prison). Shayla's fights at school were related to peer teasing, her limited array of solutions for responding to teasing, and her irritable mood much of the time (teachers described her as "on edge").

As a supplement to these MST-CAN ecological assessment procedures, the therapist conducted trauma assessments with each family member, in light of the early indications in the case that the father had been "extremely violent." Lucy had experienced multiple traumatic experiences over 10 years with her very abusive partner, including a broken jaw, being locked in a closet, cigarette burns on her legs, and sexual violence, and rated highly on trauma symptoms (e.g., re-experiencing, intrusive thoughts, avoidance of leaving the house). She also expressed a fear that her ex-boyfriend would return to the home upon release from prison, and reported ongoing verbal harassment from two of his brothers, whom she saw in her neighborhood occasionally. The children's trauma assessment revealed exposure to numerous domestic violence incidents in which they feared for their mother's life and a terrifying raid of their home by the police during which an officer shot and killed the family dog. Both children expressed symptoms of hypervigiliance (i.e., Shayla's irritability and "edginess" at school; Carlos' fears of home invasion contributed, along with his asthma, to insomnia) and rumination.

The MST-CAN therapist prioritized two main drivers of family problems, Lucy's trauma symptoms and low parenting skills. As she began to build motivation with Lucy for trauma treatment, she concurrently arranged for a meeting between Lucy and the school and discussed changes to the family's morning and evening routines to make school attendance more likely. The case manager immediately began helping Lucy find and make appointments with a physician and a dentist at times that would not conflict with the children's school attendance. Carlos' appointment for asthma was prioritized along with getting Shayla's chipped tooth fixed.

Lucy was initially reluctant to engage in Prolonged Exposure (PE) treatment for her trauma symptoms, but eventually agreed to do it "for her kids." In a given week, the therapist met with Lucy individually twice for PE sessions, once for parent management interventions, and once for family therapy sessions with the children. Family sessions focused on discussing rules and expectations for behavior, as well as ways Shayla could respond nonviolently to provocations from peers. As Lucy's trauma treatment progressed, the case manager assisted with some in vivo exposure sessions by accompanying her to sites she avoided (e.g., on public buses, a clinic where she had received stitches) and encouraging her to stay in the setting until her anxiety abated.

Once Lucy's trauma symptoms began to improve and her parenting interventions pertaining to school attendance became more consistent (e.g., she routinely rewarded the children for school attendance), the MST-CAN therapist suggested trauma treatment for the children. Given that Trauma Focused Cognitive Behavioral Therapy (TF-CBT; Cohen et al., 2006, 2012) is the gold standard treatment for children experiencing symptoms of posttraumatic stress disorder, this treatment was used with the children. Lucy agreed to this treatment direction, and the rationale for Shayla and Carlos to begin individual sessions with the therapist was discussed in family sessions. Each of the children participated separately in TF-CBT sessions and with their mother in some sessions. After several weeks, both completed the full TF-CBT protocol, with Lucy's involvement.

Meanwhile, Lucy began seeing the MST-CAN psychiatrist. Since her trauma symptoms were now greatly reduced, Lucy and the psychiatrist decided that her previous diagnosis of bipolar disorder was no longer appropriate, but that she could benefit from antidepressant medication for her remaining symptoms. Once her dose was stabilized, the psychiatrist helped Lucy find a provider in the community with whom she could continue care after MST-CAN ended. As Lucy's symptoms improved, she became more interested in seeking employment. The case manager provided extensive support in this area, including determining how much she could work without losing disability benefits, helping her identify her interests, develop a resume, and conduct online job searches at the local library.

After 5 months of treatment, the children's attendance was near 100 % per school reports (Principle 8) and much of their dental work had been completed. However, several issues remained that threatened the sustainability of the family's gains. First, the family's living situation was dangerous, since the children's father monitored the family through his brothers and associates in the neighborhood. He also sent frequent letters expressing his intention to resume living with the family upon his release, despite the fact that Lucy had sent a letter to break up with him over a year prior. The MST-CAN team connected Lucy with a victim's advocacy group who recommended several courses of action, including relocating, contacting the father's probation officer, requesting official notification of his release, and, upon notification, securing a restraining order against him. The case manager helped Lucy find a new rental property that would accept her Section 8 housing voucher and that was within a different school district for the children so that the father's monitoring of their whereabouts, which frightened them, would stop.

A second issue was that the family lacked a social support system. Lucy's estrangement from her mother was due largely to her ex-boyfriend's controlling behaviors (he wouldn't allow her to visit) and several incidents of theft and property damage he had inflicted at her mother's home. The MST-CAN therapist worked with Lucy to see the advantages of reconnecting with her mother (e.g., extended family relationships for her children, social support), supported Lucy in making the first contact, and met with Lucy and her mother on several occasions. Once Lucy's mother was convinced that Lucy was committed to staying out of her abusive relationship, she became an ally in this effort. Lucy's mother agreed to help Lucy enact the safety plan surrounding his potential release and to periodically check that Lucy was mailing his threatening letters to parole officials who would determine his release date. She also assisted the family on moving day, and began to form a bond with the children.

A final lingering issue was Shayla's insistence on having contact with her father. Her desire to write to him posed a safety threat to the family and was a source of numerous arguments with Lucy. Through family sessions Lucy was able to help Shayla understand the need for the family's safety, and an agreement was reached that Shayla was free to contact him and have a relationship with him when she turned 18. Shayla and Carlos also learned strategies for avoiding conversations with their father's brothers if they encountered them in the community.

In the last weeks of treatment, Lucy wrote clarification letters to both children, and the family shared a meaningful clarification session. Lucy reported feeling less guilty about what the children had been through and more optimistic that they would not witness more domestic violence in the future. The children were excited about their new home and were enrolled to attend summer school to make up lost credits for school promotion. Drawing upon the children's strengths and interests (Principles 2 and 6), each child was enrolled in a prosocial summer activity (art camp for Shayla, archery classes for Carlos) that was paid for by DSS. Carlos' asthma and insomnia had improved. Lucy accepted a job offer at a nursing home, and was taking the public bus without anxiety symptoms to job interviews, doctors' appointments, and her mother's house. She had plans to attend a family "parents without partners" picnic in the coming weeks with the hopes of meeting some new peers. MST-CAN closed the case after 7 months of treatment, and the family's DSS case was closed as well. At a 2-year follow-up, the family had had no new DSS referrals.

As with drivers for problem behaviors, MST-CAN therapists also identify drivers for improved behaviors. Hypothesized drivers for the improvements in the children's health and school attendance were (a) Lucy's reduced anxiety symptoms, reduced guilt about the children's past experiences, and new-found ability to leave her home; (b) Lucy's improved parenting skills, and (c) the children's improved mental health and connections with age-appropriate activities (Principle 6). The likelihood that the family's gains will be sustained over time (Principle 9) is increased due to (a) Lucy's improved social support system, (b) family's greater financial stability (Lucy working), (c) children's involvement in prosocial activities, and (d) a comprehensive safety plan to prevent future domestic violence.

Conclusion

MST-CAN is an empirically supported, evidence-based intervention for the multiple, complex problems facing families within the child protective service system who are in danger of child removal. MST-CAN is being disseminated both nationally and internationally. A key feature of MST is its emphasis on addressing known risk factors for child maltreatment comprehensively, with multiple family members receiving full courses of various treatments in most cases. Further, services are provided in community-based settings and incorporate pragmatic, empirically-supported, behaviorally-oriented intervention techniques. Importantly, these interventions are delivered in a highly integrated and time-efficient manner. Another defining feature of MST-CAN is its use of a well-conceived quality assurance and quality improvement systems to support fidelity to the treatment model. Finally, MST-CAN works closely with child protection personnel to minimize risks to child safety and to help ensure child permanency in placement.

Acknowledgments This chapter was supported by National Institute of Mental Health grant R01MH60663 to Cynthia Cupit Swenson.

References

Black, D. A., Heyman, R. E., & Slep, A. M. S. (2001). Risk factors for child physical abuse. *Aggression and Violent Behavior, 6,* 121–188. doi:10.1016/S1359-1789(00)00021-5.

Bronfenbrenner, U. (1979). *The ecology of human development: Experiments by design and nature.* Cambridge, MA: Harvard University Press.

Brunk, M., Henggeler, S. W., & Whelan, J. P. (1987). Comparison of multisystemic therapy and parent training in the brief treatment of child abuse and neglect. *Journal of Consulting and Clinical Psychology, 55,* 171–178. doi:10.1037/0022-006X.55.2.171.

Chaffin, M., Silovsky, J., Hecht, D., & Bonner, B. (2001). *Evaluation of Oklahoma Children's Services, 2001 annual report.* Unpublished manuscript, Oklahoma Department of Human Services.

Chaffin, M., Wherry, J. N., & Dykman, R. (1997). School age children's coping with sexual abuse: Stresses and symptoms associated with four coping strategies. *Child Abuse & Neglect, 21*(2), 227–240.

Cohen, J. A.. Mannarino, A. P., & Deblinger, E. (2006). *Treating trauma and traumatic grief in children and adolescents*. New York: Guilford Press.

Cohen, J. A., Mannarino, A. P., & Deblinger, E. (2012). *Trauma focused CBT for children and adolescents: Treatment applications*. New York: Guilford Press.

Cohen, S.. Mermelstein, R. J., Kamarck, T., & Hoberman, H. M. (1985). Measuring the functional components of social support. In I. G. Sarason & B. Sarason (Eds.), *Social support: Theory, research, and applications*. The Hague/Holland, the Netherlands: Martins Nexjhoff.

Crouch, J. L., Milner, J. S., & Thomsen, C. (2001). Childhood physical abuse, early social support, and risk for maltreatment: Current social support as a mediator of risk for child physical abuse. *Child Abuse & Neglect, 25*, 93–107. doi:10.1016/S0145-134(00)00230-1.

Cyr, C., Euser, E. M., Bakermans-Kranenburg, M. J., & Van Ijzendoorn, M. H. (2010). Attachment security and disorganization in maltreating and high-risk families: A series of meta-analyses. *Development and Psychopathology, 22*, 87–108.

Dinkmeyer, S.. McKay, G. D., McKay, J. L., & Dinkmeyer, D. (1998). *Systematic training for effective parenting of teens*. Circle Pines, MN: American Guidance Services, Inc.

Egeland, B. (1988). Breaking the cycle of abuse: Implications for prediction and intervention. In K. D. Browne, C. Davies, & P. Stratton (Eds.), *Early prediction and prevention of child abuse* (pp. 87–99). New York: Wiley.

Feindler, E. L. (2006). *Anger-related disorders: A practitioner's guide to comparative treatments*. New York: Springer.

Feindler, E. L., Ecton, R. B., Kingsley, D., & Dubey, D. R. (1986). Group anger-control training for institutionalized psychiatric male adolescents. *Behavior Therapy, 17*, 109–123. doi:10.1016/S0005-7894(86)80079-X.

Felitti, V. J., & Anda, R. F. (2009). The relationship of adverse childhood experiences to adult medical disease, psychiatric disorders, and sexual behavior: Implications for healthcare. In R. Lanius & E. Vermetten (Eds.), *The hidden epidemic: The impact of early life trauma on health and disease*. New York: Cambridge University Press.

Felitti, V. J., Anda, R. F., Nordenberg, D., Williamson, D. F., Spitz, A. M., Edwards, V., et al. (1998). Relationship of childhood abuse and household dysfunction to many of the leading causes of death in adults: The adverse childhood experiences (ACE) study. *American Journal of Preventive Medicine, 14*(4), 245–258.

Foa, E. B.. Hembree, E. A., & Rothbaum, B. O. (2007). *Prolonged exposure therapy for PTSD: Emotional processing of traumatic experience*. New York: Oxford University Press.

Foa, E. B., & Rothbaum, B. O. (1998). *Treating the trauma of rape: Cognitive behavioral therapy for PTSD*. New York: Guilford Press.

Gibson, D. G. (1999). *A monograph: Summary of the research related to the use and efficacy of the Systematic Training for Effective Parenting (STEP) program 1976–1999*. Circle Pines, MN: American Guidance Services, Inc.

Henggeler, S. W., Schoenwald, S. K., Borduin, C. M., Rowland, M. D., & Cunningham, P. B. (2009). *Multisystemic therapy for antisocial behavior in children and adolescents* (2nd ed.). New York: Guilford Press.

Hyman, S. M., Gold, S. N., & Cott, M. A. (2003). Forms of social support that moderate PTSD in childhood sexual abuse survivors. *Journal of Family Violence, 18*(5), 295–300.

Kilpatrick, D. G., Veronen, L. J., & Resick, P. A. (1982). Psychological sequelae to rape: Assessment and treatment strategies. In D. M. Dolays, R. L. Meredith, & A. R. Ciminero (Eds.), *Behavioral medicine: Assessment and treatment strategies* (pp. 473–497). New York: Plenum Press.

Kim, J., Cicchetti, D., Rogosch, F. A., & Manly, J. T. (2009). Child maltreatment and trajectories of personality and behavioral functioning: Implications for the development of personality disorder. *Development and Psychopathology, 21*, 889–912.

Kolko, D. J., & Swenson, C. C. (2002). *Assessing and treating physically abused children and their families: A cognitive-behavioral approach*. Thousand Oaks, CA: Sage.

Lipovsky, J. A., Swenson, C. C., Ralston, M. E., & Saunders, B. E. (1998). The abuse clarification process in the treatment of intrafamilial child abuse. *Child Abuse & Neglect, 22*, 729–741. doi:10.1016/S0145-2134(98)00051-9.

Robin, A. L., Bedway, M., & Gilroy, M. (1994). Problem solving communication training. In C. W. LeCroy (Ed.), *Handbook of child and adolescent treatment manuals* (pp. 92–125). New York: Lexington Books.

Schaeffer, C. M., Swenson, C. C., Tuerk, E. H., & Henggeler, S. W. (2013). Comprehensive treatment for co-occurring child maltreatment and parental substance abuse: Outcomes from a 24-month pilot study of the MST-Building Stronger Families program. *Child Abuse and Neglect, 37,* 596–607. doi:10.1016/j.chiabu.2013.04.004.

Schoenwald, S. K., Sheidow, A. J., Letourneau, E. J., & Liao, J. G. (2003). Transportability of multisystemic therapy: Evidence for multilevel influences. *Mental Health Services Research, 5,* 223–239.

Sidebotham, P., & Heron, J. (2006). Child maltreatment in the children of the nineties: A cohort study of risk factors. *Child Abuse & Neglect, 30,* 497–522. doi:10.1016/j.chiabu.2005.1.

Slep, A. M. S., & O'Leary, S. G. (2007). Multivariate models of mothers' and fathers' aggression toward their children. *Journal of Consulting and Clinical Psychology, 75*(5), 739–751.

Springer, K. W., Sheridan, J., Kuo, D., & Carnes, M. (2007). Long-term physical and mental health consequences of childhood physical abuse: Results from a large population-based sample of men and women. *Child Abuse & Neglect, 31,* 517–530. doi:10.1016/j.chiabu.2007.01.003.

Swenson, C. C., Schaeffer, C. M., Henggeler, S. W., Faldowski, R., & Mayhew, A. (2010). Multisystemic therapy for child abuse and neglect: A randomized effectiveness trial. *Journal of Family Psychology, 24,* 497–507.

Tuten, M., Jones, H. E., Schaeffer, C. M., Wong, C. J., & Stitzer, M. L. (2012). *Reinforcement-based treatment (RBT): A practical guide for the behavioral treatment of drug addiction.* Washington, DC: American Psychological Association.

Webster-Stratton, C., Mihalic, S., Fagan, A., Arnold, D., Taylor, T., & Tingley, C. (2001). *Blueprints for violence prevention, Book Eleven: The incredible years: Parent, teacher, and children training series.* Boulder, CO: Center for the Study and Prevention of Violence.

Part VI
Dissemination and Implementation

You have read about the ten EBTs in this volume, each representing one of four different age categories across the childhood years: infancy, young children, school-aged children, and adolescence. You have no doubt realized that the research supporting these interventions makes it clear that they have the potential for making positive change in the lives of maltreated children. But, as we noted earlier, having the EBTs established scientifically is only half the battle. Therapists who provide services for maltreated children have to be able to provide these EBTs effectively in order to achieve the promised positive outcomes. Training therapists to use the EBTs effectively and facilitating their growth and sustainment in community mental health settings is the other half of the battle. For this reason we included the following chapters on dissemination and implementation of EBTs.

In the two chapters following the descriptions of the interventions for different ages of children, we provide a framework for understanding why dissemination and implementation are important topics for those interested in EBTs. Chapter 14, "Taking It to the Street: Disseminating Evidence-Based Practices" gives the reader a framework for understanding the training process, and how the EBT developers described in this volume have trained clinicians to provide their intervention. In Chap. 15, we elaborate on the process of implementation and the difficulty EBT developers have achieving and maintaining treatment fidelity, in "The Bridge from Research to Practice – Just Leap Across the Last Bit."

Chapter 14
Taking It to the Street: Disseminating Empirically Based Treatments (EBTs)

Susan Timmer and Anthony Urquiza

There are many children and families adversely affected by child maltreatment: thousands of children experiencing child sexual abuse, child physical abuse, and neglect every day (U.S. Department of Health and Human Services, Administration for Children and Families, Administration on Children, Youth and Families, Children's Bureau, 2011). Much of this volume has detailed the impact of maltreatment on the developing child, followed by multiple interventions that have strong empirical support in alleviating child mental health symptoms, improving parent-child relationships, and improving the overall health of the child. The chapters describe the severity and risk associated with child maltreatment, and highlight the treatment needs of children who have been maltreated or exposed to domestic violence. We have also have read through ample evidence that many empirically based treatment programs are effective in alleviating a fairly wide range of mental health problems in maltreated children. Reflecting upon this information, one can't help but be impressed by the fact that we have an excellent selection of interventions for treating maltreated children with mental health symptoms, improving both child and family functioning. But are the people in need receiving these treatments?

Many scholars have discussed the gap between the advances in research on mental health interventions and their use by clinical practitioners (for a review, see McHugh & Barlow, 2010). One of the primary consequences of this gap is client lack of access to evidence-based mental health care (President's New Freedom Commission on Mental Health, 2004). With health care costs increasing, and one out of every five children under the age of 18 years in the United States having a diagnosed mental health disorder, it is even more important for children

S. Timmer, Ph.D. (✉) • A. Urquiza, Ph.D.
CAARE Diagnostic and Treatment Center, Department of Pediatrics, University of California at Davis Children's Hospital, 3671 Business Dr., Sacramento, CA 95820, USA
e-mail: susan.timmer@ucdmc.ucdavis.edu; anthony.urquiza@ucdmc.ucdavis.edu

S. Timmer and A. Urquiza (eds.), *Evidence-Based Approaches for the Treatment of Maltreated Children*, Child Maltreatment 3, DOI 10.1007/978-94-007-7404-9_14, © Springer Science+Business Media Dordrecht 2014

to be able to access effective mental health services. In the past, one reason children in need were not receiving these treatments was because mental health clinicians had not been trained to provide them, or had not been trained competently (McHugh, Murray, & Barlow, 2009). In response to a call for disseminating EBTs (e.g., Insel, 2009; President's New Freedom Commission on Mental Health, 2004), government and state agencies, as well as private foundations, have created financial and regulatory incentives and mandates supporting their use (e.g., California Institute of Mental Health [CIMH], 2011; McHugh & Barlow, 2010; Wonderlich et al., 2011). With the promise of better outcomes and financial incentives, practitioners may perceive added value in the investments associated with adopting evidence-based practices. However, the most recent information available to us suggests that EBTs are still underutilized (Cohen, Mannarino, & Rogal, 2001; Shafran et al., 2009). Few clinical training programs provide training for their students in EBTs (Sigel & Silovsky, 2011; Weissman et al., 2006); and dissemination in clinical practice settings have shown modest effects (e.g., Goisman, Warshaw, & Keller, 1999; Stewart & Chambless, 2007; Weersing & Weisz, 2002). We must assume that the same enthusiasm and attention to the details involved in the development of EBT protocols have not been accorded to understanding how people learn and maintain therapeutic skills (Fixsen, Naoom, Blase, Friedman, & Wallace, 2005).

At least up until the last several years, clinicians were most likely to receive training by reading manuals or attending brief workshops conducted by an expert trainer (Dimeff et al., 2009). These methods represent what the founders of "implementation science" – Fixsen and colleagues (2009) – describe as a "passive process," relying on clinicians to absorb the information provided and find a way to use it effectively. Interestingly, evaluation research has found that these strategies have shown little ability to increase therapists' proficiency (Dimeff et al., 2009; Miller, Yahne, Moyers, Martinez, & Pirritano, 2004). Possibly as a result of these ineffective training methods, results of the National Comorbidity Survey Replication showed that nearly a third of all mental health treatment consisted of complementary and alternative medicine treatments (Wang et al., 2005) – evidence that clinicians are not practicing EBTs, even if they are learning them. As a result, along with responding to the greater the demand for training in EBTs, we have begun to pay more attention to the process and outcomes of training. This move is consistent with what Fixsen would call the "to" in "Research to Practice" (Fixsen et al., 2009). Implementation scientists, studying how to effectively "plant" and "grow" EBTs in organizations and systems, recommend using more active and interactive implementation strategies, and maintaining strict fidelity rather than "adapting" and "adopting" as others have recommended (e.g., Rogers, 2003). This chapter will briefly describe the core implementation components set forth by Fixsen and his colleagues in their 2005 monograph (Fixsen et al., 2005), which reviewed 30 years of research on the implementation of many different evidence based programs. This will be followed by a summary of the training models used by the EBTs included in this volume of work and how they have used these core implementation components.

Implementing EBTs: Training and the Developmental Loops of Implementation

Successful implementation involves many more components than simply training selected staff to deliver a specific intervention. If the goal of implementing an EBT is to incorporate the intervention into the existing framework of the agency, then there are multiple components that need to occur prior to actual training, as part of the core training, and after completion of training. For example, prior to actual core training, an agency needs to examine the fit between the population they serve and the various interventions, how the intervention will be integrated into existing systems, and procedures for determining treatment selection. Also, for an agency or organization, implementing an EBT does not stop at simply learning how to provide the intervention. Once therapists know how to follow an intervention's protocol, and achieve positive outcomes, implementation efforts become more focused on sustaining the practice with fidelity over time and retaining trained staff. Considering the fact that staff turnover rates can easily exceed 25 % in community mental health agencies (Gallon, Gabriel, & Knudsen, 2003; Glisson, Dukes, & Green, 2006), sustaining an EBT can mean being in a state of constant training or staff EBT skill acquisition. Recognizing the fluidity of the EBT implementation process, most treatment developers and EBT trainers have acknowledged the need to support treatment fidelity by holding yearly conferences, institutes, or regional workshops, and publishing books and other supportive material. In an effort to support program sustainability, some EBT trainers have developed training models in which experienced EBT providers in an agency are encouraged and supported in their efforts to train other therapists in their agencies to effectively provide treatment – a Trainer of Trainer (ToT) model. The value of a ToT training model is that it provides a mechanism for sustaining treatment within an agency – as new staff join the agency they can be trained by the ToT. Additional benefits include having a recognized 'expert' on site to be a resource for the program, developing a 'cultural' or therapeutic milieu for the intervention within the agency, and assigning responsibility for quality assurance and fidelity assessments. A downside to this model may be the risk that the therapists who are trained by the ToT may not be as adept at training, and therefore the next generation of treatment providers would not be adequately trained, which would result in diminished treatment fidelity and presumably effectiveness in subsequent generations of therapists trained at the agency. However, preliminary research findings examining the effectiveness of ToT models are encouraging. An initial feasibility study of three generations of PCIT therapists showed no decay in the magnitude of parents ratings of improvements in problem behaviors, and in changing parents' interaction patterns from pre- to post-treatment (Urquiza, Timmer, & Girard, 2011), suggesting that the ToT model may help keep some EBT programs healthy (i.e., strong adherence to treatment protocols), while yielding positive client outcomes. However, few interventions use a ToT model. ToT models are not suitable for "individual" learners using an educational model in which an individual goes to a place of learning for information. It is most suitable when an intervention is designed to train one type of provider (i.e., therapists) and is implemented on a somewhat broader scale, such as an agency, or County mental health providers, where people may come and go, but there is a great need for the program to remain intact. Even so, most EBT developers retain firm control over who conducts their training, using only identified and approved trainers who have been specifically certified by the treatment developers. While this serves the purpose of insuring a strong training regimen with close fidelity to the treatment protocol, this also may further limit client access to the intervention.

Core Implementation Components

Fixsen and colleagues (2005) identified seven core components of implementation, which they call "implementation drivers" (i.e., factors that determine the nature and quality of the implementation). In a nutshell, these drivers are staff selection, pre-service & in-service training, ongoing coaching and consultation, staff evaluation, decision support data systems, facilitative administrative support, and system interventions. Some of these components driving the implementation are engaged before the implementation takes place, some are engaged during the implementation to support the training process, and some are engaged during the implementation process with primary focus towards sustaining the program after the initial training is completed. We will define and discuss these terms as they relate to the training efforts of the EBTs described in this volume. Table 14.1 lists the different EBTs, their training models, and characteristics of their implementation.

Pre-implementation

Some EBT trainers disseminate their interventions to individuals, and some implement interventions on a larger scale: to agencies, counties, even states and countries (Kazak et al., 2010). Trainers that focus on training individual mental health practitioners (i.e., therapists in private practice) have little concern about the context in which the intervention is provided. Their focus is typically on the skill acquisition of the provider during the training period. However, EBT trainers and their trainees that are attempting to implement an EBT in an organization or some type of larger mental health system (e.g., county or state mental health programs, hospitals) pay more attention to its supportive qualities. Some EBT trainers assess an organization's readiness to adopt an EBT as part of their practice before beginning training. Before training begins, the trainer will meet with administrators and training coordinators to determine whether the organization has a *Facilitative Administration* – an administration that provides positive leadership by setting policies and procedures that support the level of organization and oversight required by an EBT. The trainer attends to the culture and climate of the organization, to determine whether the potential trainees are

Table 14.1 Information on dissemination characteristics of selected EBTs

EBT	Staff selection (minimum provider qualifications)	Description of training model	Trainers	Pre-implementation	Therapist competence and treatment fidelity
Child Parent Psychotherapy (CPP)	Master's degree professionals in psychology, or social work with parent and child mental health experience Trainees in psychiatry or mental health services If weekly clinical supervision in CPP available: Unlicensed clinicians Those with no previous experience with CPP	Initial 3-day workshop Additional quarterly (three more times in a year) 2-day workshops Bi-monthly telephone-based case consultation of ongoing treatment cases involving children aged 0–5 who have experienced a trauma Learning collaborative model also available	Various trainers. UC San Francisco Child Trauma Research Program and on-site Contact: Chandra Ghosh Ippen, PhD Chandra.ghosh@ucsf.edu	Organizational readiness and capacity assessment	The child-parent psychotherapy (CPP) knowledge test (Ghosh Ippen 2008) designed to test trainees knowledge about CPP
Attachment & Biobehavioral Catchup (ABC)	No specific training or educational requirements for practitioners Commitment to 1 year of training	Initial training: 2–3 days to introduce theoretical and empirical basis of ABC, session content, specific principles and techniques used to facilitate caregivers' use of ABC target behaviors Weekly supervision with ABC trainers for at least 1 year	Training at University of Delaware Supervision through videoconferencing Contact: Caroline Roben, PhD croben@psych.udel.edu		Monitor, increase, and measure fidelity by coding the quality and quantity of parent coach comments in session in relation to targeted caregiver parenting behaviors
Triple P (PPP)	A professional qualification in a human services discipline	A series of accredited training courses for professionals offer training in various levels of intervention: 2–5 day training plus 1 day accreditation depending on level of intervention Courses are skills-based and involve training in required theoretical and professional skills: didactic, video and live demonstrations of strategies, role play in small groups, feedback, clinical problem solving exercises, and readings	Training at Triple P America's Head Office in Columbia, SC and various organizations for individual training Multilevel agency trainings available	Assessment of organization's readiness to implement PPP include: Organizational commitment Support staff willing to attend training Willing to provide supervision Availability of funds to ensure use of practitioner and parent resources Manager briefings to ensure support	A competency-based accreditation process requires practitioners to demonstrate their proficiency in program delivery and their knowledge and understanding of the principles upon which the program is based. Triple P America provides a certificate of accreditation Fidelity checklists

(continued)

Table 14.1 (continued)

EBT	Staff selection (minimum provider qualifications)	Description of training model	Trainers	Pre-implementation	Therapist competence and treatment fidelity
Incredible Years (IY)	Master's degree professionals in psychology, or social work with parent and child mental health experience	Initial trainings are 3-day, 21 h – mix of video modeling, group discussion, role play practice, direct teaching. Follow up is phone consult, video review of actual work, in person coaching of actual work	Training in Seattle, WA or on-site Contact: Lisa St. George, Administrative Director, lisastgeorge@incredibleyears.com	The Agency Readiness Questionnaire – Launching The Incredible Years Programs	Fidelity checklists process for accreditation that is performance and proficiency based
Parent-child Interaction Therapy (PCIT)	Master's degree professionals in psychology, or social work with child mental health experience Trainees in psychiatry or mental health services Understanding of behavioral techniques Unlicensed clinicians if weekly clinical supervision in PCIT available	Varies by trainer UC Davis PCIT Training Center Model: 10 h PCIT for Traumatized Children Web Course (ucdavis.pcit.edu) Post web course skill building (8 h) 96–120 h coaching live clients until one client completes PCIT Learning collaborative training model available through PCIT of Carolinas Didactic training with videoconferencing supervision available at Child Mind Institute, NY, NY	Various trainers. See www.pcit.org or pcit.ucdavis.edu UC Davis Training: On-site or via telehealth UC Davis ToT Training model trains & supports experienced PCIT trainers in agencies training other agency staff	Varies by trainer Program development part of UC Davis PCIT training model: Assess and consult on staff selection, referral stream, internal referral process, documentation and measurement requirements, time commitment expectations	Use therapist competency checklists during training or to assess competence Use session therapist fidelity checklists Trainer fidelity checklist available from UC Davis PCIT Training Center

| Multidimensional Treatment Foster Care-Preschool (MTFC-P) | **Vary by team position:** **Program supervisor** Master's in a clinical field Experience in behavior management Supervisory skills, organized Available 24 h a day, 7 days a week **Foster parent consultant/ recruiter/trainer** Knowledge of foster parents Prior experience as a foster parent preferred **Family therapist** Master's in a clinical field Knowledge of behavioral parenting techniques preferred **Playgroup leader** Bachelor's level education in a relevant field **Skills trainer** Bachelor's level education in a relevant field **PDR-caller** Experienced (ex-) foster parent preferred **Foster family** Basic understanding of child development and foster care Relaxed with a good sense of humor desirable **Consulting psychiatrist** For prescribing and managing medication | Pre-implementation: educate stakeholders about MTFC-P and implementation process Develop an implementation plan and timelines Implementation: staff attends a 4-day training session at the model site in Eugene, Oregon (5 days for Program Supervisors) Clinical training sessions are scheduled quarterly for replacement staff and new implementation teams | Training in Eugene, Oregon Contact: Gerard Bouwman, President TFC Consultants, Inc. gerardb@mtfc.com | Prospective programs are given the MTFC-P Feasibility Information & Review and the MTFC-P Site Readiness Questionnaire, which are completed in the program development phase | Initial certification good for 2 years, and subsequent certification for 3 years The certification applications are evaluated by the Center for Research to Practice, which is separate from TFC Consultants providing the consultation and training TFC Consultants conduct periodic reviews of MTFC-P programs |

(continued)

Table 14.1 (continued)

EBT	Staff selection (minimum provider qualifications)	Description of training model	Trainers	Pre-implementation	Therapist competence and treatment fidelity
Trauma-Focused Cognitive Behavioral Therapy (TF-CBT)	Master's degree professionals in psychology, or social work with child mental health experience	*TF-CBTWeb*, a 10-h basic web-based training (www.musc.edu/tfcbt) Introductory overview: 1–8 h Basic training: 2–3 days Ongoing phone consultation (twice monthly for 6–12 months): groups of 5–12 clinicians receive ongoing case consultation to implement *TF-CBT* for patients in their setting Advanced Training: 1–3 days	Various trainers National Conferences; CARES Institute, Allegheny General Hospital and onsite by request	Organizational Readiness and Capacity Assessment	Measures of fidelity
Alternatives for Families-Cognitive Behavioral Therapy (AF-CBT)	Master's degree professionals in psychology, or social work with child mental health experience General training in cognitive behavioral or behavioral techniques Unlicensed clinicians if weekly clinical supervision in AF-CBT available	Trainings tailored to the needs of the program, but include the following components: Initial didactic workshop training (3 days) Follow-up case consultation calls during "action plan" periods (6–12 months) Review of session performance samples for integrity/competency Booster re-training and advanced case review (1 day) Review of community metrics and progress report	Learning collaborative approach provided on a flexible basis (i.e., in a local or individual agency or in context of a regional program or training institute.) Contact: David J. Kolko, PhD kolkodj@upmc.edu		

Multisystemic Therapy-Child Abuse & Neglect (*MST-CAN*)	Requirements vary by position: *MST-CAN* **Supervisor**: Master's degree and license in clinical field Experience in managing severe family crises, family therapy and CBT for PTSD Knowledge of mandated abuse reporting laws and child welfare system *MST-CAN* **Therapist**: Master's degree in clinical field Knowledge of family violence, child development, and child welfare system Social skills to engage families Experience in crisis intervention *MST-CAN* **Crisis Caseworker**: Bachelor's degree Knowledge of employment seeking, budgeting, housing, and child development Experience in the child welfare system *MST-CAN* **Psychiatrist**: Board certification eligibility in Child and Adolescent Psychiatry	All trainees complete the Standard MST 5-day orientation. Then each team member completes a 4-day *MST-CAN* specific training and 4 days of training in adult and child trauma treatment. All training is open to CPS caseworkers who will be working with the *MST-CAN* team After start-up, training continues through weekly telephone consultation, and through quarterly on-site booster trainings (1½ days each). The *MST-CAN* supervisor is trained to implement a manualized MST supervisory protocol. Assistance in organizational matters is available as needed	At MST Services, Inc. in Charleston, SC, or on site Agencies licensed by MST Services Inc. as Network Partner Organizations also provide the MST 5-day orientation training (http://www.mstservices. com/5-day_orientation. php) Contact: Joanne Penman joanne. penman@mstservices. com	MST Services has developed site assessment tools that review of the feasibility of the program, goals, and guidelines for implementation and program practice requirements that must be met. Furthermore, each site must pass a formal Site Readiness Review conducted on site	*Therapist Adherence Measure-Revised (TAM-R)*: evaluates a therapist's adherence to the *MST-CAN* model as reported by the primary caregiver of the family *Supervisor Adherence Measure (SAM)*: evaluates the *MST-CAN* Clinical Supervisor's adherence to the MST model of supervision *Consultant Adherence Measure (CAM)*: The *MST-CAN* Therapists and *MST-CAN* Supervisors are responsible for completing this questionnaire

(continued)

Table 14.1 (continued)

EBT	Staff selection (minimum provider qualifications)	Description of training model	Trainers	Pre-implementation	Therapist competence and treatment fidelity
	Knowledge of mandated abuse reporting laws, relevant ethical guidelines and laws concerning clinical situations Experience with child and adult populations, trauma treatment, local organizations and systems				
Dialectical Behavioral Therapy	Graduate degree in mental health profession with child mental health experience General background training in behavioral therapy is important Unlicensed providers with weekly clinical supervision in DBT	Trainings tailored to the needs of the program; but include the following components: 10 day Dialectical Behavior Therapy Intensive Training™: Part 1: 5 day didactics Post Part 1: 6 month team-based self-study curriculum and as needed expert consultation Part 2: 5 day clinical case and program consultation Additional training beyond the Intensive Training for DBT® with Adolescents: 2 day workshop: DBT with Adolescents: Helping Emotionally Dysregulated and Suicidal Teens As needed clinical case and program consultation by DBT® expert	For academic programs: University of Washington Behavioral Research & Therapy Clinics (BRTC) – http://blogs.uw.edu/brtc For clinicians & agencies: Behavioral Tech, LLC – www.behavioraltech.org	Individual Clinicians: Individual Therapy Survey (ITS) DBT Provider Questionnaire (PQ) Copenhagen Burnout Evidence-Based Practice Attitude Scale (EBPAS) University of Washington Clinical Influence (UWCIS) Organizational Readiness: Texas Christian University Organizational Readiness for Change- Staff (TCU ORC-S) Team Needs Assessment (TNA) Barriers to Implementation (BTI) Program Elements of Treatment (PETQ) Self-study curriculum	University of Washington DBT® Adherence Rating Scale

NCCTS   The National Center
         for Child Traumatic Stress

Sample Organizational Readiness and Capacity Measure

Organizational Readiness and Capacity Assessment[1,2]

This readiness assessment is intended to help your agency identify issues that are known to impact readiness for adoption of a new practice. Circle the number that corresponds to how ready you believe your agency is to address the issue described in each statement. An action plan is included to help you determine how your agency can increase readiness for successful adoption of a new practice.

	Not at all Ready	About 25% Ready	About 50% Ready	About 75% Ready	Totally Ready
Clients					
1. Clients are currently able to be screened for trauma-related symptoms that could qualify them for the new practice.					
2. We already have many clients who will benefit from the new practice based on their clinical presentation, diagnosis, and histories.					
Leadership/Clinicians/Staff					
3. Clinicians in our agency agree with the rationale for using the new practice.					
4. Agency and clinical leadership actively support the adoption of the new practice for reasons clinicians can share.					
5. We have on staff seasoned professionals to whom clinicians look to for support, consultation, and guidance					
6. All staff who will be affected by the new practice know changes are coming and are prepared to offer feedback for its success.					
7. Our agency has a tradition of learning and changing so we do not become entrenched in the status quo.					
8. The clinical orientation of the new practice is not inconsistent with that of the existing staff and leadership					
9. Staff at all levels perceives the advantage of implementing the new practice.					
10. Our staff has opportunities for interaction with others in our community or around the nation who have or are currently implementing the new practice.					

Fig. 14.1 Assessment of organizational readiness, National Child Traumatic Stress Network (NCTSN)

open to learning different practices. To give you an example of the types of questions covered in a typical pre-implementation discussion, Fig. 14.1 shows the "*Assessment of Organizational Readiness*" tool developed by the National Child Traumatic Stress Network (NCTSN) and used by TF-CBT and CPP (Allred et al., 2005).

Often, EBT trainers will conduct *Pre-service or In-service Trainings* for staff and local stakeholders, to provide information about the EBT – its theoretical foundation, appropriate referral information, its effectiveness, and the intervention's potential to improve the lives of the clients. These workshops generally run from half-day to several days in length, depending on whether they are used just to build momentum and enthusiasm for the EBT training or also include some didactic training for future practitioners. In addition, pre-service/in-service workshops that include community stakeholders assist the community in understanding the new intervention (at the agency) and clarify funding and referral streams. While research has not supported using only pre-service and in-service models for training (e.g., Herschell, Kolko, Baumann, & Davis, 2010), they are noted as expedient methods for communicating information (Fixsen et al., 2009). For example, as part of their training models, MTFC-P and UC Davis PCIT Training Center conducts community presentations at agency training sites, inviting all agency staff (including administrative support staff), teachers, social workers, pediatricians, and any community stakeholder who might referral a client to the new program.

Recent years have witnessed an increase in the availability of web-based fundamental training in different EBTs (e.g., TF-CBT training at http://tfcbt.musc.edu/; PCIT training at pcit.ucdavis.edu; DBT and other therapies at http://behavioraltech.org/ol), a strategy found to be significantly more effective than manuals and workshops (Dimeff et al., 2009). Web-based trainings allow participants to acquire skills and information at their own rate, can be interactive, and provide a standardized amount and depth of information. The primary purpose of these fundamental pre-service and in-service trainings, whether given by an expert in person or web-based, is to prepare staff for the new culture of the EBT and build a commitment to its rigors. Staff enthusiasm and commitment to the EBT and stakeholders who are cheerleaders for its adoption are important drivers of successful implementation (Fixsen et al., 2005).

As part of the pre-implementation discussion, EBT trainers also discuss with administrators the external systems needed to support the organization's adoption of the EBT: funding and referrals. This may include clarifying funding streams, identifying fundable diagnostic and insurance codes, and delineating grant and service contract inclusion criteria. Additionally, developing a steady stream of appropriate referrals supports the effective use of the EBT; which often involves educating both community members and agency staff. Further, agencies with multiple EBTs may need to identify which of the EBTs is most appropriate for a specific client – as some maltreated children have common and overlapping sets of symptoms (Sedlar, Thomas, & Blacker, 2010). Without clients and a potential for funding EBT services, organizations may need a *Systems Intervention* to insure that the training will prosper and the program will thrive. Trainers may even postpone training until referral and funding problems have been resolved. To give an example, as Swenson and Schaeffer describe in their chapter in this volume, MST-CAN has very strict requirements for implementation so that it can be delivered with fidelity (i.e., the way it was conducted in research trials where outcomes were attained). Agencies seeking to implement MST-CAN must complete a site assessment with an MST-CAN program developer. To be a licensed program, they must complete goals and guidelines, and a feasibility checklist and agree to the terms of MST-CAN implementation such as collaborative relationships, established referral criteria, established program clinical goals, a team structure, and an agreement to implement the program fidelity requirements. There must also be evidence of an effective working relationship with key stakeholders such as Child Protective Services, and evidence of these stakeholders' commitment to the training.

Staff selection is the process by which a decision is made concerning which staff members are best suited to learn an intervention (Fixsen et al., 2005). Treatment developers and EBT trainers often set guidelines for academic qualifications, experience, and/or licensure; and these guidelines are generally based on the degree of clinical responsibility a job function requires. Apart from these basic guidelines, there is limited understanding regarding which therapist characteristics are best suited to learn to deliver an EBT. Some people find it easier to adopt certain interventions than others; and, some may be more willing to move beyond their current 'therapy belief system,' to develop different ways of thinking about mental health treatment, and client symptoms. Also, some therapists may be more willing to accept the challenge associated with new skills acquisition – which often involves not doing something well during the process of mastering the new skill. Currently, there are no clear guidelines or evidence as to which therapists will be more likely to be more successful at acquiring skills in an EBT training program, or who will adhere to protocol and provide higher quality services in the long run. While the notion that some individuals within an organization may be more open to innovation (i.e., "early adopters" as discussed by Rogers, 2003), it is not clear to what degree this thinking applies to implementation of new EBTs. While treatment developers and trainers can give advice on staff selection, it is often the organization that makes the final decision about who will participate.

Some of the EBTs presented in this volume have well-scripted tasks for clinicians to follow during training, and do not require adherence to certain knowledge bases and theoretical foundations. Most training programs are skill-based, recommending a knowledge of child development, effective parenting, and clinical experience with the population for which the EBT has been developed (e.g., A history of treating traumatized children – TF-CBT; a history of involvement with parenting programs for PPP, PCIT, IY), but do not require specific training in the treatment approach to qualify for training (see Table 14.1). Trainers often maintain that therapists with a variety of different knowledge bases and theoretical foundations can all learn to provide their respective interventions effectively, but must show a willingness and commitment to training for approximately a year in order to successfully master the intervention. Many, but not all, of these interventions are provided by master's degree professionals in psychology or social work with parent and child mental health experience and training, or trainees in psychiatry or mental health services, such as social work, marriage and family therapy, or pre-doctoral interns. According to information listed on the California Evidence Based Clearinghouse (CEBC) website (www.cebc4cw.org), unlicensed clinicians have provided most of these interventions, as well as those with no previous experience with the intervention (California Evidence-Based Clearinghouse for Child Welfare [CEBC], 2012). There are a few exceptions to this description: MST-CAN and MTFC-P. MST-CAN and MTFC-P, and DBT are interventions that require a team to implement. In these cases, the treatment developers are quite specific about the staff characteristics that insure success in implementation. Both of these two training purveyors have sets of criteria for staff members that the implementation sites use.

Implementation-Supporting the Training Process

Ongoing Coaching and Consultation is the mechanism that Fixsen et al. (2005) identified as primary way practitioners learn a new intervention. While in the past, the primary method of training was for an expert to conduct a 2-day workshop presenting information about how to provide an intervention, this method has generally been found to be an ineffective way to transfer information (Herschell et al., 2010). Interestingly, educational researchers have long subscribed to the value of coaching as a powerful mechanism of changing practice (Fixsen et al., 2009). Bruce Joyce & Beverly Showers studied the effectiveness of different methods of teacher trainings and found that 5 % teachers who learned a skill, 10 % of those who also saw it modeled, 20 % of those who practiced it during the training, and 90 % of teachers who were coached on the job, actually incorporated what they learned into their practice (Showers & Joyce, 1996). Possibly because implementation scientists in the field of psychology discovered these findings and championed this approach, over the past decade or so, all of the EBTs described in this volume have adopted some ongoing, practice oriented training or coaching. Their ongoing coaching ranges in intensity from periodic phone conferences, review of video recordings, to video conferencing or telehealth technology discussions, to live coaching either on-site or via telehealth technology. There are a few studies investigating the relative effectiveness of one type of coaching over another, but this area of research is fairly new. Scientists at Oklahoma conducted a randomized controlled trial comparing the effectiveness of phone consults with telehealth in training agencies in PCIT in the state of Washington. Their results showed advantages of telehealth coaching over phone consultations (Funderburk et al., 2011). Telehealth equipment allows trainers to see what their trainees are doing in the moment, and provide feedback while parts of sessions are fresh in their mind. However, telehealth equipment is costly and its accompanying training is also generally more costly, as it is more time and energy intensive than a training using periodic phone conferences for consultation.

A meta-analysis of cognitive-behavioral programs examining predictors of effective treatment, found that greater fidelity to the treatment model predicted better outcomes (Landenberger & Lipsey, 2005). For this reason, and possibly to retain a sense of "EBT identity" (i.e., knowing what specific practices define and do not define a particular EBT), trainers are appropriately concerned with training in a way that emphasizes the need to maintain fidelity to the treatment model. In response to a brief survey of our contributors on training processes, several acknowledged that one concern they had about training was whether the model was practiced with fidelity after the initial training (UC Davis PCIT Training

Center, 2012). Trainers and treatment developers handle their concerns about treatment fidelity and maintaining effectiveness by building in some type of *Staff Performance Assessment.* This is an assessment of the use of skills and outcomes that are taught and coached in the EBT training (Fixsen et al., 2009). The ABC Intervention Group instituted a practice of reviewing and coding each session's parent coaching, to insure consistent quality of treatment provision. The UC Davis PCIT Training Group developed coach coding forms and benchmarks for assessments, and forms for providers to record client outcomes in order to have a mechanism for coaches and trainers to track treatment fidelity and effectiveness. The UC Davis PCIT Training Group found that practitioners are not usually very enthusiastic about tracking outcomes; as this requires additional time in their already busy schedules. However, when there is a valued incentive for tracking outcomes, for instance if it is linked to public acknowledgment of expertise (e.g., identified as experienced in a new work setting, or eligible to be a trainer), then practitioners appear to be more motivated and organized about documentation.

Implementation-Supporting Program Endurance

Taken together, the implementation drivers that support successfully setting up and engaging in EBT training are also integral to building the longevity of the program. For example, administrative commitment and financial support of EBTs and their attending protocols (e.g., use of specific standardized measures, ongoing group supervision, EBT-specific continuing education) are integral to their ongoing sustainment, as are continuing referral streams and funding. In addition to these components, *Decision Support Data Systems,* are a way of measuring and providing information to organizational administration that helps them to make good strategic decisions, such as adjusting clinic procedures to improve the quality of client retention, or improve communication among service providers. These measures can include quality improvement characteristics, program fidelity, and consumer outcomes. Some of the EBTs described in this volume are actively engaged in working with organizations to maintain the quality of their programs. In particular MST-CAN and MTFC-P, whose programs are intertwined with those of their local stakeholders (e.g., CPS, adoptions) actively monitor program outcomes. Triple P took a public health approach in implementing their multilevel program across 18 counties in South Carolina (Prinz, Sanders, Shapiro, Whitaker, & Lutzker, 2009). They instituted data systems to support decision-making at a state level, monitoring the effects of a population-level implementation on statewide maltreatment rates, child out of home placements, and emergency room visits for maltreatment-related injuries. They considered factors such as the objectivity of the measures, the standardization of the data across counties and systems, and the value of change in the indicators.

Summary of Dissemination Efforts

As the authors have described in their respective chapters, all ten of the EBTs have proven to be as successful in practice (i.e., community mental health agencies) as they were in the research setting. The EBT trainers use several different training models, varying in the amount of and type of contact the trainer has with the trainee. EBT trainers vary considerably in the degree to which they use different pre-implementation drivers. They also vary in the degree to which they provide fidelity standards, and require ongoing assessment and fidelity after the initial training and accreditation.

The next step on this journey involves getting practitioners – whether in private practice or affiliated with large agencies – to use these effective interventions. The current challenge is to examine current barriers to implementation – so that maltreated children across the country will have access to an effective intervention to alleviate their mental health problems.

If we are to ensure that practitioners of EBTs continue to provide the same quality of care, in ways that resemble the original EBT, we will all (treatment developers, trainers, and practitioners) need to design ways to track treatment success and quality of care. We also need to continue to find ways to maintain interest and commitment to continued systematic provision of high quality EBT services. While there continue to be barriers to access to EBTs (e.g., limited number of therapists who deliver EBTs, limited number of trainers to teach EBTs, relatively high cost of training, shifting mental health service system delivery systems to incorporate EBT protocols such as pre/post-treatment assessments, intervention fidelity checks, EBT-focused continuing education), the field has made slow, but remarkable progress over the last decade.

References

Allred, C., Markiewicz, J., Amaya-Jackson, L., Putnam, F., Saunders, B., Wilson, C., et al. (2005). *The organizational readiness and capacity assessment*. Durham, NC: UCLA-Duke National Center for Child Traumatic Stress.

California Evidence-Based Clearinghouse for Child Welfare [CEBC]. (2012, December 3). Retrieved from www.cebc4csw.org/search/

California Institute of Mental Health [CIMH]. (2011). *Los Angeles County Department of Mental Health prevention and early intervention (PEI): Evidence-based practices, promising practices, and community defined evidence practices, Resource guide 2.0*. Retrieved from http://file.lacounty.gov/dmh/cms1_159575.pdf

Cohen, J. A., Mannarino, A. P., & Rogal, S. (2001). Treatment practices for childhood posttraumatic stress disorder. *Child Abuse & Neglect, 25*, 123–135.

Dimeff, L. A., Koerner, K., Woodcock, E. A., Beadnell, B., Brown, M. Z., Skutch, J. M., et al. (2009). Which training method works best? A randomized controlled trial comparing three methods of training clinicians in dialectical behavior therapy skills. *Behavioural Research and Therapy, 47*, 921–930.

Fixsen, D., Blase, K., Naoom, S., & Wallace, F. (2009). Core implementation components. *Research on Social Work Practice, 19*(5), 531–540.

Fixsen, D. L., Naoom, S. F., Blase, K. A., Friedman, R. M., & Wallace, F. (2005). *Implementation research: A synthesis of the literature* (FMHI #231). Tampa, FL: University of South Florida, Louis de la Parte Florida Mental Health Institute, The National Implementation Research Network.

Funderburk, B., Bard, E., Nelson, M., Shanley, J., Ware, L., Gurwitch, R., et al. (2011). *Remonte real-time consultation for training PCIT*. Paper presented at the 2011 Biennial International Parent-Child Interaction Therapy Convention, Gainesville, FL.

Gallon, S. L., Gabriel, R. M., & Knudsen, J. R. W. (2003). The toughest job you'll ever love: A Pacific Northwest treatment workforce survey. *Journal of Substance Abuse Treatment, 24*, 183–196.

Ghosh Ippen, C. (2008). *Child parent psychotherapy (CPP) knowledge test*. San Francisco, CA. Unpublished instrument.

Glisson, C., Dukes, D., & Green, P. (2006). The effects of the ARC organizational intervention on caseworker turnover, climate, and culture in children's service systems. *Child Abuse & Neglect, 30*, 855–880.

Goisman, R. M., Warshaw, M. G., & Keller, M. B. (1999). Psychosocial treatment prescriptions for generalized anxiety disorder, panic disorder and social phobia, 1991–1996. *The American Journal of Psychiatry, 156*, 1819–1821.

Herschell, A., Kolko, D., Baumann, B., & Davis, A. (2010). The role of therapist training in the implementation of psychosocial treatments: A review and critique with recommendations. *Clinical Psychology Review, 30*, 448–466.

Insel, T. R. (2009). Translating scientific opportunity into public health impact: A strategic plan for research on mental illness. *Archives of General Psychiatry, 66*(2), 128–133.

Kazak, A. E., Hoagwood, K., Weisz, J. R., Hood, K., Kratochwill, T. R., Vargas, L. A., et al. (2010). A meta-systems approach to evidence based practice for children and adolescents. *American Psychologist, 65*(2), 85–97.

Landenberger, N. A., & Lipsey, M. W. (2005). The positive effects of cognitive-behavioral programs for offenders: A meta-analysis of factors associated with effective treatment. *Journal of Experimental Criminology, 1*, 451–476.

McHugh, R. K., & Barlow, D. H. (2010). The dissemination and implementation of evidence-based psychological treatments. *American Psychologist, 65*(2), 73–84.

McHugh, R. K., Murray, H. W., & Barlow, D. H. (2009). Balancing fidelity and adaptation in the dissemination of empirically-supported treatments: The promise of transdiagnostic interventions. *Behaviour Research and Therapy, 47*, 946–953.

Miller, W. R., Yahne, C. E., Moyers, T. B., Martinez, J., & Pirritano, M. (2004). A randomized trial of methods to help clinicians learn motivational learning. *Journal of Consulting and Clinical Psychology, 72*(6), 1050–1062.

President's New Freedom Commission on Mental Health. (2004). *Report of the President's New Freedom Commission on Mental Health*. Retrieved from http://www.mentalhealthcommission. gov/reports/FinalReport/toc.html

Prinz, R., Sanders, M., Shapiro, C., Whitaker, D., & Lutzker, J. (2009). Population-based prevention of child maltreatment: The U.S. Triple P System population trial. *Prevention Science, 10*, 1–12.

Rogers, E. M. (2003). *Diffusion of innovations* (5th ed.). New York: Free Press.

Sedlar, G., Thomas, J., & Blacker, D. M. (2010, October). *Treatment selection for traumatized children: PCIT or TF-CBT?* 10th annual conference on parent-child interaction therapy, Davis, CA.

Shafran, R., Clark, D., Fairburn, C., Arntz, A., Barlow, D., Ehlers, A., et al. (2009). Mind the gap: Improving the dissemination of CBT. *Behavior Research and Therapy, 47*, 902–909.

Showers, B., & Joyce, B. (1996). The evolution of peer coaching. *Educational Leadership, 53*(6), 12–16.

Sigel, B., & Silovsky, J. (2011). Psychology graduate school training on interventions for child maltreatment. *Psychological Trauma: Theory, Research, Practice, and Policy, 3*(3), 229–234.

Stewart, R. E., & Chambless, D. L. (2007). Does psychotherapy research inform treatment decision in private practice? *Journal of Clinical Psychology, 63*, 267–281. doi:10.1002/jclp.20347.

U.S. Department of Health and Human Services, Administration for Children and Families, Administration on Children, Youth and Families, Children's Bureau. (2011). *Child maltreatment 2010*. Available from http://www.acf.hhs.gov/programs/cb/stats_research/index.htm#can

UC Davis PCIT Training Center. (2012). *EBT training report: Summary of survey responses*. Unpublished report, UC Davis Children's Hospital, Sacramento, CA.

Urquiza, A. J., Timmer, S. G., & Girard, E. (2011). *Dissemination of parent-child interaction therapy: Test of a ToT training model*. Poster presented at the 2011 global implementation conference, Washington, DC.

Wang, P. S., Lane, M., Olfson, M., Pincus, H. A., Wells, K. B., & Kessler, R. C. (2005). Twelve month use of mental health services in the USA: Results from the National Comorbidity Survey Replication. *Archives of General Psychiatry, 62*, 629–640.

Weersing, V. R., & Weisz, J. R. (2002). Community clinic treatment of depressed youth: Benchmarking usual care against CBT clinical trials. *Journal of Consulting and Clinical Psychology, 70*(2), 299–310.

Weissman, M. M., Verdeli, H., Gameroff, M. J., Beldsoe, S. E., Betts, K., Mufson, L., et al. (2006). National survey of psychotherapy training in psychiatry, psychology, and social work. *Archives of General Psychiatry, 63*, 925–934.

Wonderlich, S., Simonich, H., Myers, T., LaMontagne, W., Hoesel, J., Erickson, A. L. (2011). Evidence-based mental health interventions for traumatized youth: A statewide dissemination project. *Behaviour Research and Therapy, 49*(10), 579–587.

Chapter 15
The Bridge from Research to Practice – Just Leap Across the Last Bit

Susan Timmer and Anthony Urquiza

If the set of ten evidence-based interventions described in this volume is representative of all such treatments, what could the future bring but increasing quality and access to mental health services for children? Many developers and researchers have listened to complaints about the generalizability of evidence-based treatments (EBTs), establishing their effectiveness in practice settings and conducted the research that demonstrates that effectiveness (e.g., Hurlburt, Nguyen, Reid, Webster-Stratton, & Zhang, under review; Prinz, Sanders, Shapiro, Whitaker, & Lutzker, 2009; Timmer, Urquiza, Zebell, & McGrath, 2005; Toth, Rogosch, Manly, & Cicchetti, 2006). Other interventions were established in "real world" settings, treating the most difficult cases, in difficult circumstances, like ABC (Chap. 4 by Dozier, Meade, & Bernard, this volume), MTFC-P (Chap. 9 by Gilliam & Fisher, this volume), TF-CBT (Chap. 10 by Mannarino, Cohen, & Deblinger, this volume), AF-CBT (Chap. 11 by Kolko, Simonich, & Loiterstein, this volume), MST-CAN (Chap. 13 by Swenson & Schaeffer, this volume), and DBT (Chap. 12 by Berk, Shelby, Avina, & Tangeman, this volume). There have been complaints that outcome research focuses on narrow reductions of symptom severity rather than change that reflects meaningful differences in clients' lives (Kazdin, 2008) or change on a neurological or biological level that may have some meaning on a developmental trajectory (Curtis & Cicchetti, 2007). In response, some evidence based practice (EBT) researchers have demonstrated changes in children's attachment organization (e.g., Bernard et al., 2012), parent and child emotional availability (Timmer et al., 2011), re-allegations of abuse (Chaffin et al., 2004), reducing out of home placements (Swenson, Schaeffer, Henggeler, Faldowski, & Mayhew, 2010). In order to establish "multilevel change," researchers have showed the relationship between

S. Timmer, Ph.D. (✉) • A. Urquiza, Ph.D.
CAARE Diagnostic and Treatment Center, Department of Pediatrics, University
of California at Davis Children's Hospital, 3671 Business Dr., Sacramento, CA 95820, USA
e-mail: susan.timmer@ucdmc.ucdavis.edu; anthony.urquiza@ucdmc.ucdavis.edu

S. Timmer and A. Urquiza (eds.), *Evidence-Based Approaches for the Treatment
of Maltreated Children*, Child Maltreatment 3, DOI 10.1007/978-94-007-7404-9_15,
© Springer Science+Business Media Dordrecht 2014

treatment participation and change in cortisol levels (Dozier, Bernard, Bick, & Gordon, 2012, cited in Dozier et al., this volume), and normalization of diurnal cortisol patterns (Fisher, Stoolmiller, Gunnar, & Burraston, 2007), though they do not measure cortisol levels as a rule during treatment. The sum of these studies suggest that EBT researchers are committed to giving real meaning to the positive outcomes they have found, giving life to the changes in scale scores on standardized assessments they also report. While the improvements in the quality of EBT outcome research certainly reflect a response to legitimate criticisms about the quality and meaningfulness of RCTs for clinical practice, some of the effort researchers have made also must be related to the understanding that they are dependent on the practitioners to prove the merit of their intervention. Once researchers enter the world of clinical practice in the service of maltreated children, the issues become more complex. There is the complexity of EBT researchers relying on the clinical judgments of therapists working in community mental health agencies to demonstrate the robustness of their intervention.

As we saw in the previous chapter's table describing training procedures, the EBTs discussed here did not limit training to any particular type of therapist. We conclude that the interventions were designed for any therapist to use effectively, given their interest and commitment. Considering the generic qualifications for these EBTs, it is easy to forget that their effectiveness depends on therapists' clinical judgment. Clinical judgment, defined as a way of conceptualizing a client's case and making decisions about treatment is viewed warily by treatment developers, for it has not fared well in evaluations over the years (Kazdin, 2008). Some treatment developers try to control the effects of therapists' clinical judgment on their protocols by simplifying directions, manualizing the treatment, hoping to give the therapist as much training as possible to take their judgment out of the equation of effectiveness. But there really is no possible way that a treatment developer can imagine all possible crazy scenarios that might occur in the therapy room. At some point a therapist will have to "tailor" the intervention to the needs of the client. In a discussion of the tension between clinical research and practice, Kazdin notes that in spite of the problems that "tailoring" causes the measurement of EBT effectiveness, researchers give practitioners very little help or structure for making these difficult decisions. Why wouldn't treatment developers organize "tailoring" as they organized their protocol? The answer is likely varied, but it is certainly partly related to the difference between "tailoring" and "adapting" treatment protocols.

Therapists "tailor" a protocol to the needs of a client. Since each client's needs are unique, in theory, each "tailoring" should also be unique and thus difficult to anticipate. Hence one doesn't tailor a protocol to a class of clients, since by definition a "class" has shared characteristics. One "adapts" to a class of clients. Once therapists "adapt" a protocol, however, they are providing a different treatment, not the treatment supported by the RCT. In sum, unless a systematic tailoring is supported by an RCT, a treatment developer would not be likely to incorporate a practice recommendation into protocol. Even if a tailoring technique were supported by an RCT, a treatment developer might not accept it if the technique were not consistent with his or her theoretical approach.

This reluctance to guide therapists' decision-making with respect to tailoring can have unanticipated consequences. Consider the fact that there are many EBTs and therapists may receive training on more than one intervention. Therapists make clinical judgments about how to "tailor" EBTs, sometimes using strategies from another EBT to bridge a perceived limitation in the first. For example, a PCIT therapist told us about a 5-year old boy and his mother who had been exposed to severe domestic violence that she was treating. The boy seemed agitated and easily emotionally dysregulated in clinic sessions, so the therapist (also trained in TF-CBT) decided that to make progress in PCIT, she needed to introduce "feeling identification" into the fabric of treatment. During check-in at the beginning of the session, the therapist introduced this concept and decided to regularly ask about their feeling states. At times during coaching, when the therapist perceived the need, she would identify for the parent the child's feeling state, and coach the parent to mention something about it. This strategy is decidedly outside the protocol of both PCIT and TF-CBT, but a legitimate tailoring technique. However, the therapist believed that it worked so well for her that she wanted to use it with all her clients that had been exposed to domestic violence. The therapist's enthusiasm for a tailoring strategy that worked for her should be both expected and understandable, as an outgrowth of clinical judgment. But, this kind of creativity is more likely to make EBT researchers shiver in their boots.

In addition to therapists' judgment shaping the content of an intervention, clinical judgment may also determine client progress in treatment. When progress is based on clinical judgment, there is a concern that therapists may see what they want to see based on the quality of their relationship with the client rather than on the client's improvement, in the same way that a culturally insensitive interventions might cause therapists to select and work on treatment goals that reflected their own cultures rather than that of the client (Comas Diaz, 2006). As a way to combat possible negative effects of clinical judgment on outcomes, an EBT might incorporate assessment tools into the treatment protocol to guide therapists' judgment and actions (as in the case of PCIT, DBT, and MTFC-P), use a curriculum (as in the case of ABC, Triple P, or IY), or a semi-structured curriculum with benchmarks (as in the case TF-CBT). However, even incorporating assessments into a treatment protocol does not insure that therapists will pay attention to them

The availability heuristic is a social psychological principle that tells us that when people make judgments about the probability of events, that they will use information that comes most easily to mind, following the logic of "if you can think of it, it must be true" (Tversky & Kahneman, 1973). In our experience, therapists fall prey to the availability heuristic by giving more weight to what they see and hear in front of them in interactions with clients than they do results of standardized assessments when making clinical decisions. Their own observations are more "available" to them, so they seem truer than results of standardized assessments. And as a result they may discount the results of assessments or forget to administer them altogether. In the anecdote related above with the therapist using TF-CBT strategies in PCIT, for example, the therapist was not able to substantiate her belief that her creative strategy was successful with any objective assessments, nor was she able to reconstruct exactly what she did or the effect that she had by reviewing videotapes. We advised her to systematically assess the effects of her strategy before recommending its use to other clinicians and praised her for her cleverness.

With so many EBTs with similar theoretical foundations (e.g., positive parenting techniques) being used for maltreated children, it could be difficult for therapists to keep protocols straight. For example, in Los Angeles County, one of the largest county mental health systems in the United States, providers can bill for any of 32 different EBTs (Los Angeles County Department of Mental Health, 2012). Distinctive strategies for managing difficult child behavior that one treatment developer believes to be important may be forgotten or ignored if it is not supported in other protocols. In an advanced PCIT training in Seattle, Washington, in 2012, the trainer commented on parents counting out loud when giving a warning to go to time out: "It may be effective parenting, but it's not PCIT." Using this kind of "because I said so" distinction may not be helpful in the long run. When giving therapists rules to guide their behavior, it is important to give an overarching principle that identifies a goal to help guide decision-making (e.g., Welch, 2002) so that therapists can develop "meta-competences" – a higher level of competence associated with understanding a model's theory and application, and the ability to work flexibly with the model (Roth & Pilling, 2007).

To sum up, EBT researchers have been slow to acknowledge the power of individuals and their clinical judgment to influence the effectiveness of their intervention and its adoption by the clinical field. It is possible for individuals to have a positive, creative influence on EBTs, with systematic assessment. EBT researchers could benefit from incorporating implementation realities into their protocol, acknowledging, guiding, and supporting clinical decision-making, and showing an understanding of the environment in which these decisions are made: the community mental health agency. While some of the inconsistency in the effectiveness of implementing EBTs (e.g., Weersing & Weisz, 2002) can be attributed to not understanding the "human factor," there is considerable research that suggests that organizational social construct – culture, climate, and work attitudes play an influential role in the effectiveness of EBT implementation (e.g., Glisson et al., 2008).

In an effort to comprehend the community mental health setting, it is useful to remember a few facts about volume and types of clients that therapists see in community mental health practice, in addition to a description of the kinds of therapists who see them. According to the Child Maltreatment 2010 report (U.S. Department of Health and Human Services, Administration for Children and Families, Administration on Children, Youth and Families, & Children's Bureau, 2011), approximately 60 % of maltreated children are referred for some kind of child welfare services, including mental health treatment. An earlier study investigating the mental health needs of children involved with child welfare showed that nearly half of children had clinically significant emotional or behavioral problems (Burns et al., 2004). Most maltreated children receiving mental health services are eligible to receive treatment through publicly funded mental health service systems (Burns et al.), Agencies that provide mental health services for their child welfare population are likely to be state or county departments of mental health, or non-profit community mental health agencies that are supported by county, state, or federal matching funds. These agencies typically have high levels of staff turnover, and particularly among the front line workers, showing evidence of 'burnout' (Paris & Hoge, 2010). Additionally, while state licensing regulations require that a licensed mental health professional be responsible for every case, in our experience visiting hundreds of agencies across the State of California and throughout the United States, clients treated in public mental health systems appear most likely to be seen by unlicensed staff, with varying amounts of administrative and clinical oversight. This is not to suggest that these licensed staff members are poor mental health providers, but they are less experienced in providing mental health services and may have less understanding of the effects of maltreatment on children, and confronted with complex and distressing clinical problems. Thus, between therapist burnout, the inconsistent work environment caused by turnover, and the deficit in emotional resources caused by therapists' inexperience, it may be difficult for maltreated children to get the full benefit of empirically based treatments staff have been trained to provide.

Community mental health agencies vary in size and health, but whether large or small, are generally dependent on staff work effort to make their budgets. For most mental health programs, work effort is determined by an examination of the number of staff work hours, caseload sizes, and productivity expectations (which are often calculated by therapist treatment hours or billable minutes). Healthy organizations have lighter productivity requirements, smaller caseloads, and build in training time. Less healthy organizations demand more from their staff, or may try different strategies to reduce overhead. Often, the balance of agency fiscal health rests on exhausting staff through having too large of a caseload, or too severe of a productivity expectation – and attempting to generate sufficient income to maintain staff salaries. In this balance, needing too high of a work effort from staff to keep the doors open can create an unhealthy work climate: staff may feel resentful about the pressure to produce and the lack of support, perceiving that the quality of care they provide is less important to the agency than the quantity of billing. High productivity requirements may also make it difficult for therapists to provide quality services, possibly diminishing their sense of gratification from helping clients. There is a thin profit margin separating healthy from less healthy organizations. Budgets and contracts are executed from year to year, dependent on state and local funding, and agency administrators never exactly know whether they will be able to cover the costs of salaries from 1 year to the next.

With this brief description of community mental health agencies' resources, hopefully the reader will understand how important each billable minute is to their overall bottom line. The cost of contracting with EBT trainers is high. When an agency's administrators decide to spend them money and have therapists trained in an EBT, they are likely imagining that having these skills will increase their marketability, their revenue stream, and their ultimate organizational health. It is doubtful that they have any idea how much training time will detract from productivity, or how much time it will take to maintain an EBT as a viable program in their agency. While EBTs can bring about many positive changes in an organizations' culture – such as feeling empowered by the success of the services provided, mandating systematic assessment – it can also increase the workload for trainees or reduce productivity. If the reduction in productivity is unanticipated, increasing the workload for trainees, then their commitment to training may also shrink – as the training values (e.g., quality is important) are not well-supported by organizational need (e.g., quantity is mandated). At the 2012 Annual UC Davis PCIT Conference, Lucy Berliner gave a keynote, speaking about the future of EBTs. Her comments illustrate some of the difficulties community mental health agencies have implementing EBTs:

> Well, can we really have five different supervision groups and fidelity monitoring schemes? … I am a mental health center. I mean [we] might be small, but we have to deal with all of this. And I'm like, "Forget it. That's not feasible." And you get these people sitting in the universities, and literally, they will say things like, "Well, that's just what you have to do." And I'm like, "Really? I'll tell you we can outlast you in not doing something if it isn't feasible." (Berliner, 2012)

Future Directions and Policy Implications

Hopefully the descriptions of the limitations and promises of mental health treatment in community mental health agencies resound in the ears of funders and policy makers. The cost of training is greater than the amount of money an agency must pay to an EBT expert. There are real initial investments agencies must make in terms of productivity that will not likely be realized for at least a year. Interestingly, a recent (2012) training project implementing PCIT in Los Angeles County funded by First 5 LA included monies for LA County Department of Mental Health to reimburse agencies for the lost productivity hours needed for effective training. While the outcomes of this strategy remains to be documented, we believe this is a needed step for successfully implementing an EBT in a County Mental Health System.

Many implementation scholars have argued for the importance of conducting research on the mechanisms of change and identifying core components of EBTs (e.g., Fixsen, Blase, Naoom, & Wallace, 2009; Fixsen, Naoom, Blase, Friedman, & Wallace, 2005; Herschell, Kolko, Baumann, & Davis, 2010; Kazdin, 2008). We affirm this need, giving credit to Deblinger and her colleagues for beginning this effort in TF-CBT research (Deblinger, Mannarino, Cohen, Runyon, & Steer, 2011). EBT researchers need to understand better the limits of their intervention's effectiveness and publishing these results – including difficult-to-swallow research, like "this CAN work for this type of client, but maybe only in certain circumstances." This is sometimes difficult, because it runs counter to our desire to believe the best of our respective programs.

In our opinion, agencies that understand the role their organization plays in the implementation of EBTs are indeed more successful in their implementation, as a considerable body of literature suggests (e.g., Glisson et al., 2008). EBT trainers need to be deliberate about educating agencies about the process of pre-implementation, helping the administrative staff understand the sacrifices they may have to make to insure long-term success providing EBTs. Trainers and researchers of EBTs could also be more helpful in recommending staff for training. UC Davis PCIT Training Center has made recommendations like, "therapists that are in the process of learning another EBT should probably not be selected for training in a second;" and, "interns who will leave in 8 months should not be the sole recipients of EBT training, because in 8 months the agency will need to train an entirely new set of therapists at great cost and expense." While these are common sense recommendations, EBT researchers could investigate predictors of training success. We all (EBT researchers, trainers, agency administration, therapists) need to embrace the idea that systematic evaluation is a reflection not of therapist ability, but as a way of contributing to our knowledge about the limits of EBTs. The heart and soul of Empirically Based Practice is the assurance that some strategy we use to treat maltreated children and their families should work. If it doesn't work we need to pick apart and examine the whole system.

References

Berliner, L. (2012). PCIT in context: EBP for the future. Keynote address delivered at the UC Davis annual PCIT conference, 2012. Davis, CA. http://www.youtube.com/watch?v=EBX9v60u9T0

Bernard, K., Dozier, M., Bick, J., Lewis-Morrarty, E., Lindhiem, O., & Carlson, E. (2012). Enhancing attachment organization among maltreated infants: Results of a randomized clinical trial. *Child Development, 83*, 623–636.

Burns, B., Phillips, S., Wagner, H. R., Barth, R., Kolko, D., Campbell Y., et al. (2004). Mental health need and access to mental health services by youths involved with child welfare: A national survey. *Journal of the American Academy of Child & Adolescent Psychiatry, 43*(8), 960–970.

Chaffin, M., Silovsky, J., Funderburk, B., Valle, L. A., Brestan, E., Balachova, T., et al. (2004). Parent–child interaction therapy with physically abusive parents: Efficacy for reducing future abuse reports. *Journal of Consulting and Clinical Psychology, 72*(3), 500–510.

Comas Diaz, L. (2006). Latino healing: The integration of ethnic psychology into psychotherapy. *Psychotherapy: Theory, Research, Practice, Training, 43*(4), 436–453.

Curtis, W. J., & Cicchetti, D. (2007). Emotion and resilience: A multi-level investigation of hemispheric electroencephalogram asymmetry and emotion regulation in maltreated and non-maltreated children. *Development and Psychopathology, 19*(3), 811–840.

Deblinger, E., Mannarino, A. P., Cohen, J., Runyon, M. K., & Steer, R. A. (2011). Trauma-focused cognitive-behavioral therapy for children· Impact of the trauma narrative and treatment length. *Depression and Anxiety, 28*, 67–75. doi:10.1002/da.20744.

Dozier, M., Bernard, K., Bick, J., & Gordon, M. K. (2012). *Normalizing the diurnal production of cortisol: The effects of an early intervention for high-risk children.* Unpublished manuscript, University of Delaware, Newark, DE.

Fisher, P. A., Stoolmiller, M., Gunnar, M. R., & Burraston, B. O. (2007). Effects of a therapeutic intervention for foster preschoolers on diurnal cortisol activity. *Psychoneuroendocrinology, 32*, 892–905. doi:10.1016/j.psyneuen.2007.06.008.

Fixsen, D., Blase, K., Naoom, S., & Wallace, F. (2009). Core implementation components. *Research on Social Work Practice, 19*(5), 531–540.

Fixsen, D. L., Naoom, S. F., Blase, K. A., Friedman, R. M., & Wallace, F. (2005). *Implementation research: A synthesis of the literature* (FMHI #231). Tampa, FL: University of South Florida, Louis de la Parte Florida Mental Health Institute, The National Implementation Research Network.

Glisson, C., Landsverk, J., Schoenwald, S., Kelleher, K., Hoagwood, K., Mayberg, S., et al. (2008). Assessing the Organizational Social Context (OSC) of mental health services: Implications for research and practice. *Administration and Policy in Mental Health, 35*, 98–113.

Herschell, A., Kolko, D., Baumann, B., & Davis, A. (2010). The role of therapist training in the implementation of psychosocial treatments: A review and critique with recommendations. *Clinical Psychology Review, 30,* 448–468.

Hurlburt, M. S., Nguyen, K., Reid, J., Webster-Stratton, C., & Zhang, J. (2013). Efficacy of the Incredible Years group parent program with families in Head Start who self-reported a history of child maltreatment. *Child Abuse & Neglect, 37*(8), 531–543. doi:10.1016/j.chiabu.2012.10.008

Kazdin, A. (2008). Evidence-based treatment and practice: New opportunities to bridge clinical research and practice, enhance the knowledge base, and improve care. *American Psychologist, 63*(3), 146–159.

Los Angeles County Department of Mental Health. (2012). *Mental Health Services Act: Annual update, Fiscal Year 2012–2013.* http://file.lacounty.gov/dmh/cms1_179197.pdf. Retrieved 18 Dec 12.

Paris, M., & Hoge, M. A. (2010). Burnout in the mental health workforce: A review. *Journal of Behavioral Health Services and Research, 37*(4), 519–528.

Prinz, R., Sanders, M., Shapiro, C., Whitaker, D., & Lutzker, J. (2009). Population-based prevention of child maltreatment: The U.S. Triple P System Population Trial. *Prevention Science, 10,* 1–12.

Roth, A. D., & Pilling, S. (2007). *The competences required to deliver effective cognitive and behavioural therapy for people with depression and with anxiety disorders.* Available from http://www.dh.gov.uk/prod_consum_dh/groups/dh_digitalassets/@dh/@en/documents/digitalasset/dh_078535.pdf. Retrieved 18 Dec 12.

Swenson, C. C., Schaeffer, C. M., Henggeler, S. W., Faldowski, R., & Mayhew, A. (2010). Multisystemic therapy for child abuse and neglect: A randomized effectiveness trial. *Journal of Family Psychology, 24,* 497–507.

Timmer, S., Ho, L., Urquiza, A., Zebell, N., Fernandez y Garcia, E., & Boys, D. (2011). The effectiveness of Parent-child Interaction Therapy with depressive mothers: The changing relationship as the agent of individual change. *Child Psychiatry & Human Development, 42*(4), 406–423.

Timmer, S., Urquiza, A., Zebell, N., & McGrath, J. (2005). Parent-child interaction therapy: Application to physically abusive and high-risk dyads. *Child Abuse & Neglect, 29,* 825–842.

Toth, S. L., Rogosch, F. A., Manly, J. T., & Cicchetti, D. (2006). The efficacy of toddler-parent psychotherapy to reorganize attachment in the young offspring of mothers with major depressive disorder: A randomized preventive trial. *Journal of Consulting and Clinical Psychology, 74*(6), 1006–1016.

Tversky, A., & Kahneman, D. (1973). Availability: A heuristic for judging frequency and probability. *Cognitive Psychology, 5*(1), 207–233. doi:10.1016/0010-0285(73)90033-9.

U.S. Department of Health and Human Services, Administration for Children and Families, Administration on Children, Youth and Families, Children's Bureau. (2011). *Child maltreatment 2010.* Available from http://www.acf.hhs.gov/programs/cb/stats_research/index.htm#can

Weersing, V. R., & Weisz, J. R. (2002). Community clinic treatment of depressed youth: Benchmarking usual care against CBT clinical trials. *Journal of Consulting and Clinical Psychology, 70*(2), 299–310.

Welch, D. (2002). *Decisions, decisions: The art of effective decision-making.* Amherst, NY: Prometheus Books.

Author Bios

Claudia Avina, Ph.D. is a licensed clinical psychologist, specializing in work with children and adolescents. She received her doctorate from the University of Nevada, Reno, and completed postdoctoral training in the Child and Adolescent Psychiatry program at Harbor-UCLA Medical Center, focusing on DBT and child trauma. She also served as a Research Psychologist and Project Director for a clinical research study aimed at reducing health risk behaviors among depressed adolescents in a primary care setting, as part of the Youth Stress and Mood Program at UCLA. She has extensive clinical and research experience working with youth diagnosed with mood and anxiety disorders. More recently, she has specialized in the delivery of cognitive-behavioral treatments and Dialectical Behavior Therapy (DBT) for suicidal adolescents. She currently serves as a Project Director and DBT therapist for the CARES Study, a multi-site, randomized controlled trial examining the effectiveness of DBT with suicidal teens.

Michele S. Berk, Ph.D. is a licensed clinical psychologist, Associate Professor of Psychiatry, and Director of the Adolescent DBT Program at Harbor-UCLA Medical Center. She earned her bachelor's degree at the University of California, Berkeley and her Ph.D. at New York University. She completed a post-doctoral fellowship with Dr. Aaron T. Beck at the University of Pennsylvania. The focus of her research is on psychotherapy approaches for suicidal behavior. She is currently a Principal Investigator on a multi-site, randomized clinical trial of DBT with adolescents, in collaboration with Dr. Marsha Linehan. She was recently awarded the Young Investigator Award from the Los Angeles Biomedical Research Institute at Harbor-UCLA. Dr. Berk is the founder of the adolescent DBT program at Harbor-UCLA, which serves suicidal and self-harming adolescents in the county system. She has also provided numerous trainings on DBT and other CBT approaches to clinicians working in Los Angeles County.

S. Timmer and A. Urquiza (eds.), *Evidence-Based Approaches for the Treatment of Maltreated Children*, Child Maltreatment 3, DOI 10.1007/978-94-007-7404-9,
© Springer Science+Business Media Dordrecht 2014

Kristin Bernard, Ph.D. is assistant professor at Stony Brook University, having received her Ph.D. from the University of Delaware in 2013. She completed an internship at University of Illinois-Chicago in 2013. Kristin is interested in the effects of early adversity (e.g., maltreatment, foster care, institutional care) on children's development of behavioral and neurobiological regulation, as well as the buffering effects of early interventions, caregiver commitment, and attachment quality for these children. She is also involved in efforts to disseminate the interventions, including training and supervision of new parent trainers.

Judith A. Cohen, M.D. is a Board Certified Child & Adolescent Psychiatrist, Medical Director of the Center for Traumatic Stress in Children & Adolescents at Allegheny General Hospital (AGH) in Pittsburgh, PA, and Professor of Psychiatry at Drexel University College of Medicine. Dr. Cohen is one of the co-developers of Trauma-Focused Cognitive Behavioral Therapy (TF-CBT). Together they have written the book *Treating Trauma and Traumatic Grief in Children and Adolescents*. Since 1983, Dr. Cohen has been funded by more than a dozen federally supported grants to conduct research related to the assessment and treatment of abused and traumatized children. Dr. Cohen was the first author of ISTSS's first edition of published guidelines for treating childhood PTSD, and co-editor of the second edition of this book. Dr. Cohen is the Principal Author of the Practice Parameters for the assessment and treatment of childhood Posttraumatic Stress Disorder published by the American Academy of Child & Adolescent Psychiatry (AACAP). AACAP awarded her its 2004 Rieger Award for Scientific Achievement. Dr. Cohen has published and taught extensively related to the assessment and treatment of childhood trauma.

Esther Deblinger, Ph.D. is a licensed clinical psychologist and professor at the University of Medicine and Dentistry of New Jersey–School of Osteopathic Medicine. She is co-founder and co-director of the New Jersey Child Abuse Research Education and Service (CARES) Institute, which is a member center of the National Child Traumatic Stress Network (NCTSN).

Dr. Deblinger has conducted extensive clinical research examining the mental health impact of child abuse and the treatment of PTSD and other abuse-related difficulties. She has authored numerous scientific articles and book chapters, and published four books including, *Treating Sexually Abused Children and Their Nonoffending Parents: A Cognitive Behavioral Approach*.

Dr. Deblinger is one of the co-developers of Trauma-Focused Cognitive-Behavioral Therapy (TF-CBT). In 2001, TF-CBT was given an "Exemplary Program Award" by the US Department of Health and Human Services, Substance Abuse and Mental Health Services Administration. In 2004 it was named a Best Practice by the Kauffman Best Practices Task Force of the NCTSN, and was given the highest classification for an evidence based practice by the US Department of Justice sponsored report, Child Physical and Sexual Abuse: Guidelines for Treatment.

Mary Dozier, Ph.D. is the Amy E. du Pont Chair of Child Development at the University of Delaware. She is the Principal Investigator of the school's Infant

Caregiver Project. Her interests in understanding connections between experience, brain development, and behavior have led to the ABC Intervention, a practical application of findings from years of research.

Since coming to Delaware in 1994, Mary has studied the development of young children who are neglected and young foster children. She has developed training programs for the caregivers of these children, with efficacy trials funded by the National Institute of Mental Health. Mary was promoted to Associate Professor in 1996, Full Professor in 2004, and Amy E. du Pont Chair of Child Development in 2004. She is the recipient of the Bowlby-Ainsworth Award for Translational Research on Adoption. She serves as a regular member of an NIMH study section and is on several editorial boards.

Phillip A. Fisher, Ph.D. is a Professor of Psychology (clinical) at the University of Oregon and a Senior Scientist at the Oregon Social Learning Center (OSLC). He is also Science Director for the National Forum on Early Childhood Policy and Programs and a Senior Fellow at the Center on the Developing Child, both based at Harvard University. Dr. Fisher's work on children in foster care and the child welfare system includes (a) basic research characterizing the effects of early stress on neurobiological systems such as the HPA axis and areas of the prefrontal cortex involved in executive functioning; (b) the development of preventive interventions, including the Multidimensional Treatment Foster Care Program for Preschoolers (MTFC-P) and the Kids in Transition to School Program (KITS); and (c) the dissemination of evidence-based practice in community settings.

Lindsay A. Forte is the Parent-child Interaction Therapy (PCIT) Training Coordinator at the UC Davis CAARE Diagnostic & Treatment Center. She has Bachelor's degrees in Psychology and Human Development from UC Davis, and is pursuing a Master's in Child Development at UC Davis. At the CAARE Center, Lindsay coordinates PCIT training of agencies across the country, and is active in disseminating information about PCIT services to clients and clinicians alike. She also manages the PCIT website, National Listserv, and agency database, while acting as a resource for trainees and those interested in PCIT. Her interests in child development and evidence-based practice drive her to help agencies implement treatments that will be available to at-risk children and caregivers that need them most

Kathryn S. Gilliam is a doctoral student in clinical psychology at the University of Oregon. She earned her undergraduate degree in Neuroscience from the University of Michigan. Her research interests in translational developmental neuroscience involve better understanding the effects of early life stress on underlying physiological systems and the brain. Specifically, she is interested in elucidating how different forms of maltreatment (e.g., abuse vs. neglect) may differentially impact the neuro-endocrine stress system and how these effects unfold developmentally over time. She is also interested in the mechanisms by which interventions such as Multidimensional Treatment Foster Care for Preschoolers (MTFC-P) affect positive change in the stress system and child outcomes more broadly.

Nicole Hollis, Ph.D. is a lecturer in Human Development in the Department of Human Development and Ecology at UC Davis. She earned her B.S. in Human Development and in Biological Sciences, her M.S. in Child Development, and her Ph.D. in Human Development at UC Davis. Dr. Hollis's dissertation focuses on assessing risk markers for and outcomes of child maltreatment and the effectiveness of Parent-child Interaction Therapy (PCIT) as an intervention to improve child externalizing behavior and parent-child relationships for maltreated children. Dr. Hollis is currently studying the differential effects of PCIT on mothers' perceptions of improvement in their maltreated children's externalizing problem behavior based on mothers' reports of their own depressive symptoms, cumulative risk models for the occurrence of maltreatment, and the effects of psychological control by parents and siblings.

David J. Kolko, Ph.D., ABPP, is a Professor of Psychiatry, Psychology, Pediatrics, and Clinical and Translational Science, at the University of Pittsburgh School of Medicine. He is Director of the Special Services Unit at Western Psychiatric Institute and Clinic, a program devoted to the development and dissemination of evidence-based practices for children/adolescents served in diverse community settings or systems including juvenile justice, child welfare, pediatric primary care, and mental health. Dr. Kolko served two terms on the Board of Directors of the American Professional Society on the Abuse of Children, was Co-Chair of its Research Committee, and received its Research Career Achievement Award for 2001. Much of his current work is directed towards the dissemination and evaluation of "Alternatives for Families: A Cognitive Behavioral Therapy" (AF-CBT; www.afcbt.org). A book co-written with Dr. Cindy Swenson, *Assessing and Treating Physically Abused Children and Their Families: A Cognitive-Behavioral Approach* (2002, Sage Publications, Thousand Oaks, CA) describes AF-CBT.

A sample of Dr. Kolko's clinical research activities and articles may be found online at http://www.pitt.edu/~kolko

Anna Loiterstein, B.S. is a graduate of Carnegie Mellon University with a Bachelor of Science in Psychology. She will attend a doctoral program in child clinical psychology at Yeshiva University.

Anthony P. Mannarino, Ph.D. is the Director of the Center for Traumatic Stress in Children and Adolescents and Vice Chair, Department of Psychiatry, Allegheny General Hospital, Pittsburgh, PA. He is also Professor of Psychiatry at the Drexel University College of Medicine. Dr. Mannarino has been a leader in the field of child traumatic stress for the past 25 years. He has been awarded numerous federal grants from the National Center on Child Abuse and Neglect and the National Institute of Mental Health. Dr. Mannarino has received many honours for his work, including the Betty Elmer Outstanding Professional Award, the Model Program Award from the Substance Abuse and Mental Health Services Administration for "Cognitive Behavioral Therapy for Child Traumatic Stress." Dr. Mannarino has recently completed 2-year terms as the President of APSAC. He is one of the co-developers of Trauma-Focused Cognitive-Behavioral Therapy (TF-CBT).

Elizabeth Meade joined the Infant Caregiver Project in 2011 as a graduate student in the Clinical Science Program at the University of Delaware. Before joining the lab, she received her B.A. in Psychology from Stanford University in 2009 and worked as a research assistant at Brown University for 2 years. Her research interests include efficacy, effectiveness and dissemination of the parent training interventions, as well as moderating factors that influence the interventions success with different families.

John A. Pickering is a Ph.D. scholar at The University of Queensland, where he also earned his undergraduate degree. He has been a research associate at the Parenting and Family Support Centre for over 5 years, with his primary research focussed on ways of destigmatizing the notion of parents seeking parenting support and enhancing population-level impact of parenting intervention. He is a trained and accredited Triple P practitioner.

Vilma Reyes, Psy.D. is a licensed clinical psychologist who provides Child-parent Psychotherapy and coordinates community-based mental health outreach services and evaluation at the University of California, San Francisco, Department of Psychiatry in the Child Trauma Research Program.

She has over 11 years of experience providing community based services to children birth to five and their families and offering trainings about early childhood and the impact of trauma to community providers. Dr. Reyes is bilingual and bicultural and specializes in working with low income Latino immigrant families.

Matthew R. Sanders, Ph.D. is a Professor of Clinical Psychology and Director of the Parenting and Family Support Centre at the University of Queensland. As the founder of the Triple P-Positive Parenting Program, Professor Sanders is considered a world leader in the development, implementation, evaluation and dissemination of population based approaches to parenting and family interventions. Triple P is currently in use across many countries worldwide. Professor Sanders' work centres on research and dissemination efforts geared towards delivering effective, evidence-based parenting intervention at a population level.

Cindy M. Schaeffer, Ph.D. is a child-clinical psychologist and Associate Professor of Psychiatry within the Family Services Research Center at the Medical University of South Carolina. She completed her doctorate at the University of Missouri, a child-clinical internship at the University of Maryland Baltimore, and a post-doctoral fellowship in prevention science at the Johns Hopkins Bloomberg School of Public Health. Her areas of expertise include juvenile offending, substance abuse, child maltreatment, adolescent peer relationships, and family-based interventions. She is a developer of Multisystemic Therapy-Building Stronger Families (MST-BSF), designed to serve families involved in the child protective service system for the co-occurring problem of parental substance abuse and child maltreatment. Dr. Schaeffer is the author of numerous scientific articles and one book entitled, *Reinforcement-Based Treatment for Substance Use Disorders: A Comprehensive Behavioral Approach.*

Janine Shelby, Ph.D. is the Director of Child Trauma Clinic at Harbor-UCLA and an Associate Professor in the Geffen School of Medicine at UCLA. She completed her doctoral work at the University of Miami, and then specialized in Child and Adolescent Psychology during her post-doctoral fellowship at Harbor-UCLA Medical Center. Dr. Shelby served as President of the Association for Play Therapy Foundation, Consultant to the National Center for Child Traumatic Stress, and Clinical Director of the Rape Treatment Center at Santa Monica-UCLA Medical Center. She has assisted in numerous, world-wide humanitarian relief efforts. She has published and presented extensively on the integration of developmentally sensitive and evidence-based treatments for traumatized youth.

Heather Simonich, M.A. earned her Master's Degree in Counseling Psychology from Ball State University in Muncie, Indiana. She is a Research Coordinator and Psychological Assessor at the Neuropsychiatric Research Institute in Fargo, North Dakota. She is the recipient of the 2012 Bush Fellowship Award. She currently serves as the Project Coordinator for the Treatment Collaborative for Traumatized Youth and has received advanced training in evidence-based practices for treating childhood trauma, including Alternatives for Families: A Cognitive Behavioral Therapy (AF-CBT). She routinely provides training and consultation to child-serving organizations on the topic of child traumatic stress. As a Licensed Professional Counselor, she maintains a clinical practice serving traumatized children and their families.

Cynthia Cupit Swenson, Ph.D. is a Clinical Psychologist and Professor at the Family Services Research Center in the Department of Psychiatry and Behavioral Sciences of the Medical University of South Carolina. She is developer of the Multisystemic Therapy for Child Abuse and Neglect treatment model based on a 5-year NIMH-funded randomized clinical trial. She is also a model developer for Multisystemic Therapy – Building Stronger Families (MST-BSF), a treatment model for families experiencing co-occurring child maltreatment plus parental substance abuse. She has conducted research in the child abuse and neglect area nationally and internationally for over 20 years. In addition, Dr. Swenson has authored many journal articles and recent books on treatment for physical abuse, youth substance abuse, and treating community violence and troubled neighborhoods. She is also involved in community development and health projects in Ghana, West Africa.

Keegan R. Tangeman, Psy.D. is a licensed clinical psychologist, specializing in work with children and adolescents. He received his doctorate from Pepperdine University. Dr. Tangeman completed postdoctoral training in Child and Adolescent Psychiatry at Harbor-UCLA Medical Center, where he specialized in child and adolescent trauma and DBT with adolescents. While at Harbor-UCLA, he served as the Assistant Director of the adolescent DBT program, and was the founder and director of the Behavior Assessment and Treatment clinic for youth with disruptive behavior disorders. He is currently the director of mental health services at STAR of California, where he oversees community mental health treatment as well as a clinical training program. Dr. Tangeman maintains faculty positions at both Harbor-UCLA Medical Center and Pepperdine University and serves as a Project Director and DBT therapist for the CARES Study, a multi-site, randomized controlled trial examining the effectiveness of DBT with suicidal adolescents.

Susan Timmer, Ph.D. is a research scientist at the CAARE Diagnostic and Treatment Center and PCIT Training program manager at the PCIT Training Center at University of California Davis Children's Hospital. She is also a faculty member of the Human Development Graduate Group at UC Davis, and Clinical Assistant Professor in the Department of Pediatrics, at the UC Davis Children's Hospital. Dr. Timmer was a co-developer of the PCIT for Traumatized Children Web Course (pcit.ucdavis.edu). Her research focuses on evaluating the dissemination and implementation of PCIT, as well as its effectiveness. She also investigates parent-child relationship processes in the context of children's experience of maltreatment.

Anthony Urquiza, Ph.D. is a clinical psychologist, professor in Pediatrics, and Director of both the CAARE Center and the UC Davis PCIT Training Center. He earned undergraduate and graduate degrees at the University of Washington and completed an internship at Primary Children's Medical Center in Salt Lake City, Utah. The CAARE Center provides medical evaluations, psychological assessments, and a range of mental health treatment services primarily for abused and neglected children. During the last two decades Dr. Urquiza has been adapting Parent-child Interaction Therapy (PCIT) to families involved in child welfare systems (i.e., physically abusive families, foster families, adoptive families) and community mental health clinics. He is currently involved in dissemination and implementation services research, including a PCIT dissemination/implementation training project, which has trained more than 130 community mental health agencies throughout the United States and internationally.

Patricia Van Horn, Ph.D. is a licensed clinical psychologist, Clinical Professor in the Department of Psychiatry at the University of California San Francisco, Associate Director of the Child Trauma Research Program, and Director of the Division of Infant, Child, and Adolescent Psychiatry at San Francisco General Hospital. Her research is with children under six who have witnessed domestic violence, investigating the effects of witnessing violence on the functioning of the children, as well as the efficacy of a relationship-based model for treating the children and their mothers. Her training activities include the creation of a curriculum for the divorcing parents of infants and toddlers, a training curricula about child trauma for domestic violence advocates, and a training manual for child-parent psychotherapy. She has provided training in child-parent psychotherapy to clinicians in 27 states and Israel.

Carolyn L. Webster-Stratton, Ph.D., FAAN is Professor Emeritus and founding director of the Parenting Clinic at the University of Washington. She is a licensed clinical psychologist and nurse practitioner. Over the past 30 years, she has conducted numerous randomized control group studies evaluating the effectiveness of The Incredible Years Parent, Teacher and Child Series for promoting children's social and emotional competence, school readiness skills and preventing conduct problems in high risk populations. She has also evaluated a treatment version of this series for reducing conduct problems in children diagnosed with oppositional defiant disorder, conduct disorder and ADHD.

The Incredible Years Series that she has developed, researched and refined over many years include separate training workshops, comprehensive intervention manuals, books and DVDs for use by trained therapists, group leaders and teachers.

She has published numerous scientific articles and chapters as well as books for parents, therapists, teachers, and children.

Index

CPSIA information can be obtained at www.ICGtesting.com
Printed in the USA
LVOW10*0222021015

456648LV00008B/39/P